"Lipsitt has meticulously detailed the evolution of a field that has influenced all of medicine. His unique and pioneering role is carefully researched and incorporates philosophy, psychology, clinical experience, and humor, detailing the contributions of those who brought together medicine and psychiatry in an engaging and illuminating work."

Carol C. Nadelson, MD, Professor of psychiatry,
Harvard Medical School, Department of Psychiatry,
Brigham and Women's Hospital, Boston, MA

"A masterful, authoritative, and often inspiring account of the conceptual and organizational development of consultation-liaison psychiatry. Don Lipsitt turns to philosophy, history, case vignette, and personal narrative to characterize the reach of a concept and practice, from ancient medicine to Obamacare and beyond."

Peter D. Kramer, MD, author of *Ordinarily Well: The Case for Antidepressants*, Emeritus Clinical Professor of psychiatry
and human behavior, Brown University, Providence, RI

"Don Lipsitt has succeeded in writing the definitive history of consultation-liaison psychiatry in a lucidly written, scholarly manner. This masterpiece reflects his 60 years of academic leadership in this psychiatric subspecialty. His passion for his own clinical and academic work serves as a model for students, residents, and fellow physicians. This grand opus is must reading for primary care physicians as well as psychiatrists, social workers, nurses, and clinical psychologists."

Stephen C. Scheiber, MD, Adjunct Professor,
Department of Psychiatry and Behavioral Medicine,
Medical College of Wisconsin, Milwaukee, WI

"*Foundations of Consultation-Liaison Psychiatry* is a must-read and will be of interest to all within and beyond the fields of medicine, including students, trainees, social workers, teachers, psychologists, and art therapists. C-L psychiatry has changed the practices of patient diagnosis, assessment, and treatment to save lives and recommend more accurate and successful treatment results. Lipsitt's knowledge, skills, and dedication make the book a challenge and a joy to read."

Leah J. Dickstein, MD, MS, Professor Emerita and
former Associate Dean for Student Affairs, as well as faculty and
student advocacy, University of Louisville,
Department of Psychiatry and Behavioral sciences

FOUNDATIONS OF CONSULTATION-LIAISON PSYCHIATRY

Foundations of Consultation-Liaison Psychiatry: The Bumpy Road to Specialization documents the development of consultation-liaison psychiatry from its inception to the present. The book draws on contributions from philosophy, physiology, psychoanalysis, epidemiology, and other disciplines to define the broad scope of the field. Distinctions and similarities between consultation-liaison psychiatry and psychosomatic medicine will be of interest to psychiatrists, social workers, and health psychologists, as well as students, residents, and fellows pursuing careers in these disciplines.

Don R. Lipsitt, M.D., is professor of clinical psychiatry at Harvard Medical School and a past president of the International College of Psychosomatic Medicine. The founder of two journals on consultation-liaison psychiatry, he is the recipient of several lifetime achievement awards for contributions to the field. The Academy of Psychosomatic Medicine has inaugurated the "Don R. Lipsitt Award for Achievement in Integrated and Collaborative Care."

FOUNDATIONS OF CONSULTATION-LIAISON PSYCHIATRY

The Bumpy Road to Specialization

Don R. Lipsitt

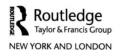

Routledge
Taylor & Francis Group

NEW YORK AND LONDON

First published 2016
by Routledge
711 Third Avenue, New York, NY 10017

and by Routledge
2 Park Square, Milton Park, Abingdon, Oxon, OX14 4RN

Routledge is an imprint of the Taylor & Francis Group, an informa business

© 2016 Taylor & Francis

Library of Congress Cataloging-in-Publication Data
Names: Lipsitt, Don R., author.
Title: Foundations of consultation-liaison psychiatry : the bumpy road to specialization / Don R. Lipsitt.
Description: New York, NY : Routledge, 2016. | Includes bibliographical references and index.
Identifiers: LCCN 2015039739 | ISBN 9781138906273 (hbk : alk. paper) | ISBN 9781138906259 (pbk : alk. paper) | ISBN 9781315695600 (ebk)
Subjects: LCSH: Consultation-liaison psychiatry.
Classification: LCC RC455.2.C65 L57 2016 | DDC 616.89—dc23
LC record available at http://lccn.loc.gov/2015039739

ISBN: 978-1-138-90627-3 (hbk)
ISBN: 978-1-138-90625-9 (pbk)
ISBN: 978-1-315-69560-0 (ebk)

Typeset in Bembo
by Apex CoVantage, LLC

Printed and bound in the United States of America by Publishers Graphics, LLC on sustainably sourced paper.

CONTENTS

PREFACE

When one has reached an understanding of what materials are furnished by the world around about him, and what resources he can hope for inside himself, it still remains for him to appraise the past as it is left to operate in the present, to understand it, to appropriate it, and to become its master.

—*John Herman Randall, Jr., 1940, p. 6*

The idea for this book has been a long time incubating. In 1982, JoAnn Miller of Basic Books and H. Keith H. Brodie, at the time president of the American Psychiatric Association (APA), had asked me to produce a book exploring the history of consultation-liaison (C-L)[1] psychiatry and its controversies and prospects. Time had a way of passing, and the landscape changed. New commitments took interested people in new directions: I was immersed in running a department, and, by the time I had furnished an outline, the book company had changed and the interested editor had moved on. Finally, with the passage of time, the field has become infinitely more nuanced (some say "organized"), now designated as a subspecialty aspect of psychosomatic medicine. The time seems right to take a panoramic view of consultation-liaison psychiatry, its foundations, and its stuttering journey toward specialization.

In the 1960s, fresh from a two-year research fellowship at the National Institute of Mental Health (NIMH), I joined the psychiatry staff of Boston's Beth Israel Hospital to complete my residency training. Interest in applying psychiatric knowledge to medical care and training won me appointment as director of Medical Psychology and the Psychiatric Consultation Service. The title seemed a bit ambiguous to me, but I adapted to it with only minimal uneasiness; the "medical psychology" part of the program, a British designation, reflected the

European influence brought to the department by Harvard's first woman professor and department chair, psychoanalyst Grete L. Bibring, a former student of Freud. Since I had also done major graduate work in psychology, the title seemed reasonably compatible with me. But as years passed, I became more accustomed to the commonly used term "consultation-liaison psychiatry"; it described an aspect of psychiatry with the lofty aspiration of bringing the application of psychological, psychiatric, and psychoanalytic insights to the well-being of patients, and the instruction of the physicians who attended them.

While inherently descriptive of its purpose, and even rhythmically appealing, the uneasy acceptance in both psychiatry and medicine of C-L psychiatry has been a constant thorn in the side of those who practice it. Further complicating its definition has been its mutable relationship with psychosomatic medicine, seen by some to be the "practical arm" of the latter field, by others to be interchangeable with it, and by yet others to be a misrepresentation of it. A past president of the American Psychosomatic Society (APS), in his annual address, bemoaned the possibility that the public would think of C-L psychiatry as "all there is" (to psychosomatic medicine) (Graham, 1979).

Throughout the history of psychiatry, there have been "specializers" and "generalizers," depending upon one's preference for either strengthening psychiatry as a distinct separate entity or absorbing it into medicine as an integrated endeavor. As a long-term observer and occasional participant in the agitations over the definition, name, roots, and future of C-L psychiatry, I have come to that point where it seems useful to reach for an "understanding of what materials are furnished by the world about [us]." This, I believe, can be done by exploring the foundations of the field in as broad a scope as time, space, and energy permit. In this endeavor, appreciation of past history can reward us with perspective on where we have come and where we might be going in the future. According to Randall (1940):

> A tracing of the history of the birth and growth of these [ideas] should make it easier to achieve a sense of the relevance of ideas to their setting, of their validity in the terms of the environment which developed them, and of their utility only so long as that environment still nurtures them.
>
> *(pp. 5–6)*

Arguably, C-L psychiatry—embracing medicine, neurology, and psychiatry, as well as a variety of other disciplines—is the most inclusive, eclectic subspecialty of all psychiatry. Psychiatrists who identify themselves as specializing in C-L activities are among the busiest practitioners in the profession. More than merely closeted psychotherapists or ward doctors, they are the peripatetic members of the field, most often traveling to the neighborhoods where patients and their doctors reside, on the services of medical, surgical, obstetric, pediatric, and neurological departments or on the outpatient environs of those same disciplines. Much less structured or theory based than office psychotherapy, C-L psychiatry must be flexible, adroit, available, and tolerant of ambiguity, resistance, and uncertainty.

As they diligently pursue their chosen work, C-L psychiatrists must have specialized knowledge and skills that transcend the more traditional psychiatric education. They are the heirs of a vast wealth of knowledge and discovery woven, often imperceptibly, into the fabric of their art and science. As such, the C-L psychiatrist has a comprehensive approach to care of the sick in body and mind, in contrast to a psychiatry that focuses more exclusively on the disturbances of mind. Before the days of psychopharmacology, psychiatrists trained largely to provide psychotherapy on either an individual or a group basis. After 1955, there was a trend toward greater pharmacological practice and a decreasing interest in psychotherapy—other health professionals including social workers and psychologists also absorbed more of the therapist's role, leaving the "medically oriented" aspects to psychiatrists. The consulting psychiatrist remains closest to medicine, utilizing all the skills and approaches that acknowledge social, biological, and psychological aspects of a person's being.

As psychosomatic medicine flourished between the 1920s and 1940s, advocates proclaimed that it would become the "new medicine." Controversy over whether C-L psychiatry should or should not be a field of specialization has swirled at least since the 1960s. In 1968, Schwab, author of the first handbook of consultation psychiatry, wrote that "psychiatric consultation work should not generate a subspecialty . . . . [T]he term is only descriptive of psychiatric activities with patients who complain of somatic distress or seek the help of physicians, surgeons, or general hospitals for treatment." "The consulting psychiatrist," he stated, "should be a specialist only in the sense that he is dedicated to comprehensive medicine, with a view of man as a creature of biology, a social being, and a part of his culture. . . . A psychiatric consultant is not a subspecialist" (Schwab, 1968, p. vii). It was his position that all psychiatrists should be able to incorporate consulting psychiatry in their repertoire since it represented the most general of all psychiatric training (pp. vii–viii). Schwab's incisive comments carried the weight of wisdom and probably slowed establishment of subspecialty status of the field.

Time, circumstances, and culture have brought changes to the field, as we shall describe more fully herein. The most recent and emphatic modification of Schwab's position is the certification in 2013 of psychosomatic medicine by the American Board of Medical Specialties, the seventh specialty of psychiatry to be so accredited. By rejecting C-L psychiatry as a specialty in favor of psychosomatic medicine, the board has arguably contributed to, rather than diminished, the ongoing confusion that swirls around both domains. Most C-L psychiatrists continue to regard themselves as practitioners of that "discipline" rather than of psychosomatic medicine.

The Book

This book is designed to trace the meanderings of the field of C-L psychiatry, with its twists and turns, the controversies, the stumbles and starts accompanying early evolution of the field—"to appraise the past as it is left to operate in the present"

(Randall, 1940, p. 6). Its winding road to its current designation and the contributions to its formalized status are explored. Following sometimes tortuous paths may take us on many detours and byways. Pursuit of interesting sidelines may be only the whim and experience of the author, hopefully to be tolerated (even if disputed) by the interested reader. Readers at any juncture may justifiably question the relevance of any particular line of exploration as it evolves. The appearance of extraneous detail may at times appear excessive but is included to reflect the often marked serendipitous nature of developments in the field.

Unlike a growing number of publications on the psychiatric and psychological aspects of medical illness, this book is not a "how-to" treatise. Nor will it be a handbook, "casebook," or encyclopedic coverage of the field. As an inquiry into the relationship of one aspect of psychiatry to the rest of medicine, it will nonetheless serve as a textbook and reference for those who wish to understand the development, definition, and application of both psychosomatic principles and consultation-liaison psychiatry to the broader field of medicine as it is encountered in today's world.

Contemporary books on C-L psychiatry tend increasingly to resemble "medical" textbooks, reviewing all illness categories and the special concerns of the psychiatrist in those entities. Book chapters typically adopt headings of specialized disciplines of, for example, gynecology, endocrinology, orthopedics, surgery, and medicine, as well as special situations such as abortion, addiction, life-threatening illness, or the ostomy patient. Although this practice may optimistically imply a welcomed "final" absorption of psychiatry into medicine, this book will not follow that trend; while C-L psychiatry is solidly grounded in medicine, it is not to be assumed that the C-L psychiatrist must know all about medicine or surgery any more than we expect nonpsychiatrist physicians to know all about psychiatry.

In its current form, C-L psychiatry is heir to prominent vestiges of philosophy, psychology, psychoanalysis, psychophysiology, general hospital psychiatry, psychotherapy, psychosomatic medicine, and epidemiology. The book navigates the confluence of these tributaries as they flow into the mainstream of medicine. The profusion (and confusion) of terms like medical psychology, psychiatric medicine, behavioral medicine, biobehavioral medicine, biopsychosocial medicine, general hospital psychiatry, consultation psychiatry, liaison psychiatry, medical-surgical psychiatry, primary care psychiatry, (stress psychiatry?), and others reflect not only the multifactorial aspect of the field but perhaps also a glaring need within the profession to establish its identity and to acknowledge its constant attempts at "remedicalization"; this enduring process began as early as the 1920s and reached its greatest intensity in the 1970s with the increased prominence of primary care medicine.

Exploring the historical contributions to C-L psychiatry calls up reference to Zilboorg (1941), who, in his important history of medical psychology, states: "We proclaim the merits of the past to emphasize the greater merits of the present" (pp. 19–20). He makes the assumption that we discard old ideas with some contempt but also nostalgia, only to return to them later in the role of "collectors," ready now to admire the once-scorned object and to find in it newly assigned and possibly greater value (p. 19). In this role as collector, I endeavor in this book to explore and assess the value of ideas past that have had some impact on today's subspecialization of C-L psychiatry.

To avoid the unevenness that often characterizes many multiauthored books, this one is single authored, so that its unevenness, as it occurs, will be attributed to one author, whose reliability will rise or fall on the success of the endeavor. Although I write as a psychiatrist and psychoanalyst, I know from experience the importance of the team in consultation-liaison work; the "patient" being consulted often encompasses a whole system of settings, staff, family, and others involved in the sick patient's world.

The book especially targets physicians electing psychiatry as their professional discipline or area of scholarly interest as well as psychiatric educators, residency training directors, and department chairpersons. However, it is also intended as a resource for teachers and clinicians in psychiatric nursing, social work, and psychology, especially those preparing for work in general medical settings. The book proposes to be, as well, a practical reference for medical students, medical house officers, and trainees in family medicine and primary care who seek a holistic, humanistic dimension to their medical interests and pursuits. Researchers in the history of psychiatric, psychological, and social intervention in medical illness will find ample reference here. As a standard reference for the field of C-L psychiatry, availability in medical libraries will facilitate the preparation of those interested in being credentialed as specialists in the new field called psychosomatic medicine.

Organization of the Book

The book begins with a broad view of C-L psychiatry's fundamental concept: to narrow if not close the sometimes wide gap between psychiatry and medicine. References to "gap" in one aspect or another will appear throughout the text. Setting the stage for what follows, the opening prologue on struggles in the field is reprinted here with permission of the American Psychiatric Press, from *American Psychiatry After World War II (1944–1994)*, edited by Menninger and Nemiah (2000); it serves as a kind of "executive summary" of what is to follow.

The remainder of the book selectively amplifies these struggles in five sections: Section I, "Seeds and Roots," explores origins of the concept and application of consultation and liaison, with contributions from Cannon, Pavlov, Freud, and others in disciplines of philosophy (psychology), physiology, psychoanalysis, psychosomatic medicine, and epidemiology to the field of C-L psychiatry in their attempts to explain and breach the "mysterious leap" from psyche to soma and to restore medicine and psychiatry to their holistic relationship. Section II, "Crises and Benefactors," expounds on the vital affirmative role of foundation funding in the evolution and very survival of the field, and it describes the fiscal problems of the field throughout its history. Section III, "The Process of Specialty Recognition," addresses the formative elements, including meetings, "politics," and organizational efforts in the process of seeking specialization in C-L psychiatry, hopefully to assure its sustainability, culminating in recognition of psychosomatic medicine as the seventh psychiatric specialty. And section IV, "Post-Specialization," assesses the current status and future prospects of C-L psychiatry, and it questions whether specialization is a boon or bane. Confirming that money alone is not sufficient for survivability of the field, the book concludes with an appendix of a partial list of individual contributors to C-L psychiatry and a personal reminiscence of the author's reflections as a C-L psychiatrist. Tables and index follow. References and notes are included in each chapter rather than compiled at book's end.

My wish is that the reader will find the same excitement and curiosity I experienced as a resident when my senior mentor first took me to the medical ward to answer a colleague's request for consultation. Since time was less precious than it is today, he showed me how to review the patient's record and how to speak to the house officer and the nurse attending the patient before going to the bedside to interview and assess the patient, keeping in mind the question posed by the consultee. It was an inspiring demonstration of how psychiatry could enhance a patient's comfort, comprehensive care, and staff collaboration toward a holistic approach to medicine.

Now, as a putative "component" of psychosomatic medicine, C-L psychiatry concerns itself with transactions of medicine and psychiatry where they meet at the "interface"; tracing its historical development encounters a labyrinth of intertwined resources in medicine, philosophy, psychology, psychiatry, and other disciplines. Interested readers may wish to consult other "foundational" books such as those by esteemed predecessors (Cobb, 1952; Christie & Mellett, 1981; Nemiah, 1961) who have added knowledge in our field.

Note

1 I use C-L to abbreviate consultation–liaison psychiatry, while the literature reveals other variations. My rationale for this preference is explained in my paper *Hyphen or Slash? Coming of Age* (Lipsitt, 1991), in which consultation and liaison are viewed as concurrent and not as either/or.

References

Christie, M.J., & Mellett, P.G. (1981). *Foundations of Psychosomatics*. New York, NY: John Wiley & Sons.

Cobb, S. (1952). *Foundations of Neuropsychiatry*. Baltimore, MD: Williams & Wilkins.

Graham, D.T. (1979). Presidential address—1979. What place in medicine for psychosomatic medicine? *Psychosomatic Medicine, 41,* 357–367.

Lipsitt, D.R. (1991). Hyphen or slash? Coming of age. *General Hospital Psychiatry, 13,* 149.

Lipsitt, D.R. (2000). Psyche and soma: Struggles to close the gap. In R. Menninger & J.C. Nemiah (Eds.). *American Psychiatry After World War II (1944–1994)*. (pp. 152–186). Washington, DC: American Psychiatric Press.

Nemiah, J.C. (1961). *Foundations of Psychopathology*. New York, NY: Oxford University Press.

Randall, J.H., Jr. (1940). *The Making of the Modern Mind*. Cambridge, MA: The Riverside Press.

Schwab, J.J. (1968). *Handbook of Psychiatric Consultation*. New York, NY: Appleton-Century-Crofts.

Zilboorg, G. (with Henry, G.W.). (1941). *A History of Medical Psychology*. New York, NY: W.W. Norton & Co.

ACKNOWLEDGMENTS

Tradition has it that most books contain a statement of acknowledgement. No one arrives at the authorship of a book without considerable input and influence from a large circle of others, whether one wishes to own one's participation or not. This acknowledgement is longer than most since it is probably the last book-length project I will undertake.

Seeds and roots begin of course with parents Anna and Joseph, and to them I owe not only my beginnings but also lifelong support for all that I am. Their unwavering insistence that "education is the best investment" kept me at the endeavor, even when other diversions beckoned. I am the fortunate benefactor of excellent teachers from secondary through graduate school, capped with medical education at University of Vermont College of Medicine. An award for an essay on doctor-patient relationships imprinted on me an indelible curiosity about how doctors treat patients (in every sense of the word!). It has imbued my entire career.

Teachers during master's studies at Boston University were a premed launch into the psychology field, with influential course instruction from Milton Greenblatt, M.D., and Edward Bibring, M.D., who ignited my interest in psychiatry and psychoanalysis.

I lovingly dedicate this book to Merna, my wife and lifelong intellectual companion, whose humor, compassion, and tolerance have been so sustaining. I regret that she has been unable to enjoy (or bear, with my complaining) this last endeavor with me. Previous collaborative enterprises have worked so well: two talented, music-making, wise, empathic, and humorful sons, Eric and Steven, experts in giving and taking criticism, life joys that have helped maintain my compass. Now their own families of Brenda, Jonah, Mara, Daria, and Caleb bring new joy. The loving competitiveness of four accomplished brothers—Paul, Lewis, Cyrus, and

Peter—cannot be dismissed, since they have been the longest cherished acquaintances of my life.

My career has been shaped in large sense by the support of my three career chiefs: Milton Rosenbaum, M.D., chairman of the Department of Psychiatry at New York's Einstein College of Medicine; Joel Elkes, M.D., director of the William Alanson White Neuropsychopharmacologic Research Center at St. Elizabeths Hospital and National Institute of Mental Health in Washington; and Grete L. Bibring, M.D., chief of psychiatry at Harvard's Beth Israel Hospital.

I am especially grateful to colleagues Stephen Green, Ronald Pies, and Carol Alter, who have given unstintingly of their time to critique individual chapters, and I thank them for their keen observations and suggestions, although final flaws continue to rest with me.

I am indebted to Irene Lipowski for allowing me access to important biographical materials about her husband, Zbigniew J. Lipowski.

My many chats with old college friend Sydney Wolfe Cohen have been inspirational, and from him I have learned that index is not just a finger.

There are those who have contributed in other ways, and I acknowledge my indebtedness to them:

Carole Berney, whose intelligence, creativity, and wisdom through 36 years of co-editorship saved me from many an embarrassing pitfall.

ZJ ("Bish") Lipowski was a good friend, colleague, and editorial collaborator, whose many contributions to the field of consultation-liaison psychiatry are unparalleled and continue to teach me.

The hundreds of patients, students, residents, and fellows who have put their trust in me over the years have been the best teachers of my craft. I have profited from and enjoyed the colleagueship of Drs. Robert Joseph, Donald Meyer, and Malkah Notman for the many years in our Somatization Work Group. Parts of this book have undoubtedly osmotically emerged from lively discussion with those colleagues.

Graciela Rivas's loving care of Merna has allowed me writing time with full confidence that Merna is in expert hands.

And I am, of course, unexpectedly indebted to the three Princes of Serendip for spicing up life with surprises.

There are those I miss: the companionship of good friend Ted Nadelson, whose wisdom and wit made our parallel careers in consultation-liaison psychiatry, research, and chairmanships of psychiatry departments a constant (often laughable) pleasure. Rich Feinberg's zany humor and word play through internship helped us both get through the experience. Rich Glass's kindness and stability helped sustain us through the early childhood years of Eric and Steven.

And, of course, once again, I thank nephew Daniel Lipsitt for his computer expertise, rescuing parts of this book from disappearing into a black hole (for better or worse!).

Finally, as with all books, without the benefit of a special group of people, books, including this one, would never see the light of day. I am greatly indebted to the Routledge staff, from George Zimmar, who encouraged me to pursue, and supported me in, this project, to the shepherding through the production process by Meira Bienstock, Zoey Peresman, Dan Khan, and Tina Cottone.

I am glad to bring this book to a close; to begin to get back to a normal life, to my wife, to my grown sons and their families; to restore time robbed by my intense involvement in finally getting this 30-year project off my desk. Our dining table is once again available for its intended purpose.

Regarding source material for the book, I have benefited greatly from Dorothy Levenson's superb history of the American Psychosomatic Society, *Mind, Body and Medicine*; Ron Chernow's *Titan* has been a rich resource about the Rockefeller family; de Mandeville's *Treatise of the Hysterick and Hypochondriak Passions* has been a rare historical find.

Permission to use my chapter "Psyche and Soma: Struggles to Close the Gap" is gratefully acknowledged. In Menninger, R.W., & Nemiah, J.C. (Eds.). (2000). *American Psychiatry After World War II, 1944–1994.* (pp. 152–186). Washington, DC: American Psychiatric Publishing, Inc.

Other major references of source material, include the following:

Gifford, G.E., Jr. (1978). *Psychoanalysis, Psychotherapy and the New England Medical Scene, 1894–1944.* New York, NY: Science History Publications.

Rosenzweig, S. (1994). *The Historic Expedition to America (1909): Freud, Jung and Hall the King-maker.* St. Louis, MO: Rana House.

Readers interested in further elaboration of ideas expressed here are invited to view other of my writings:

1- From alienist to collaborator: The twisting road to consultation-liaison psychiatry. In Bloch, S., Green, S.A., & Holmes, J. (Eds.). (2014). *Psychiatry: Past, Present and Prospect.* (pp. 196–218). Oxford, UK: Oxford University Press.

2- Psychosomatic medicine: History of a "new" specialty. In Blumenfield, M., & Strain, J.J. (Eds.). (2006). *Psychosomatic Medicine.* (pp. 3–20). Philadelphia, PA: Lippincott Williams & Wilkins.

3- Psychotherapy. In Wise, M.G., & Rundell, J. (Eds.). (2002). *Textbook of Consultation-Liaison Psychiatry: Psychiatry in the Medically Ill.* (pp. 1027–1051). Washington, DC: American Psychiatric Publishing, Inc.

PROLOGUE

The Gap

Preamble: *As a clinical discipline allied with psychiatry, consultation-liaison psychiatry is heir to the perennial struggles of clinicians in medicine to "close the gap," establish "bridges," or "integrate" complementary elements. Awareness that our perceptual mechanisms are inclined to fill in the blanks has fostered a whole school of psychology called Gestalt, adherent to the principle that the whole is greater than the sum of its parts. The dictum that "nature abhors a vacuum (*horror vacui)*" has a long and controversial history dating at least to 485 BC, when Parmenides averred that a void cannot exist, that unfilled spaces go against the laws of nature. Perhaps a primitive fear that one might carelessly fall in a hole induces a wish to eliminate such a threat.*

Whatever the source, gaps attract the attention, curiosity, thinking, and innovation of philosophers, theologians, mathematicians, physicians, psychologists, physiologists, clinicians, physicists, laypeople, and sundry other thinkers to "close the gap." Gaps in knowledge exist in every field, and it is their presence that sparks curiosity about them and the essential need to fill or eliminate them.

Our interest here is to survey the ways in which gaps between psyche and soma have contributed to the evolution of the clinical disciplines called consultation-liaison psychiatry and psychosomatic medicine, the hyphen in each serving as proxy for the many unknowns yet to be discovered.

As a background to our exploration, we begin with the chapter "Psyche and Soma: Struggles to Close the Gap," reprinted here from American Psychiatry after World War II (1944–1994), *edited by Menninger and Nemiah (2000), with permission of the American Psychiatric Press. The remainder of the book endeavors to assess the foundations of the field and their ultimate summation in specialty status.*

Reference

Lipsitt, D.R. (2000). Psyche and soma: Struggles to close the gap. In R.W. Menninger & J.C. Nemiah (Eds.). *American Psychiatry After World War II (1944–1994)*. (pp. 152–186). Washington, DC: American Psychiatric Press.

PSYCHE AND SOMA

Struggles to Close the Gap

During the very years that the winds of war were stirring in Europe, American psychiatry was on the threshold of some of its most important advances. The late 1920s and most of the 1930s saw a number of major moves to "remedicalize" psychiatry. It was not that anyone actually denied that psychiatry was a branch of medicine, but the relationship was always a bit shaky and unsteady, like a person attempting to balance on one foot. The tenuous tie has ranged all the way from a declaration that mental illness is a myth totally unrelated to medicine (Szasz, 1961) to predictions that all mental illness will one day be explainable in Virchovian cellular terms. Denigrators of the medical foundation of psychiatry also persist in pronouncements that other nonmedical specialists can competently fulfill needs for mental health services.

It is sometimes forgotten—by laypersons and medical professionals alike—that psychiatry claims medicine as its parent. The self-conscious tentativeness with which that birthright is held is reflected in allusions to the "battered child" of medicine (Greenblatt, 1975), in references to psychiatry's "identity crises" (Bandler, 1965; Braceland, 1969), and in debates as to whether psychiatry is mostly art or mostly science and whether it is the purveyor of humaneness and compassion or a specialty with precise diagnoses and treatments. The relationship was perhaps most seriously questioned by the proposal that psychiatry did not require medical training as a requisite for its practice (Romano, 1970).

Historical driftings apart of psychiatry and medicine intermittently prompt the rallying cry to "bridge the gap," whether between psychiatry and medicine or between mind and body. Outgrowths of these efforts punctuate the psychiatric literature as attempted "bridgings" through developments in psychosomatic medicine, models of "comprehensive medicine," and regular calls for more holistic or integrated medical care. Psychiatry as a profession, of course, has always asserted its desire to see the patient as a whole, as an individual whose mind and body coexist in various degrees of harmony or discord—a wish observed more in the philosophical breach than in the clinical reality.

In fact, it was the psychoanalysts, the psychosomaticists, and—since the late 1930s—the consultation-liaison psychiatrists who most avidly chose to "ride this horse." The following is a statement by Winnicott (1966) regarding the likelihood of combined soma-care and psyche-care:

> Some practising doctors are not really able to ride the *two* [author's empha-sis] horses. They sit in one saddle and lead the other horse by the bridle or lose touch with it. After all, why should doctors be more healthy in a psychiatric sense than their patients? They have not been selected on a psy-chiatric basis. The doctor's own dissociations need to be considered along with the dissociations in the personalities of the patients. (p. 510)
>
> In more recent years, health psychologists and behaviorists of all stripes have elected to mount the beasts, although some would appear to take their risks bareback, as it were.

My intent in this chapter is to take the measure of these efforts at bridging what Freedman (1992) calls "the to and fro" of trends in the medicalization, demedical-ization, and remedicalization of psychiatry. Strivings toward an integrated, holistic approach to the care of the sick and an understanding of the well have indeed had an erratic and sometimes paradoxical course, with forward movement not uncom-monly accompanied by equal and opposite forces.

In a confluence of events between the First and Second World Wars, Ameri-can psychiatry saw the budding of fruitful growth in psychosomatic medicine, consultation-liaison psychiatry, and general hospital psychiatry. It is useful to trace the twists and turns of psychiatry from prewar beginnings to postwar modifica-tions in each of these intertwined areas, the better to assay the impact of World War II on psychiatry's relationship to general medicine. Excellent reviews exist of the history of psychosomatic medicine (Kimball, 1970; Leigh & Reiser, 1977; Lipowski, 1977; Reiser, 1974; Wittkower, 1960), consultation-liaison psychiatry (Greenhill, 1977; Lipowski, 1983, 1986; Schwab, 1989), and general hospital psy-chiatry (Greenhill, 1979; Lebensohn, 1980; Lipsitt, 1983); therefore, only those salient features of each that elucidate the vicissitudes of the perennial mind-body controversy are highlighted here.

Beginnings

A brief historical survey places this struggle (to close the gap) in the proper his-torical context to illuminate the developmental patterns in the whole tapestry.

American psychiatry was born of a free and independent spirit that cherished the hard-won rights of strong-willed individuals. Benjamin Rush, a signer of the Declaration of Independence and a physician, wrote *Medical Inquiries and Observations on the "Diseases of the Mind"* (1812), a work that "for many years . . . remained the only textbook on mental diseases in America" (Binger, 1966, p. 274). Rush regarded each person as a unified being, with mind and body indivisibly related (Rush, 1812/1988). For this epochal work and his innovative treatments, many of which would be considered retrospectively primitive and even physically inhumane, he was declared the Father of American Psychiatry (Binger, 1966). In 1844 a group of 13 superintendents of American insane asylums met to ponder their moral and medical obligations to the mentally ill of a young nation, even as they "warehoused" patients at great remove from the rest of medicine, their families, and their communities. Because there was not yet any credentialing of psychiatrists, all were rightfully general physicians, and their respectful obeisance to medicine was reflected in the new name taken in 1892 by this special interest group: American Medico-Psychological Association,[1] to become the American *Psychiatric* Association in 1921.

The Swing of the Pendulum

As psychiatry adopted the stance and trappings of a specialty differentiated from the rest of medicine, it constantly risked obscuring its parenthood. Nonetheless, some powerful tropism constantly struggled to reestablish the bond between mind and body and between psychiatry and medicine.

Throughout the latter decades of the nineteenth century, luminaries such as Pliny Earle (1868), a uniquely designated professor of psychological medicine, and John Gray (1869), then editor of the *American Journal of Insanity,* called for the incorporation of psychological medicine into the teaching and practice of medicine before there were departments or curricula of psychiatry or even a body of knowledge that could be identified as the psychology of medicine.

Ignoring the urging of such influential physicians, the newborn psychiatry seemed to stray increasingly from its base in medicine. Describing efforts of psychiatrists in the second half of the nineteenth century to restore the renegade psychiatry to its rightful holistic-medical home, Lipowski (1981) wrote that "a struggle to end the separation of psychiatry and the rest of medicine had begun" (p. 889). In a "pep talk" in 1894 to the attendees of the fiftieth annual meeting of the American Medico-Psychological Association, S. Weir Mitchell reprimanded psychiatrists for ignoring their medical roots. "His sharp critique," according to Lipowski (1981), "helped accelerate the trends aimed at ending the isolation of psychiatry from the rest of medicine and from science and at bringing psychiatric services physically closer to other medical ones" (p. 890). In spite of Lipowski's optimistic spin on this event, Mitchell's reproach would be echoed over and over in subsequent decades by many eminent professionals in both the written and spoken word.

Adolf Meyer and William Alanson White

Whether by response to Mitchell's reprimand or merely by the natural swing of the developmental pendulum, psychiatry at the turn of the century did begin creeping back to its medical domicile. Assisting in this reconciliation were the psychobiological teachings of both Adolf Meyer and William Alanson White. Although Swiss by birth and training, Meyer was typically American in his commitment to the individual, to freedom, and to democratic values; his focus on "the person" in his teaching and practice was quite at home in the United States. His ideas did much to hold mind and body together in an integrated perspective on health and disease, and he had a major influence on the early development of American psychiatry. Open to many ideologies and eclectic in his outlook, he advocated a commonsense approach that led many skeptics to an appreciation of psychiatry's relationship to medicine (Lief, 1948).

White (1936) also reiterated, with more of a psychoanalytic predilection, the imperative that both medicine and psychiatry must strive for a synthesis of mind and body to maximize benefits to the patient and humanity as a whole. But, he said, "the real difficulty here is in translating psychological mechanisms into terms that are immediately comprehensible to those who have been engaged in studying the usual problems of what I call by contrast somatic medicine" (p. 189). Even monists have difficulty avoiding dualistic explanations! However, Meyer's emphasis on "the person" converged nicely with White's (1936) concept of "the organism-as-a-whole" to stress the need to abandon "the either-or way of thinking of parts of the organism, to the both-and way of thinking of the organism in its different aspects" (p. 193). The emergence of these ideas seemed to crest not long after the First World War, with a similar parallel trend following the Second World War. It may be assumed that the ravages and dehumanization of war in each instance brought a conflation of humanistic and socially responsible ideas intended to reaffirm the wholeness and goodness of the individual.

Dawn of the Twentieth Century

At the cusp of the twentieth century, then, much was happening in America and elsewhere that would influence the vacillations of psychiatry in its relationship to medicine. Sigmund Freud had discovered the unconscious and was embellishing a new and creative way to understand human behavior, motive, and drive. With its focus on the mind and its intricate workings, Freud's approach was thoroughly individualistic. It was hardly surprising that it met with greater receptivity in the United States than in Europe.

Concurrent developments in psychoanalysis, psychosomatic medicine, general hospital psychiatry, and consultation-liaison psychiatry in the early decades of the twentieth century had a powerful impact on the bridging of psychiatry and medicine. Although these fields of interest overlapped considerably as they evolved, they will be explored somewhat discretely to assess their respective contributions to the to and fro of psyche and soma in their complex efforts at synthesis.

Psychosomatic Medicine

The Mysterious Leap

The beginnings of psychosomatic medicine are attributed to the German physician Heinroth in 1818, but its roots in America were distinctly psychoanalytic and psychodynamic.[2] A number of Freud's disciples and students, escaping Hitler and the war, sought safe haven personally and professionally in the United States, where they applied their psychoanalytic knowledge to studies of a variety of physical disorders. Freud himself never alluded to "psychosomatic" medicine, yet he urged others to use psychoanalytic concepts to clarify the relation of physiological and endocrinological events to mental phenomena, and his transplanted students faced the challenge with great élan. The concept of conversion seemed a particularly propitious starting place to study the mysterious leap from mind to body.

Freud essentially renounced his roots in medicine, denied the importance of medical training in the study of psychoanalysis, and adopted a virtually total reductionistic view of the human organism; nonetheless, it was his innovative work that provided the tools for one of the most important epochs of rapprochement of mind and body through subsequent psychosomatic research. As chronicled by Felix Deutsch (1959), Freud "never gave up the hope that some time in the future there must be a comprehensive fusion of both the biological and psychological concepts." According to Deutsch, Freud "always adhered to a 'universal monism'" (p. 9).

Certainly other nonpsychoanalytic work had contributed considerably to psychosomatic medicine. The work of Pavlov and Cannon, for example, provided original psychophysiological insights. Also, Flanders Dunbar had already laid the foundation for a popular acceptance of psychosomatic medicine through her text on the subject (Dunbar, 1935), but the movement acquired its major thrust and prestige from the methodologically impressive researches of psychoanalysts such as Franz Alexander and his associates in the Chicago Psychoanalytic Institute. The founding of the American Psychosomatic Society by prominent psychoanalysts and of the journal *Psychosomatic Medicine* by Dunbar in the late 1930s presaged a bright future for this new field of endeavor. Carrying the torch of "integrated medicine," the editors of the first issue of the journal (1939) stated their intention "to endeavor to study in their interrelation the psychological and physiological aspects of all normal and abnormal bodily functions and thus to integrate somatic therapy and psychotherapy" (p. 3). The editors added that "psychic and somatic phenomena take place in the same biological system and are probably two aspects of the same process" (Editorial note, 1939, p. 4). Later acknowledgment of environmental factors resulted in the modified statement that "the criterion of psychosomatic health is maintenance by the organism of homeostatic equilibrium within itself and within its environmental field" (Dunbar & Arlow 1944, p. 283).

Dunbar's *Synopsis of Psychosomatic Diagnosis and Treatment* (1948) emphasized combining both physiological and psychological approaches "because psychosomatic study of illness must of necessity include a combination of both techniques" (p. 18).

The belief that psychiatry was on the threshold of enlightening medicine was reflected in Alexander's (1950) comment that "the significance of psychiatry, particularly of the psychoanalytic method, for the development of medicine lies in the fact that it supplies an efficient technique for the study of the psychological factors in disease" (p. 23). As if to doubly underscore his point, he said, "it was reserved for psychiatry, the most neglected and least developed specialty in medicine, to introduce a new synthetic approach into medicine" (p. 24).

Of the challenge to psychosomatic medicine, Dunbar (1959) colorfully wrote, "the bridge, for one end of which Freud built a firm foundation, after Virchow, Ehrlich and Pasteur had established the other end, has remained with a middle span which behaves like 'Galloping Gerty' [a notably long suspension bridge that galloped in the wind until it collapsed in a storm] when subjected to the aerodynamic pressure of medical controversy" (p. 6).

So exalted were the flag-bearers of this renewed effort to bridge the gap that Deutsch (1959), in a memorial presentation on Freud's one-hundredth birthday, proclaimed that "the science called 'psychosomatic medicine' has not only become a domain of psychoanalysis, but almost deserves the name of 'psychoanalytic medicine'" (pp. 9–10).

A celebration of the influence of psychosomatic medicine on the rest of medicine was evident in the 1942 publication of Christian's fourteenth edition of Osler's *Principles and Practice of Medicine,* which devoted the entire first chapter to "Psychosomatic Medicine." Bringing psychiatry and psychoanalysis to the bedside of patients with physical illness in the general hospital setting was a giant step forward for psychosomatic research.

Although born in Europe, psychosomatic medicine, as elaborated in the United States, was as American as apple pie. Stressing as they did the humanistic side of medicine and the preeminence of the individual even in the diseased state, both Alexander and Dunbar promoted a medicine that had great appeal. Alexander stressed the importance of intrapsychic conflict in the choice of disease, whereas Dunbar subscribed to the etiological significance of specific personality profiles. Such psychologizing of medicine had, for at least several decades, greater appeal than the medicalizing effects on psychiatry of the introduction of such organic techniques as electroconvulsive treatment, insulin coma, and psychosurgery of the early 1930s (Alexander & Selesnick, 1968).

By the 1950s, psychosomatic medicine began to shift more toward the study of disease as an adaptive process in response to stress (e.g., Engel, 1962; Kubie, 1953; Selye, 1966; Wolff, 1950). Attention to aspects of coping abilities, adaptational responses, and environmental stimuli (in addition to internal defenses) represented a significant broadening of the research base of psychosomatic medicine and demonstrated a closer link with clinical application.

Interestingly, even as Alexander's specificity theory and Dunbar's personality profiles had fallen into disfavor, the compelling correlation of personality factors or characterological traits with specific disease processes resurfaced in the highly popular studies of cardiovascular disease in individuals with Type A personalities (Friedman & Rosenman, 1959). In this regard, it is important to heed the warning of psychosomaticists that in rejecting some of the early tenets and theories of psychosomatic research, the baby not be discarded with the bath water. Dunbar herself felt that theories were merely transient, to serve their heuristic purpose, and were to be subsequently revised or discarded when new facts were discovered.

The Effects of War

What, then, was the impact of World War II on psychosomatic medicine and the integration of psyche (psychiatry) and soma (medicine)? It is difficult to define precisely how psychosomatic medicine was affected by or involved in the events of the war years, although there seems little doubt that psychiatry's capital was significantly enhanced. Freud had noted, in a letter to Ernest Jones during the First World War, that "science sleeps" (Gay, 1988, p. 351), and this characterization did seem to apply to those researchers who were called into military service to aid the war effort. In her introduction to the *Synopsis,* Dunbar (1948) observed the following:

> Physicians who have done experimental investigation have been severely hampered; if they were in the armed services, by being unable to publish; if they were in civilian practice, by lack of facilities to carry out their projects to a scientifically accepted conclusion.
>
> *(p. 16).*

The primary task of military psychiatrists was the clinical care of inductees and the wounded. Whatever research was done was that which was most clearly identified with the war effort, which meant, essentially, weapons development. The exigencies of war did not facilitate pursuit of research in the military beyond fundamental statistical and clinical reports. There is no persuasive evidence that researchers in psychosomatic medicine exploited wartime situations to promote research objectives, except for one study of duodenal ulcer by Weiner and associates (Weiner, Thaler, Reiser & Mirsky, 1957). These researchers reported on more than 2,000 army inductees separated of necessity from their families. They were screened to test the multifactorial hypothesis that those who were hypersecretors of pepsinogen who experienced conflict about separation and dependency would be most likely to develop duodenal ulcer under the stress of military training. Significantly accurate predictions based on psychological data identified which hypersecretors would develop active ulcers. This landmark double-blind study demonstrated that psychological factors were necessary but not sufficient to account for the etiology of a psychosomatic disorder.

Other aspects of the war's impact on psychiatry (if not psychosomatic medicine per se) are addressed by sociologist Paul Starr (1982). He suggests that events of World War II did enhance psychiatry's postwar currency and that the need for control in the military "made it a proving ground for the psychological professions" (p. 344). A Division of Neurology and Psychiatry was created to psychologically test, screen, and treat all mentally disturbed servicemen. According to Starr (1982), "more than 1 million men were rejected from military service because of mental and neurological disorders, and another 850,000 soldiers were hospitalized as psychoneurotic cases during the war" (p. 344).

These statistics were not lost on the public and politicians after the war, when the resources for training, education, and treatment reached a zenith in the history of psychiatry. The war increased the army's need for psychiatrists from its total of 25 in 1940 to almost 2,500 at the height of the war. Dr. William Menninger, a psychoanalyst, was promoted to the rank of brigadier general, the highest rank ever held by a psychiatrist.

Although there was little opportunity (or need) for psychoanalytic treatment in military settings, the conceptual orientation of Menninger and other psychoanalytically trained psychiatrists imbued treatment with a psychodynamic cast, a veritable sea change from the earlier descriptive psychiatry of the First World War. The many psychiatrists and psychoanalysts recruited for military duty were challenged to modify psychoanalytic and psychodynamic treatment approaches. Herbert Spiegel, from his experience and observations as an army psychiatrist in World War II, defined a number of criteria that distinguished candidates who were responsive to short-term or brief interventions, and thus returnable to combat, from those whose mental disorders were irreversible under conditions of combat (Spiegel, 1944). Those early observations were of seminal importance to the foundations of today's approaches to brief psychotherapy.

The literature published on wartime psychiatry between 1940 and 1948 (Lewis & Engle, 1954) consisted largely of descriptive reports of clinical encounters in a variety of hospital and clinical settings. As one might expect, it was a rare report that suggested utilization of in-depth interventions. Indeed, it was often cautioned that such techniques ran the risk of increasing disability in the short run. However, conversion disorders, somatization, and other psychosomatic perturbations were much better understood as complex reactions that could be addressed with short-term crisis interventions, hypnosis, and focused psychodynamic treatment. But even in cases of conversion disorder, the preferred treatment was suggestion, reassurance, "coercion," and sodium pentothal or amytal for diagnostic as well as therapeutic purposes.

Nonetheless, the collective clinical reports provided insight into treatment needs, epidemiological observations, and general conclusions about differences in mental manifestations by soldiers in both world wars. For example, "soldier's heart" was said to have decreased between the two wars, whereas gastrointestinal disorders were noted to have increased significantly, and even traumatic neuroses showed a decrease when clear diagnostic criteria were used (Solomon, 1947; Spitz, 1944, p. 561).

The most frequently occurring symptoms in military life were gastrointestinal, cardiovascular, rheumatic, and allergic. The prevalence of these disorders probably provided the impetus for much postwar research. The importance of studying individual differences was underscored by Sontag (1948), who wrote:

> The wards full of military personnel in Army hospitals during World War II emphasize dramatically the difference between individuals in their emotional and physiological responses to stress. Psychosomatic disturbances represented a large proportion of Army casualties, and while vast differences existed in the experience of soldiers, these differences in experience did not by any means account for the variations in their proneness to the development of disturbances of physiological function, or to state it more concisely, in their somatizing of emotions.
>
> *(p. 38)*

William Menninger (1945) reported a survey of 11 general hospitals showing that 24% to 40% of patients with cardiovascular disorders and 20% to 30% of patients with gastrointestinal disorders were "functional." Because these data were based on reports by internists, Menninger assumed that the numbers would have been much higher if reported by psychiatrists. In a subsequent article, Menninger (1947) emphasized the need of the average physician to learn that the "functional illness" is quite as interesting as the "organic type of problem" if proper treatment of the "organ neuroses" (p. 95) was to take place in medical wards. Menninger saw the army as an ideal opportunity to urge psychiatrists in supervisory positions to promote policies and practices "for the largest single group of doctors in the world" (p. 97). A technical medical bulletin, *Neuropsychiatry for the General Medical Officer,* was distributed to all military physicians (Lewis & Engle, 1954).

After the war, cumulative military experience resulted in accounts such as William Menninger's (1948a) *Psychiatry in a Troubled World* and Grinker and Spiegel's (1945) *Men Under Stress.* The latter described the influence of the war on psychosomatic medicine as follows:

> The war has hastened the development of psychosomatic medicine because the severe stresses which it has imposed on the fighting men have brought into the clinical symptomatology of war neuroses thousands of emotionally induced physical disturbances. Hundreds of doctors have witnessed this

phenomenon at first hand and have learned of the relationship between psychological causes and physical effects. They are eager to learn further details of etiology and methods of treatment, for they know therein lies the future of medicine.

(Grinker & Spiegel, 1945, p. 252).

The problems of stress in combat in relation to psychosomatic medicine were extensively reviewed and presented at a symposium cosponsored by the Division of Medical Sciences of the National Research Council and the Army Medical Services Graduate School of the Walter Reed Army Medical Center (1953); this was one of several postwar symposia and included such noted teachers and researchers as John Whitehorn, I. Arthur Mirsky, Hudson Hoagland, Curt Richter, Albert Glass, Douglas Bond, David Rioch, John Spiegel, Harold Wolff, Theodore Lidz, Jurgen Ruesch, Henry Brosin, Alfred Stanton, David Hamburg, Henry Beecher, and Daniel Funkenstein.

Postwar Developments

Wartime psychiatry certainly encompassed a great deal more than psychosomatic medicine and had a profound influence on the developmental pathways that psychiatry would follow in subsequent years. According to Oken (1983), the immediate postwar years saw "the ties between psychiatry and medicine . . . strengthened amid great intellectual excitement" (p. 26). Psychiatrists experienced collaboration not only with medical specialists but also with social workers and psychologists, whose team efforts were critical in rehabilitation programs. Psychoanalysts like Alexander and French (1946) stressed the importance of modifying psychoanalytic techniques for more contemporary application. Abraham Kardiner's psychoanalytic monograph (1941) on war neuroses provided a solid foundation for research on traumatic neuroses (and subsequently on posttraumatic stress disorder).

The stage was set for a better-than-ever rapprochement between psychiatry and medicine, fertilized by the common war experiences of physicians. Of these heady times, William Menninger (1948b) wrote, "psychiatry . . . probably enjoys a wider popular interest at the present time than does any other field of medicine" (p. 2).

Many physicians were switching to psychiatry, with their retrofitting paid for by government funding. According to Starr (1982), the National Institute of Mental Health (NIMH), established by law in 1946 and inaugurated in 1949, was the second and fastest growing division of the National Institutes of Health (NIH). It was especially striking that this rampant growth should occur during the very years that Albert Deutsch (1948) revealed the deplorable state of the nation's mental institutions in his scandal-provoking book *The Shame of the States.* But this negative publicity only seemed to galvanize Congress to pass the National Mental

Health Act of 1946, providing funds for research, training, and special programs such as child psychiatry and suicide prevention. Graduating medical students were attracted in great numbers to residencies in psychiatry not only because it seemed an exciting, emerging field but also because residency stipends, bolstered by government funding, were larger in this medical specialty.

The collective experience of wartime psychiatry (Lewis & Engle, 1954) contained the seeds for vigorous growth of general hospital and consultation-liaison psychiatry: conditions referred to as *effort syndrome, combat fatigue, battle exhaustion, soldier's heart,* and *shell shock* were observed to be complex medical-psychiatric conditions; somatic complaints called attention to somatization as a preeminent expression of anxiety, personality disorder, and neurosis and signaled a need for further postwar explorations; multidisciplinary approaches to emotional rehabilitation through group therapy, occupational therapy, activity therapy, and other "mental hygiene programs" were seen to reduce hospitalization; the realization that combat psychiatric casualties could be treated in medical settings suggested broader application of newer psychiatric techniques in general hospital settings; the efficacy of prompt, early, brief emergency interventions with combatants at battle sites encouraged their further elaboration and application in civilian settings; and the importance of education in psychological factors of illness for all physicians was sharply heightened. The "salvage" value of psychiatry, as demonstrated on the battlefield, had obvious ramifications for community mental health programs.

An explosion of events in the immediate postwar years put psychiatry at the height of its trajectory: the Hospital Survey and Construction Act (Hill-Burton) of 1946 increased the number of hospitals by hundreds; medical schools received research grants that increased the number of clinicians and researchers in medical schools and general hospitals; the American Medical Association inaugurated a Council on Mental Health; state legislatures expressed concern for mental health problems; educational materials on mental illness proliferated; and opportunities for private practice flourished. New general hospitals increased opportunities for general hospital and consultation-liaison psychiatry, whereas medical schools facilitated more sophisticated psychosomatic research.

Although allocation of time for psychiatry in medical school curricula proceeded at a very temperate pace, there was considerable postwar enthusiasm for the education of nonpsychiatrist physicians in the theory and practice of psychosomatic medicine. Whether this zeal was shared equally by teachers and students is difficult to say, but postgraduate courses, seminars, and workshops on "psychotherapeutic medicine" proliferated (Levine, 1949; Witmer, 1947), increasing interaction between psychiatrists and their nonpsychiatrist colleagues.

Before the war, psychosomaticists held a strong conviction that learning how to work simultaneously with matters of the mind and of the body would result in an integrated, holistic approach to the care of the patient. If, it was thought, physicians with a constricted, reductionist focus on diseased organs could be opened up to the complexities and challenges of the psychosomatic approach, patients would benefit and physicians would be gratified. After World War II, this pedagogical excitement began to make its thrust even more zealously against the prevailing dualistic medicine. For a group of psychosomaticists, many of whom had psychoanalytic training, this seemed to be the "teachable moment" for many returning physicians who had seen the extent of psychiatric disability in military inductees.

Gathering in Hershey, Pennsylvania, in February 1945, several former military psychiatrists and educators met under the auspices of the National Committee for Mental Hygiene and the Commonwealth Fund (Witmer, 1947) to consider the needs of physicians who would be called on in their practices to treat veterans with a variety of psychoneurotic reactions. Because there were insufficient psychiatrists to treat the large numbers of patients with psychosomatic symptoms, it was agreed that general physicians would have to bear the major burden of the task. Hence a postgraduate course in psychotherapeutic medicine was taught in two weeks of April 1946 at the University of Minnesota.

In the introduction to the course, Geddes Smith stated that although physicians had always had their share of depressed and anxious patients complaining of a wide variety of physical ailments, "it took the war and its psychiatric casualties to spotlight their need" (cited in Witmer, 1947, p. 1). The teaching staff comprised a veritable Who's Who of American psychiatry, including Douglas Bond, Henry Brosin, Donald Hastings, M. Ralph Kaufman, and John M. Murray, all newly returned from military duty. Of them, Smith said they "felt that psychiatry had something that could and must be shared with general medicine and recognized the urgent need of collaboration from general medicine in the care of the psychoneuroses" (cited in Witmer, 1947, p. 3).

This ambitious undertaking encountered all the expected impediments, including the hardship of trying to weave the elements of the doctor–patient relationship, a "listening" (instead of a "doing") stance, and a new way of taking a history into a too well learned focus on organic medicine. According to Smith, "patients with proven physical lesions and emotional handicaps challenged the doctors' ability to hold the two aspects of medicine in balance" (cited in Witmer, 1947, p. 21). It was nonetheless felt by instructors and participants alike that some new appreciation of the dynamic value of the doctor-patient relationship emerged, and the interaction of emotional stress and physical illness was acknowledged as "real." This educational experiment, unfortunately lacking follow-up data, established a template in 1945 for many subsequent courses in "office psychiatry." More recently, the benefits of teaching nonpsychiatrist physicians how to detect and treat emotional disorders in general practice have been called into question by outcome studies showing low levels of recognition and diagnosis and inadequate therapeutic success (Perez-Stable, Miranda, Munoz & Ying, 1990).

Although psychosomatic medicine may not have fulfilled its promise to realign psychiatry with medicine, it certainly contributed greatly to the new respect for and acceptance of psychiatry after the war. It also established a foundation for important research in subsequent decades into illness as a multidetermined phenomenon, with social, cultural, predispositional, genetic, immunological, viral, hormonal, endocrinological, neurological, relational, and other significant contributors (Weiner, 1977). Important studies have been undertaken in such areas as the relationship of illness to bereavement (Parkes, 1972), hopelessness (Engel, 1967; Schmale, 1972), life change (Rahe, 1977), Relationships (Ackerman, Hofer & Weiner, 1975), inability to express emotions *(alexithymia)* (Nemiah, Freyberger & Sifneos, 1976), and transduction (Cameron, Gunsher & Hariharan, 1990; Chalmers, 1975). The techniques, methodology, and sophisticated hypothesizing of Psychosomatic research have kept the journal *Psychosomatic Medicine* one of the most widely cited journals in the research world, although its scope has broadened remarkably since its founding in 1939.

But perhaps one of the most substantive achievements of wartime psychiatry was to attract those psychiatrists from remote asylums and state hospitals and the "ivory towers" of psychoanalytic institutes back to the mainstream of both psychiatry and medicine. The heightened attention on the general hospital as the site of postwar psychiatric treatment set the stage for the aggressive growth of consultation-liaison psychiatry.

Consultation-Liaison Psychiatry

Psychosomatic Medicine's Foot Soldier

Even as psychosomatic research in the 1960s and 1970s turned more toward the study of social and environmental stimuli as they affected illness expression, its partial success in realigning psychiatry and medicine was a boon to the development of consultation-liaison psychiatry and general hospital psychiatry. Consultation-liaison psychiatrists were a receptive phalanx prepared to build on the commitment to teaching demonstrated by psychosomaticists discharged from the military. With the postwar enthusiasm for training physicians, people such as M. Ralph Kaufman, Sidney Margolin, and Lawrence Kubie quickly made their imprint on psychiatric services in the general hospital (Kaufman & Margolin, 1948; Kubie, 1944).

In spite of organized psychiatry's on-again, off-again engagement with medicine, that small but specialized branch referred to as consultation-liaison (C-L) psychiatry appeared to march steadily to a sometimes different drumbeat. Derived from its collective progenitor of psychosomatic medicine, psychoanalysis, and psychophysiology, C-L psychiatry—the pragmatic, clinical arm of psychosomatic theory and research—seemed to endure even when its antecedents intermittently fell out of favor. What might account for this steadfastness?

This branch of psychiatry was more practical than theoretical or investigatory. Physicians, when stymied by efforts to make sense of nonanatomical physical presentations, perhaps found it useful and more acceptable to turn to psychiatric colleagues for relief of their frustration and help with their patients. Acting as the clinical messenger of psychosomatic medicine, C-L psychiatrists nevertheless had no evangelical intent to persuade nonpsychiatrist physicians of the psychogenesis of illness, an apparent tenet of earlier studies in psychosomatic medicine.

Since its earliest beginnings, the focus of C-L psychiatry has been on the emotional *reactions* of medical-surgical patients. Its service delivery nature was designated as *consultation,* and the more educational part was characterized as *liaison.* The combined activities of the hyphenated term represent, according to Greenhill (1977), the "organizational structure within which the delivery of mental health services to the medically and surgically ill takes place" (p. 115). The C-L psychiatrists have been psychosomatic medicine's pedagogical disseminators of information about the integrative aspects of somatopsychic and psychosomatic conditions, the critical impact of the patient-doctor relationship on the outcome of medical intervention, and the potential of a biopsychosocial perspective (Engel, 1977) for enlarging the scope of medicine. Like other attempts to offer an antidote to the divisive effects of a mind-body dualism, C-L psychiatry subscribed to a more-or-less holistic approach. Always ready to adopt a flexible assimilationist role, it learned to speak the language of medicine and neurology without totally relinquishing its own identity.

Barrett (1922) was most likely the first to use the term *liaison* to allude to psychiatry's relationship to medicine and social problems. Subsequently Pratt (1926), a Boston physician and member of the National Committee for Mental Hygiene, anticipated that psychiatry would become "the liaison agent" to bring together the many clinical aspects of patient care; it was his belief that psychiatry would become "the integrator that unifies, clarifies and resolves all available medical knowledge concerning that human being who is the patient, into one great force of healing power" (p. 408).

In 1929 Henry outlined the concept of liaison psychiatry in the following words:

> On the staff of every general hospital there should be a psychiatrist who would make regular visits to the wards, who would direct a psychiatric outpatient clinic, who would continue the instruction and organize the psychiatric work of interns and who would attend staff conferences so that there might be a mutual exchange of medical experience and a frank discussion of the more complicated cases.
>
> *(p. 496).*

The equation of liaison with the teaching component of consultation-liaison psychiatry appears prominently in evidence here.

Following soon after Henry's publication, Franklin Ebaugh (1932), a member of the National Committee for Mental Hygiene, described "the crisis in psychiatric education" (p. 707), and the *New England Journal of Medicine* anticipated a "new era in psychiatry" (Editorial, 1933, p. 98) in which physicians would be taught a more humanistic approach to medical practice. But it was Billings (1939), a psychiatrist at Colorado General Hospital, where Ebaugh was professor of psychiatry, who actually used the term *psychiatric liaison* to characterize the educational relationship of psychiatrists to interns in the general hospital setting (Billings, 1936). Billings (1966) also described the essential aims of a liaison service in terms that are relevant to this day:

1) to sensitize the physicians and students to the opportunities offered them by every patient, no matter what complaint or ailment was present, for the utilization of a common sense approach for the betterment of the patient's condition, and for making that patient better fitted to handle his problems—somatic or personality—determined by both;
2) to establish psychobiology as an integral working part of the professional thinking of physicians and students of all branches of medicine;
3) to instill in the minds of physicians and students the need the patient-public has for tangible and practical conceptions of personality and sociological functioning.

(p. 20).

In part, it was Billings's intent not only to improve physicians' attitudes toward emotional aspects of illness, but also to counteract the false ideas, misunderstandings, and myths that hampered the patient's receptivity to appropriate (psychological) help from the physician.

Even before World War II, liaison psychiatry rode the educational wave of psychiatric reform. There is widespread agreement that the remarkable expansion of C-L psychiatry would not have occurred had it not been for Alan Gregg's pioneering vision and committed support (Summergrad & Hackett, 1987). He had studied with Francis Weld Peabody, Walter Cannon, James Jackson Putnam (the earliest proponent of psychoanalysis in America and chief of neurology at Massachusetts General Hospital), and other prominent teachers of his day. Gregg, director of the Rockefeller Foundation's Medical Sciences Division, believed that "once the etiology of the major acute medical illnesses, such as infectious disease, had been determined and treatments derived, the treatment of psychiatric disorders would become of greater urgency" (Summergrad & Hackett, 1987, p. 442).

Rockefeller Foundation support in the amount of $11 million from 1933 to 1941 for psychoanalysis, academic psychiatry centers, psychosomatic research, and fields related to psychiatry (e.g., neurology, psychology, neuroanatomy) created a rich matrix in which C-L psychiatry would be nurtured, first by the general funding from the NIMH shortly after the war and again in the 1970s by the Psychiatry Education Branch of the NIMH under James Eaton's direction. The infant nourished by Rockefeller funding required continuous feeding if it was to survive. Because the liaison, or teaching, component of the young specialty had been the most touted but the least capable of ultimate self-support, the issue of reimbursability for the work of C-L psychiatrists took center stage in the next few decades.

Postwar Advances

The postwar decades were a golden age for C-L psychiatry, although different institutions variously emphasized one side or the other of the hyphenated label to characterize their particular bias. Oken (1983) has pointed out that the designation of *consultation-liaison services* is often indiscriminate, sometimes implying the existence of a liaison component where none exists.

One of the best postwar examples of a true consultation-liaison service is that initiated by Kaufman (Kaufman, 1953; Kaufman & Margolin, 1948) at Mount Sinai Hospital in New York. The liaison service at Mount Sinai Hospital benefited not only from the synthesizing creativity of Kaufman, whose roots were in medicine, psychoanalysis, and psychosomatic medicine, but also from the postwar social consciousness and largesse that permitted voluntary attending physicians to provide unpaid teaching in a clinical setting. Liaison in Kaufman's program was carried out by assignment of individual psychiatrists, most with psychoanalytic training, to identified hospital wards and services. As such, they became collaborative members of treatment teams, getting to know and becoming known by their nonpsychiatrist colleagues. Familiarity, in this case, bred not contempt but trust and mutual respect. Kaufman applied firsthand military experience to demonstrate that psychiatrists, internists, and surgeons could work effectively together when they shared a common focus.

With the establishment of a liaison service in 1946 at Mount Sinai Hospital, Kaufman (1953) optimistically said that postwar psychiatry had, for the first time, entered "into the great stream of American medicine" (p. 369). He described the new psychiatry as not just a specialty limited to diagnosing and treating mental disease, but also as extending to "the individual and the complex psychological and emotional factors which might etiologically and concurrently relate to all forms of illness" (p. 369). Without relinquishing his foundations in psychoanalysis and psychosomatic medicine, Kaufman envisioned the psychiatrist in the general hospital as the integrator and catalyst in the teaching and practice of medicine. He described liaison psychiatry as "the most significant division for the role of psychiatrists in a general hospital" (p. 370).

Kaufman delineated the essential practicalities to assure effective collegial relationships: to speak (and write) a comprehensible language that is jargon-free, straightforward, and not abstrusely psychoanalytic; to make every attempt to understand and be of practical help in the total treatment of the patient; and to honestly acknowledge one's professional identity rather than to "smuggle oneself into medicine under false colors" (p. 373). The program at Strong Memorial Hospital in Rochester, New York, allied itself with medicine, in part because George Engel, its originator, himself was an internist and psychoanalyst, but also because he (and his colleagues) believed that a better alliance was made through a medical (rather than a psychiatric) identity.

Most other programs were created by psychiatrists and departments of psychiatry. At the Beth Israel Hospital in Boston, where Kaufman had spent some time before his chairmanship at Mount Sinai, Grete Bibring, chair of the department and a former student of Freud's, had strongly nurtured the teaching opportunities of a department of psychiatry in a general hospital setting. Writing in 1951 of psychiatry's great potential for preventive work with medically ill patients, Bibring attracted faculty and trainees with similar interests, almost all with psychoanalytic training. She had the good fortune to enjoy maximum support from a physician-in-chief (Herman Blumgart) who had personal experience with psychoanalysis.

Although the psychiatric service, with attending staff and fellows assigned to specialty services, fulfilled the criteria of a true liaison service, the use of the term *medical psychology* at Beth Israel Hospital in conjunction with the consultation service was perhaps a symbolic tip of the hat to Pliny Earle (1868), who emphasized the relevance of medical psychology in the physician's education. "Consultation on questions of the management of medical and surgical patients," as described by Kahana (1959), "is most frequently, perhaps, an immediate exercise in the integration of psychological thought in medical practice" (p. 1003). This philosophy extended beyond the inpatient focus to the inauguration of an outpatient integration clinic (Lipsitt, 1964) for the care of patients with complex medical-psychiatric conditions.

Bibring was particularly steadfast in her decision not to have inpatient psychiatric beds, with "the advantage, from the teaching standpoint, of never permitting the house physician to relinquish to the psychiatrist all responsibility for the care of his patient within the hospital" (Kahana, 1959, p. 1003). Bibring's emphasis was not so much on psychiatric diagnosis as it was on understanding the nature of the patient-doctor relationship, the "normal" personality diagnosis (Kahana & Bibring, 1964), and the spectrum of psychologically informed interventions that would promote healing and avoidance of further illness.

In a seminal article in the *New England Journal of Medicine,* Bibring (1956) wrote: "The purpose of this paper is not to discuss 'psychosomatic medicine' or psychiatry as a medical specialty concerned mainly with neuroses and psychoses, but rather to delineate certain important aspects of the role of psychological thought in medical practice" (p. 75)—by which she implied psychoanalytically oriented psychology. By deemphasizing the crusade extant at the time to integrate psychiatry and medicine, and focusing instead on the bedrock of medicine—the patient in relation to the physician—Bibring found a more receptive audience for these "medicopsychological and medicopsychotherapeutic" (p. 75) (rather than psychiatric) interventions. Her concluding remarks in the 1956 article summarized her medical philosophy:

> In the doctor's work, psychological understanding is of profound importance. It enables one to gain the most helpful perspective and awareness of

one's own involvement as well as to comprehend the patient's life pattern and his basic reactions to his sickness and all it entails, including his relation to his physician. The doctor's own feeling of freedom and security provides clarity of thinking and the best potential for his intuitive diagnostic functioning. It permits him to observe the patient fully, protects him and the patient from rigid, defensive bedside manners, and secures for the patient a great feeling of safety derived from his medical care. This, in turn, evokes in the patient all his positive strength, his willingness to cooperate, and his constructive wish to get well and to do right by himself and by his doctor. Thus, the optimal psychosomatic condition is established that may make the difference between a patient who wants to live and the apathy and sabotage of the patient who lets himself die.

(p. 87).

In the 40 years since Bibring's article was published, the field of C-L psychiatry has shown a remarkable versatility in adapting to changes in medicine, the complexity of models required for different settings, and even controversy within the ranks of C-L psychiatrists themselves. But, for the most part, the objectives first delineated by Henry and Billings, enhanced by Kaufman, Bibring, Engel, and others, have shown impressive stamina and endurance.

In the 1990s, the need for clinical C-L research has been recognized and responded to (Cohen-Cole, Howell, Barrett, Lyons & Larson, 1991). Technological shifts and advances in medical practice have been met with similar shifts in the style of C-L practice. Most recently, economic and administrative pressures have skewed the focus more toward reimbursable consultation and less toward the more pedagogical parts of the enterprise, which are less likely to be compensated (Lipsitt, 1992).

It was anticipated that the primary care movement of the 1970s would increase the demand for C-L psychiatry (Lipsitt, 1980). Public Law 94–484 (1976) specified that training in primary care should include faculty with background in behavioral sciences who are active in clinical consultation and in the preparation and implementation of appropriate portions of the curriculum. It appeared that C-L psychiatry would have expanded opportunities to offer training and supervision to these programs. It would also mean a new infusion of funds to bolster academic pursuits. Some (Fink, 1978) said that anywhere from 1,000 to 10,000 additional psychiatrists would be needed to provide the necessary teaching in primary care and family medicine residencies.

But these predictions were misguided in all respects. Some programs interpreted "behavioral science" so broadly that they used either nonphysician mental health staff or none at all. The generally pessimistic outcome for psychiatry in the primary care movement is reflected in a survey (D.R. Lipsitt, 1979) of 42 primary care residents and fourth-year medical students—regarding their attitudes toward psychiatry as part of primary care—that failed to reveal a strong concern for and interest in psychological or social facets of health and illness.

Primary care residents ranked psychiatry low in significance or importance (only slightly more important than minor surgery) and did not list it as a significant part of their attraction to primary care medicine. It is just such pessimistic evidence of attempts in medical education and practice to fuse art and science, humanism and scientism, and the psyche and soma of the human condition that have augured badly for the future of a biopsychosocial approach to health care (Engel, 1977). Writing of the pitfalls of traditional medical thinking, Engel (1979) states disappointedly that "as long as physicians are imbued with the reductionism and dualism of western science, there is no way in which the conflict between psychiatry and the rest of medicine can be resolved" (p. 71).

Increasing Uncertainty Ahead

By the late 1970s, it was clear that C-L psychiatry, although having established a solid beachhead in general hospitals, was headed for shaky times. The number of C-L programs in the country had not increased in a decade (Schubert & McKegney, 1976), a smaller percentage of patients were being referred for psychiatric consultation (Wallen, Pincus, Goldman & Marcus, 1987), psychiatric residents spent less time in C-L experiences (Tilley & Silverman, 1982), and the economic forecast was for still tighter strictures.

Nonetheless, the number of psychiatrists who spent some or all of their time in C-L pursuits continued to grow through continuing remedicalization of psychiatry; by 1983, at least 25% of almost 38,000 psychiatrists nationally claimed activity in C-L psychiatry. The receptivity of the general hospital to the proven cost-effectiveness of C-L programs attracted more and more psychiatrists to that work setting.

It is of some compelling curiosity that the preoccupation of C-L psychiatrists with external factors that typically obstructed the integration of psychiatry with medicine for several decades has seemed to shift in recent years, largely to internal concern with "controversies . . . among its practitioners over the objectives they should strive for and the strategies chosen to achieve them" (Lipowski, 1986, p. 312). Having become accustomed to the halcyon years of strong NIMH support, C-L psychiatry was guilty of some wholesale disregard of important economic, political, conceptual, and organizational vectors that could affect the very viability of hard-won achievements. The ferment stirred by attention to these matters was a healthy sign of growth and stimulated productive controversy.

Questions were raised about the importance of outcome-oriented research, the source of support for fellowship training, competency-based objectives for C-L education, specialty status, and organizational membership. To be appropriately competitive in the "new" medical marketplace, C-L psychiatry would have to establish its credentials beyond anecdotal evidence of its success with and approval by its nonpsychiatrist consumers.

Dissatisfaction with the level of support from the parent organization of psychiatry, the American Psychiatric Association, catalyzed momentum among a number of smaller organizations with a significant interest in the special area of C-L psychiatry. As the economic and political vises tightened, concern was mobilized at the "crossroads" of C-L psychiatry (Lipowski, 1986; Pasnau, 1982). It was not that C-L psychiatry was subject to outside forces different from those affecting any other branch of medicine, but rather, there seemed no collective voice for what was a sometimes forgotten and difficult-to-define endeavor by a segment of psychiatrists working essentially in the general hospital setting.

To address these troublesome concerns, there was a mobilization of activity and reactivity in the service of C-L psychiatry. A number of national organizations identified their C-L interests, including the Academy of Psychosomatic Medicine, the American Association of General Hospital Psychiatrists, the American Psychiatric Association (APA), the American Psychosomatic Society, and the Association for Academic Psychiatry. The Academy of Psychosomatic Medicine, long associated with the relationship of psychiatry to general medicine, had begun to modify its structure to place greater emphasis on C-L psychiatry as its major focus. The American Association of General Hospital Psychiatrists had been representative of the broad spectrum of psychiatric services provided by psychiatry departments in general hospitals, including C-L psychiatry. The APA had always considered the importance of its own liaisons with other nonpsychiatric medical (and even nonmedical) associations. But it had not given high visibility to C-L psychiatry until 1982, when the name of the Committee on Psychiatry and Primary Care Education was officially changed to the Committee on Consultation-Liaison Psychiatry and Primary Care Education. At that time, the committee was inexplicably threatened with "sunsetting" in a restructuring of components, just when psychiatry needed to bolster its image and role in the primary care movement. A letter to the APA Board stated that "it would be anachronistic for the APA to publicly espouse the need for increased numbers of psychiatrist educators in the primary care fields and to internally bury and make less visible this important focus" (Committee on Consultation-Liaison Psychiatry and Primary Care Education, 1981). The committee survived, and in 1987 it played a major role in urging the Accreditation Council for Graduate Medical Education to adopt training requirements in C-L psychiatry for certification in psychiatry, among other significant achievements. Also of importance, the APA established an ad hoc task force to explore the development of funding mechanisms.

Since its founding in 1939, the American Psychosomatic Society was known for its commitment to the synthesis of medicine and psychiatry, but the amount of time and space devoted to basic clinical topics in both annual meetings and the journal *Psychosomatic Medicine* had given way to a major focus on basic research. Some members became disenchanted, but the late 1970s and 1980s saw a resurgence of C-L topics in research, education, and clinical experience. In addition, the American Psychosomatic Society's largest segment of membership came from the ranks of C-L psychiatrists.

In 1977 the Association for Academic Psychiatry established a special section on C-L psychiatry to meet the interests and needs of a significant number of academic psychiatrists. The minutes of a January 17, 1978, meeting describe concerns about the low level of development of C-L programs in training centers, even as there was evidence of increased interest in publications, research, innovative programs, involvement in primary care education and practice, and the funding priority that was given to C-L proposals by the Psychiatry Education Branch of the National Institute of Mental Health. It was determined that the C-L Section would focus on development of task forces to address research, education, and funding. The C-L Section promoted regional C-L groups; increased dialogue between C-L psychiatrists and other nonmedical professionals, such as health psychologists and behavioral scientists; and interacted with other organizations to promote and expand programmatic planning in liaison psychiatry. Several important C-L publications emerged from task force activities in education (Cohen-Cole, Haggerty & Raft, 1982), research (McKegney & Beckhardt, 1982), and economics or funding (Fenton & Guggenheim, 1981).

With increasing anxiety, C-L psychiatry searched for signs of its own vulnerability. Many programs had either lost funding or anticipated such loss. Difficulty in maintaining fellowships was experienced in many training centers, and economics was perhaps the major concern. It had already been realized that a research base had only recently been appreciated as essential to both program efficacy and future funding (Pincus, Lyons & Larson, 1991). Surprisingly, in 1937 Billings himself had recognized the important offset value of C-L psychiatry in his question, "What does the consideration of patients from the psychiatric aspect mean in terms of decreasing hospital days and therefore in saving dollars and cents?" (Billings, McNary & Rees, 1937, p. 242). Even earlier, Karl Menninger (1924) had alluded to the presence of psychiatric units in the general hospital as being the most economical way to address the needs of patients.

But these rare instances of economic insight were obscured by the financially secure years made possible first by the Rockefeller Foundation and then by the NIMH. The sense of security that came with external support enabled C-L psychiatrists the luxury of diminished concern for the economics of providing a valuable clinical and educational service. Considerable time could be spent in pedagogical liaison functions, for which no direct charge was made and for which no specific reimbursement, other than general funding, was received. When funding ceased, it was no longer possible to engage in business as usual. Some staunch teaching institutions even declared a surcease of all liaison functions. It was not until Levitan and Kornfeld (1981) effectively demonstrated the efficacy of C-L psychiatry that the prospects and urgency for similar research captured the attention of C-L psychiatrists.

In 1981 a small number of concerned leaders in C-L psychiatry gathered at Brook Lodge in Augusta, Michigan, to address troublesome issues. Discussion was usually lively, often productive, and sometimes acrimonious as each participant confronted the prospects of a relatively large number of programs competing for the same restricted resources. Much time was devoted to reports of the activities and experiences of a variety of programs, to strategic planning for the next decade, to exchange of information, and to discussion of how better to invite APA's interest and support.

In the next several years, three presidents of the APA were identified as C-L psychiatrists (viz., Pardes, Pasnau, Fink); the APA Committee on Consultation-Liaison Psychiatry and Primary Care Education was infused with new charges to propose curriculum objectives and to assess the relationship of C-L psychiatry to behavioral medicine; and in general, interest in C-L psychiatry among trainees and graduates fared better. It was noted that five journals[3] addressing primarily C-L topics were now available (in contrast to one or two a decade before), and that a number of books had been published on C-L psychiatry since John Schwab's (1968) pioneering *Handbook of Psychiatric Consultation.* On the programmatic side, several medical-psychiatric units were established, and a growing number of C-L outpatient clinics had made their appearance. New linkages were made with specialty areas of medicine, such as transplant units and oncology services. But on a more pessimistic note, the trend of department chairs with major research interests in biological psychiatry was to give C-L psychiatry a very low priority in some institutions where they had previously enjoyed considerable prestige. It was also reported that some hospital administrators, eager to pare their costs, did not understand the need or the place for psychiatric liaison, or if they did, they felt that nonmedical mental health professionals could provide it at lower cost. All these issues spawned interest in fellowship support, as well as possible certification and accreditation in the subspecialty of C-L psychiatry.

In 1988 representatives of several organizations met in Chicago and agreed to establish a consortium with task forces to address issues of subspecialization, fellowship training, C-L research, funding issues, and liaison networking with other groups of interested psychiatrists. Consortium members included the Academy of Psychosomatic Medicine, the American Academy of Child and Adolescent Psychiatry, the American Association of General Hospital Psychiatrists, the American Psychiatric Association, the American Psychosomatic Society, the Association for Academic Psychiatry, and the Association of Directors of Psychiatric Residency Training. Task force chairs were assigned, and a second Brook Lodge conference held in June 1989 to consider their reports. The cumulative effect of these reports was to propose a resolution as follows: 1) that consultation-liaison psychiatry be designated a subspecialty; 2) that the consortium continue for a minimum of 2 years; and 3) that during this period, two areas should be developed: a short-range plan to provide operational rules, fiscal support, and a structural organization; and long-range strategies leading toward accreditation, certification, and funding.

In spite of some expressed concern that subspecialization could risk fragmenting general psychiatry or excluding some psychiatrists from a major source of income, the resolution was accepted. Sabshin (1989), representing the APA, noted that the community mental health movement and the previous elimination of the internship for psychiatry tended to isolate psychiatry from medicine as a whole; however, it was his impression that the remedicalization of psychiatry with its new overemphasis on biological psychiatry may have caused an overcorrection. Sabshin (1989) felt that this issue of remedicalization did not affect C-L psychiatrists because they had "never become demedicalized" (p. 3).

The creative output and energy mobilized by these Brook Lodge retreats produced renewed optimism in C-L psychiatry, a field that, as of this writing, is "on hold" as a subspecialty requiring "added qualifications" for certification. The Academy of Psychosomatic Medicine has assumed a major role in this endeavor.

It has been 60 years since Billings first described liaison psychiatry. The bumps and bruises sustained since then have not deterred efforts to merge treatment of the psyche with treatment of the soma. Although the pendulum perpetually swings, its amplitude is smaller. Perhaps the major peril now is that psychiatry in the general hospital setting may lose its identity by becoming too thoroughly medicalized or by being supplanted by other professions eager to assume roles now held by physicians. One must bear in mind that it was the treatment of *psychiatric* patients in the general hospital that fertilized the growth of C-L psychiatry.

General Hospital Psychiatry

In the prewar years, had the general hospital not experienced growing receptivity to psychiatry on its premises, it is doubtful that C-L psychiatry would have flourished. Most general hospitals were not disposed to admit patients with mental illness. By default, these patients were often shunted to large, mostly rural state hospitals such as those administered by the founders of the APA. These institutions became the repositories for the seriously mentally ill, who, in part because of the psychopharmacological revolution, would not begin to be deinstitutionalized until the mid-1950s.

The first psychiatric unit was established at the Albany Hospital in New York (Mosher, 1909) at about the same time that Freud delivered his seminal lectures at Clark University in Worcester, Massachusetts. Recognizing that the custodial asylums only perpetuated the view of psychiatry as alienist and isolated from the rest of medicine, a few psychiatrists began an active campaign to reunite with medicine in settings that might reacquaint doctors of the mind with doctors of the body.

Even before the first inpatient psychiatric unit in the United States was established in a general hospital in 1902, modest efforts to treat these patients in general hospitals in their own communities is believed to have begun as early as 1755 at the Pennsylvania Hospital, where history has it that a number of beds were designated for "the reception and cure of lunatics" (Mosher, 1900, p. 325). Mosher's

(1909) avowed aims of his innovative step were 1) to provide psychiatric treatment of patients with acute mental illness; 2) to provide treatment of a quality that compared favorably with that of medical patients; 3) to reduce the stigma of sending patients away by offering treatment closer to their own communities and families; and 4) to expose both medical and nonmedical staff to training in psychiatric care—objectives ideally espoused even today.

Characterized by Lipowski (1981) as "one of the most far-reaching developments in psychiatry's history" (p. 892), this movement permitted psychiatrists interested in careers in general hospitals to interact with their nonpsychiatrist colleagues, to establish the rudiments of liaison through their interest in teaching, and to create networks for referral of private patients to build part-time psychotherapeutic practices. According to Lipowski (1981), "more than any other organizational change, that development has helped raise the standards of psychiatric patient care, training, and research and to reduce the isolation of psychiatry from progress in the rest of medicine" (p. 892).

In the early 1930s, partly catalyzed by Rockefeller Foundation support, the number of general hospitals with psychiatric units swelled from less than 10 to 153. There was a concurrent increase of "scatter beds" for psychiatric patients in general medical wards, as well as growth of C-L services.

Experience in the war with multidisciplinary approaches to emotional rehabilitation established their utility for milieu treatment or therapeutic communities on inpatient psychiatric units. Effective psychiatric interventions counteracted the distrusted stereotype of protracted, couch-bound, psychoanalytic treatment. Attitudes toward the appropriateness of psychiatric care in the general hospital were considerably altered by wartime medical experience.

Postwar Success and Failure

For reasons previously cited, psychiatry's currency with medicine once again ran high in the postwar years. A renaissance of interest in the general hospital as the proper setting for treating the majority of patients with psychiatric conditions catalyzed a burgeoning of inpatient and other psychiatric services to accomplish this purpose. By the 1970s, at least 1,000 such units had been established.

Psychiatry's successful acceptance into the general hospital was also, in some respects, a failure because of at least two major repercussions. First, except for the C-L aspects of psychiatry, the expansion of psychiatry and the uniqueness of psychiatry (compared with medicine and surgery) posed some threat to members of the hospital staff who felt that psychiatric patients would somehow change the ambiance of the hospital and even present a risk to others. Perhaps in response to such reactions, psychiatry's fate was to become compartmentalized and isolated even in the midst of other medical specialties in the general hospital. Second, if the 1940s and 1950s can be characterized as a period of the preeminence of psychiatrists, psychoanalysts, and medical psychotherapists, the 1960s, bolstered by the community mental health movement, marked the beginning of the ascendance of the nonmedical mental health professional. This trend was further nurtured by the strong democratizing influence of the multidisciplinary milieu or therapeutic community approach of general hospital psychiatric units, in which all mental health professionals often played interchangeable roles.

Rome (1965) has eloquently alluded to the vectors working to pull medicine and psychiatry apart, even as they appeared finally to have come functionally so close together. According to Rome, writing of a reaffiliation of psychiatry with medicine,

> Days, weeks, and months of face-to-face encounters inevitably conduce to a central tendency in the over-all values shared by the hitherto separate and uninfluenced specialties. Despite the very successful attempts to bring about an ever-closer rapprochement between psychiatry and medicine, however, there are still many defects in the synthesis. There are few if any who can cross discipline boundaries and function with comparable expertness. The multisecting of the patient which results requires a coordination of all the king's horses and all the king's men if it is hoped to put the patient together again. And few have the temerity even to try.
>
> *(p. 182).*

Reminiscent of Winnicott's (1966) reference to the "two horses" of psyche and soma, described earlier, Rome's articulate, perhaps pessimistic, but extraordinarily candid assessment of efforts to perceive the acceptance of psychiatric services into the general hospital as mostly a positive event contains some jarring forecasts of problems to come. If psychiatrists were lacking in scientific medicine, and if some aspects of psychiatric treatment could readily be provided by nonmedical ancillary mental health professionals, did not this indeed call into question the need for a strong medical foundation in psychiatric care?

In many respects, the hard-won rapprochement in the general hospital appeared to be more of an uneasy coexistence than a true integration. Small (1965), describing psychiatry's isolation even within the general hospital setting, wrote,

> Unfortunately, in many instances, the psychiatric unit merely exists within the framework of the general hospital and, in truth, operates an independent psychiatric hospital except for the convenience of x-ray, biochemical, bacteriological, and other laboratory services. In the same institutions the psychiatrists are considered as a group apart, or are perhaps accepted because of their knowledge of neurology rather than their potential contribution to a psychodynamic appreciation of human behavior in illness and health.
>
> *(p. 342).*

Verification of this sentiment is found in the regularity with which psychiatric services in the general hospital have been customarily assigned the most isolated and obsolete quarters.

Establishment of psychiatric units in general hospitals, especially in the late 1980s and early 1990s, was most likely more often on the basis of economic concerns than because of an administration's responsivity to community needs or some idealistic subscription to a more holistic approach to health care. Psychiatrists and other mental health professionals who have worked in general hospital psychiatric units have been aware of the extent to which they lived a fairly isolated professional life, eating together, avoiding or being excluded from most general hospital functions, and the neglect of opportunities for their own continuing medical education through attendance at medical grand rounds and the like. Beaton (1965), even as he expressed the "hope for the great return, at least in part, of psychiatry to the general hospital and to the company of its fellow disciplines in the house of medicine" (p. 351), cautioned that "to remain a doctor, [the general hospital psychiatrist] should be immersed in the maelstrom of the general hospital for his own professional good, [rather than as merely a zealous teacher bringing] his leavening influence on his colleagues in medicine" (p. 351). Furthermore, psychiatric staff in the general hospital setting have become accustomed to the corpus of humor, mocking and otherwise, directed at psychiatric patients, staff, and services within the "medical" institution. Particularly pointed barbs have been directed at talking treatment, the lack of a medical model in psychiatric ward structure, and the fact than an outsider often cannot tell the difference between staff and patients because of the absence of distinguishing medical uniforms.

Increasing Ambivalence

By 1963 the "bandwagon approach" to the establishment of psychiatric services in general hospitals was questioned as to whether it was a boon or a bane (Schulberg, 1963). The absence of useful research into the efficacy of general hospital units was noted as it was recalled that even the World Health Organization Committee on Psychiatric Treatment in 1953 had rejected popular sentiment that the general hospital was necessarily the most appropriate and desirable site for the provision of psychiatric care. It is unclear why this was so, although it is possible that competing private hospitals in both Europe and the United States did not share enthusiasm for a proliferation of specialized psychiatric units in general hospitals in the United States.

And so the pendulum continued to swing. At times, political and professional debates were suggestive of the uneasy truce of one people's attempts to peacefully coexist in another people's land. It was not surprising to hear fresh references to psychiatry's "identity crisis" (Bandler, 1965). Bandler felt that psychiatry's identity had not been well established in training programs, in medical school curricula, or even in the proper subject matter of the specialty. It appeared as though its own definition was being obscured by social, environmental, behavioral, and even political issues.[4]

Grinker (1964) referred to a psychiatry that was "riding madly in all directions" (p. 236). Although the Kennedy and Johnson administrations brought a heightened social consciousness, they were not necessarily turning to psychiatry to meet the nation's vast mental health needs. Perhaps the attitude toward psychiatry in the general hospital reflected the ambivalence about psychiatry in society generally. The psychiatric profession was portrayed (Starr, 1982) as anything but a unified discipline with the tools, knowledge, and skill to maintain its hard-won battles at remedicalization; it became a faddish pastime to categorize psychiatrists as "organicists" or "dynamicists" as a measure of their dualistic split allegiance to the tenets of medical practice (Hollingshead & Redlich, 1958).

The split in psychiatric identity was further heightened by Solomon's urging in his APA presidential speech that "our large mental hospitals should be liquidated" (Solomon, 1958, p. 7). By this time, the establishment of psychiatric services in general hospitals seemed an incontrovertible trend, and the psychiatric revolution in psychopharmacology had made it possible to consider returning many, if not all, psychiatric patients to the community. These suggestions sparked controversy that swirled around the question of appropriate treatment and care of the mentally ill for most of the 1960s.

Psychiatry's extension into social, political, economic, legal, and public health arenas drew attention to poverty and other social blights as contributors to poor mental health. The psychiatrist came to be identified more as a social engineer directing a multidisciplinary team of mental health specialists. Reference to *psychiatric treatment* began to be replaced by the less medical-sounding term *mental health services,* and *clinics* were referred to as *centers.* Nonmedical social workers, counselors, educators, and psychologists assumed a larger role in direct care, with treatment focused more in communities than in hospitals, and with psychiatrists leaving underfunded community programs for more remunerative private practice. The democratization of mental health professionalism of the milieu-oriented inpatient service was transplanted to the community mental health center. Psychiatry expanded (or diluted) its former medicalized dualism of mind and body to a more socialized triad of mind, body, and society. This shift to an emphasis on social rather than on mental dysfunction involving mind, brain, and body as a basis for mental disorder in both inpatient and outpatient settings seemed a derailment of the trend toward an integration of psyche and soma.

Although the medical setting of inpatient psychiatric units in general hospitals strengthened and maintained the psychiatrist's position as "team leader" in the multidisciplinary medical institution, this therapeutic function and leadership role were less and less distinguishable from those of nonmedical colleagues, thus threatening psychiatry's unique identity (Lipsitt, 1981). This trend fostered the notion in some that medical training was nonessential in the armamentarium of a psychiatrist. That such an outrageous conclusion actually could be proposed merely fueled the dissension and frenzy that already existed in psychiatric circles. The implementation of such a notion indeed had the potential for the ultimate demedicalization of psychiatry! Nonetheless, the announcement was made in 1969 that the American Board of Psychiatry and Neurology would not require the completion of a medical internship for eligibility in psychiatry; John Romano (1970) led the outraged charge against this "act of regression" in its apparent abandonment of medicine and responsibility for patient care as the bedrock of psychiatric training. Reasserting the psychiatrist's heritage in medicine, Romano wrote:

> The psychiatrist, as a physician, brings to the field his ancient heritage of the physician and broad experience in biology and clinical medicine, as well as in psychology and the social sciences. To reduce the dimensions of the role of the psychiatrist as physician would seriously impair his contributions as practitioner, teacher, scholar, and investigator. It is a degradation of quality.
>
> *(p. 1575).*

Within a very short time, the medical internship (although in modified form) was restored as a requirement for eligibility in psychiatry, and psychiatry once again seemed reassured of its propinquity to medicine.

A more realistic and circumscribed remedicalization began to emerge. Psychiatrists, relinquishing their preeminence as psychotherapists to nonmedical professionals, increasingly embraced those dimensions of the specialty that indeed depended on a knowledge of physical disease, pharmacology, neuroscience, and endocrinology. In part this appeared a safe haven, which unlike the large and ill-defined realm of psychotherapy, could not be invaded easily by others of lesser training, and in part it was in all likelihood a matter of economic preservation.

The formulation of a new psychiatric taxonomy (DSM-III [American Psychiatric Association, 1980] and DSM-III-R [American Psychiatric Association, 1987]) helped strengthen the medical nature of psychiatric disorder. Designation of axes as part of a complete diagnosis established some parallels with the staging and classifying of physical diseases such as cancer and cardiovascular disease and therefore garnered more credibility. Attempts to standardize diagnosis and treatment were long overdue, and thoughtful nosological revision won plaudits from many circles; it also provided the framework in which good research could take place, the better to assure psychiatry's acceptance in the new marketplace approach to cost-effective and successful treatment.

Not all psychiatrists were happy with these new medicalized guidelines; much of what distinguished psychiatry from other medical specialties (e.g., its underpinnings in dynamic psychiatry and its reliance on formulation and respect for the highly individualistic characteristics of each patient) appeared to have been abandoned for the sake of *not merely rapprochement with* medicine, but perhaps *even absorption into* medicine. It is revealing to note the return of references to the prewar term *neuropsychiatry* in the psychiatric literature and presentations.

Summary and Conclusion

Ever since psychiatry drifted from its roots in medicine, its history has been punctuated with efforts at reunion. Medicine, it was believed, should be a very human enterprise, and without psychiatry to remind it of its artful, emotional side, it would become coldly technologized and abandon its humanistic intent.

With its many approaches to and diversions from the main body of medicine, psychiatry has endured a succession of identity crises (Bandler, 1965; Braceland, 1969; Ebaugh, 1932; Grinker, 1964) and turning points (Sabshin, 1990) in its quest to rejoin mind and body; this union was thought to have been permanently severed by the teachings and writings of the seventeenth century philosopher Descartes. The task of reconnecting psyche and soma into one conceptual frame has been taken up by psychoanalysis, psychosomatic medicine, consultation-liaison psychiatry, general hospital psychiatry, and psychopharmacology, with each skewed toward a slightly different aspect of the challenge.

The literature of the profession is peppered with cautions against either-or thinking, with preferred urgings to think holistically, monistically, or biopsychosocially. The frustrated wailing of repeated near successes or utter failures can be heard in the scapegoating of Descartes as the villain, unlikely as this explanation seems (Brown, 1989). There is a perception that naming the "thing" (the mindbody connection) might make it real, although attempts at operationally combining the mind and body sometimes have the feel of two magnets approaching one another, only to abruptly swing away at the point of near contact.

Close encounters of the integrated kind were alluded to as the medicalizing or the remedicalizing (depending on timing) of psychiatry, as with electroconvulsive therapy, psychopharmacology, or neuroscience; separation from medicine, as with psychoanalysis, institutionalization, community mental health, or psychotherapy, was described as demedicalization. The rhythmic vacillations have been as regular as swings of the pendulum. Contributing momentum or drag, as the case may be, were a host of happenings—scientific, political, economic, and social, not the least of which was World War II. This cataclysmic event added thrust to the swing toward the psyche side of the arc. With a new appreciation of psychiatry's performance in the war effort, a new attitude toward the relevance of mental health for the nation, and new governmental support in the form of legislation, funding, hospital construction, and granting agencies, psychiatry flourished. Its stock with medicine was greatly enhanced, as was its alliance. Psychiatry's alliance with medicine was built on foundations of earlier but less publicly acknowledged rapprochements. After some disappointments in psychosomatic medicine's promises, psychiatry took its rightful place alongside medicine in the general hospital setting, and consultation-liaison psychiatry offered insurance against further separations.

But however fast or forcefully the pendulum swings, there can be only a visu-ally distorted perception that the gap has truly closed. It is, however, the ringing of the chimes more than the hypnotic swinging of the pendulum that attracts atten-tion. And there is much in psychiatry's bumpy history of realignment for which the bell tolls. The dilemma, however, of how to bridge the gap between psyche and soma remains, perhaps most cogently addressed by Morton Reiser (1974), who writes that

> regardless of our ultimate conviction that mind and body constitute a true functional unity, the fact remains that as observers, investigators and theo-rists, we are obliged (whether we like it or not) to deal with data from two separate realms, one pertaining to mind and the other to body. . . . There is no way to unify the two by translation into a common language, or by reference to a shared conceptual framework, nor are there as yet bridging concepts that could serve, as Bertalanffy suggests, as intermediate templates, isomorphic with both realms. For all practical purposes, then, we deal with mind and body as separate realms; virtually all of our psychophysiological and psychosomatic data consist in essence of covariance data, demonstrat-ing coincidence of events occurring in the two realms within specific time intervals at a frequency beyond chance.
>
> *(p. 479).*

Although the efforts of many neuroscientists and psychopharmacologists have shed much light on the multiplicity of ways in which the brain functions and potentially connects with the mind, we are reminded that any conceptualizing that veers too much toward the brain or too much toward the mind runs the risk of evolving into either a "mindless" or a "brainless" psychiatry (Eisenberg, 1986; Reiser, 1988). Reiser (1989), once again, sums up where we are:

> As a profession, psychiatry—fully appreciative of the rapidly expanding body of knowledge in neurobiology and its immediate practical applications in clinical psychopharmacology—has been intensively engaged in a process of "remedicalization." The impetus for this has received reinforcement from a variety of other pressures, such as new patterns of reimbursement, cost-effectiveness "criteria" and blurred professional boundaries in the field of mental health. All of this has led to major changes in patterns of mental health care and psychiatric practice, in both public and private sectors.
>
> *(p. 187).*

The tension generated in psychiatry's creative navigation of the reefs and shoals of sometimes stormy seas of psyche and soma has been very productive. If the search for a conceptual model (even if not operational) of integrated treat-ment and care had not persisted, the great advances in psychosomatic medicine, consultation-liaison psychiatry, and general hospital psychiatry might not have occurred. Psychiatry's next hurdle in keeping the study of the mind in medicine may be its response to the perturbations of managed care, managed competition, and other products of emerging health care reform.

Notes

1 The vicissitudes of "identity" may already have been hinted at in Dunbar's reference to the American Psychomedical [sic] Association in her text on psychiatry (Dunbar 1959).
2 Nemiah (Taylor, 1987) notes a (1796) poetic mention of the word *psychosomatic* in Coleridge's early works. It is believed that Dunbar (1948) was first to use the term in American literature. The term itself, first thought to supplant the word *functional,* created some dissension because it appeared to preserve the very dichotomy it was intended to mend. But it was ultimately accepted as more palatable to physicians than Meyer's suggested alternative *ergasiology* (the science of energy economy) (Lief, 1948, pp. 544–555).
3 *General Hospital Psychiatry; Journal of Psychosomatic Research; Psychiatric Medicine; Psychiatry in Medicine; Psychosomatics.*
4 It is of some speculative interest that Bandler's own virtuosity in the several aspects of 1960s psychiatry—psychoanalysis, psychiatric education, general hospital psychiatry, academic psychiatry, residency training, and community psychiatry—may have heightened his awareness of the field's search for identity.

References

Ackerman, S.H., Hofer, M.A., & Weiner, H. (1975). Age at maternal separation and gastric erosion susceptibility in the rat. *Psychosomatic Medicine, 37,* 180–184.

Alexander, F.G. (1950). *Psychosomatic Medicine: Its Principles and Applications.* New York, NY: Norton

Alexander, F.G., & French, T.M. (1946). *Psychoanalytic Therapy.* New York, NY: Ronald Press.

Alexander, F.G., & Selesnick, S.T. (1968). *The History of Psychiatry.* New York, NY: New American Library.

American Psychiatric Association. (1980). *Diagnostic and Statistical Manual of Mental Disorders.* (3rd edition). Washington, DC: American Psychiatric Association.

American Psychiatric Association. (1987). *Diagnostic and Statistical Manual of Mental Disorders.* (3rd edition, revised). Washington, DC: American Psychiatric Association.

Army Medical Services Graduate School. (1953). *Symposium on Stress.* Walter Reed Army Medical Center. Washington, DC, March 16–18.

Bandler, B. (1965). Programs for interns and residents on other services in the hospital. In M.R. Kaufman (Ed.). *The Psychiatric Unit in a General Hospital: Its Current and Future Role.* (pp. 315–331). New York, NY: International Universities Press.

Barrett, A.M. (1922). The broadened interests of psychiatry. *American Journal of Psychiatry, 2,* 1–13.

Beaton, L.E. (1965). Postgraduate education for psychiatrists. In M.R. Kaufman (Ed.). *The Psychiatric Unit in a General Hospital: Its Current and Future Role.* (pp. 350–359). New York, NY: International Universities Press.

Bibring, G.L. (1951). Preventive psychiatry in a general hospital. *Bulletin of the World Federation for Mental Health, 5,* 224–232.

Bibring, G.L. (1956). Psychiatry and medical practice in a general hospital. *New England Journal of Medicine, 254,* 366–372.

Billings, E.G. (1936). Teaching psychiatry in the medical school general hospital: A practical plan. *Journal of the American Medical Association, 107,* 635–639.

Billings, E.G. (1939). Liaison psychiatry and intern instruction. *Journal of the Association of American Medical Colleges, 14,* 375–385, 1939.

Billings, E.G. (1966). The psychiatric liaison department of the University of Colorado medical school and hospitals. *American Journal of Psychiatry, 122,* 28–33.

Billings, E.G., McNary, W.S., & Rees, M.H. (1937). Financial importance of general hospital psychiatry to hospital administrators. *Hospitals, 11,* 400–444.

Binger, C. (1966). *Revolutionary Doctor: Benjamin Rush, 1746–1813.* New York, NY: W.W. Norton.

Braceland, F. (1969). Our medical heritage. *American Journal of Psychiatry, 126,* 877–879.

Brown, T.M. (1989). Cartesian dualism and psychosomatics. *Psychosomatics, 30,* 322–331.

Cameron, O.G., Gunsher, S., & Hariharan, M. (1990). Venous plasma epinephrine levels and the symptoms of stress. *Psychosomatic Medicine, 52,* 411–424.

Chalmers, J.P. (1975). Brain amines and models of experimental hypertension. *Circulation Research, 36,* 469–480.

Christian, H.A. (1942). *Osler's Principles and Practice of Medicine.* (14th edition). New York, NY: Appleton Century.

Cohen-Cole, S., Haggerty, J., & Raft, D. (1982). Objectives for residents in consultation psychiatry: Recommendations of a task force. *Psychosomatics, 23,* 699–703.

Cohen-Cole, S.A., Howell, E.F., Barrett, J.E., Lyons, J., & Larson, D. (1991). Consultation-liaison research: Four selected topics. In F.K. Judd, G.D. Burrows, & D.R. Lipsitt (Eds.). *Handbook of Studies on General Hospital Psychiatry.* (pp. 79–98). Amsterdam: Elsevier.

Committee on Consultation-Liaison Psychiatry and Primary Care Education. (1981). *Letter.* Washington, DC: American Psychiatric Association.

Deutsch, A. (1948). *The Shame of the States.* New York, NY: Harcourt, Brace.

Deutsch, F. (1959). *On the Mysterious Leap from the Mind to the Body: A Workshop Study on the Theory of Conversion.* New York, NY: International Universities Press.

Dunbar, H.F. (1935). *Emotions and Bodily Changes.* New York, NY: Columbia University Press.

Dunbar, H.F. (1948). *Synopsis of Psychosomatic Diagnosis and Treatment.* St. Louis, MO: Mosby.

Dunbar, H.F. (1959). *Psychiatry in the Medical Specialties.* New York, NY: Blakiston.

Dunbar, H.F., & Arlow, J. (1944). Criteria for therapy in psychosomatic disorders. *Psychosomatic Medicine, 6,* 283–286.

Earle, P. (1868). Psychological medicine: Its importance as a part of the medical curriculum. *American Journal of Insanity, 24,* 257–280.

Ebaugh, F.G. (1932). The crisis in psychiatric education. *Journal of the American Medical Association, 99,* 703–707.

Editorial. (1933). The new era in psychiatry. *New England Journal of Medicine, 208,* 98–99.

Editors. (1939). Introductory statement. *Psychosomatic Medicine, 1,* 3–5.

Eisenberg, L. (1986). Mindlessness and brainlessness in psychiatry. *British Journal of Psychiatry, 48,* 497–508.

Engel, G.L. (1962). *Psychological Development in Health and Disease.* Philadelphia, PA: W.B. Saunders.

Engel, G.L. (1967). A psychological setting of somatic disease: The "giving up-given up" complex. *Proceedings of the Royal Society of Medicine, 60,* 553–555.

Engel, G.L. (1977). The need for a new medical model: A challenge for biomedicine. *Science, 196,* 129–136.

Engel, G.L. (1979). Resolving the conflict between medicine and psychiatry. *Resident & Staff Physician, 26,* 73–79.

Fenton, B.J., & Guggenheim, F.G. (1981). Consultation-liaison psychiatry and funding: Why can't Alice find wonderland? *General Hospital Psychiatry, 3,* 255–260.

Fink, P.J. (1978). Politics and funding in primary care: A look to the future. *Psychiatric Opinion, 15,* 14–17.

Freedman, D.X. (1992). The search: Body, mind, and human purpose. *American Journal of Psychiatry, 149,* 858–866.

Friedman, M., & Rosenman, R.H. (1959). Association of specific overt behavior patterns with blood and cardiovascular findings. *Journal of the American Medical Association, 169,* 1085–1096.

Gay, P. (1988). *Freud: A Life for Our Time.* New York, NY: W.W. Norton.

Gray, J.P. (1869). Insanity, and its relation to medicine. *American Journal of Insanity, 25,* 145–172.

Greenblatt, M. (1975). Psychiatry: The battered child of medicine. *New England Journal of Medicine, 292,* 246–250.

Greenhill, M.H. (1977). The development of liaison programs. In G. Usdin (Ed.). *Psychiatric Medicine.* (pp. 115–191). New York, NY: Brunner/Mazel.

Greenhill, M.H. (1979). Psychiatric units in general hospitals: 1979. *Hospital & Community Psychiatry, 30,* 169–182.

Grinker, R.R. (1964). Psychiatry rides madly in all directions. *Archives of General Psychiatry, 10,* 228–237.

Grinker, R.R., & Spiegel, J.P. (1945). *Men Under Stress.* Philadelphia, PA: Blakiston.

Henry, G.W. (1929). Some modern aspects of psychiatry in a general hospital practice. *American Journal of Psychiatry, 86,* 481–499.

Hollingshead, A.B., & Redlich, F. (1958). *Social Class and Mental Illness.* New York, NY: Wiley & Sons.

Kahana, R.J. (1959). Teaching medical psychology through psychiatric consultation. *Medical Education, 34,* 1003–1009.

Kahana, R.J., & Bibring, G.L. (1964). Personality types in medical management. In N.E. Zinberg (Ed.). *Psychiatry and Medical Practice in a General Hospital.* (pp. 108–123). New York, NY: International Universities Press.

Kardiner, A. (1941). The traumatic neuroses of war. In *Psychosomatic Medicine Monographs II-III.* (pp. 68–132). Washington, DC: National Research Council.

Kaufman, M.R. (1953). Role of the psychiatrist in the general hospital. *Psychiatric Quarterly, 27,* 367–381.

Kaufman, M.R., & Margolin, S.G. (1948). Theory and practice of psychosomatic medicine in a general hospital. *Medical Clinics of North America, 32,* 611–616.

Kimball, C.P. (1970). Conceptual developments in psychosomatic medicine: 1939–1969. *Annals Internal Medicine, 73,* 307–316.

Kubie, L.S. (1944). The organization of a psychiatric service for a general hospital. *Psychosomatic Medicine, 6,* 252–272.

Kubie, L.S. (1953). The central representation of the symbolic process in relation to psychosomatic disorders. *Psychosomatic Medicine, 15,* 1–7.

Lebensohn, Z.M. (1980). General hospital psychiatry U.S.A.: Retrospect and prospect. *Comprehensive Psychiatry, 21,* 500–509.

Leigh, H., & Reiser, M.F. (1977). Major trends in psychosomatic medicine. *Annals of Internal Medicine, 87,* 233–239.

Levine, M. (1949). *Psychotherapy in Medical Practice.* New York, NY: Macmillan.

Levitan, S.J., & Kornfeld, D.S. (1981). Clinical and cost-benefits of liaison psychiatry. *American Journal of Psychiatry, 138,* 790–793.

Lewis, N.D.C., & Engle, B. (1954). *Wartime Psychiatry.* New York, NY: Oxford.

Lief, A. (1948). *The Commonsense Psychiatry of Adolf Meyer.* New York, NY: McGraw-Hill.

Lipowski, Z.J. (1977). Psychosomatic medicine in the seventies: An overview. *American Journal of Psychiatry, 134,* 233–244.

Lipowski, Z.J. (1981). Holistic-medical foundations of American psychiatry: A bicentennial. *American Journal of Psychiatry, 138,* 888–895.

Lipowski, Z.J. (1983). Current trends in consultation-liaison psychiatry. *Canadian Journal of Psychiatry, 28,* 329–338.

Lipowski, Z.J. (1986). Consultation-liaison psychiatry: The first half century. *General Hospital Psychiatry, 8,* 305–315.

Lipsitt, D.R. (1964). Integration clinic: An approach to the teaching and practice of medical psychology in an outpatient setting. In N.E. Zinberg (Ed.). *Psychiatry and Medical Practice in a General Hospital.* (pp. 231–249). New York, NY: International Universities Press.

Lipsitt, D.R. (1979). Unpublished manuscript: Survey of 42 primary care residents and 4th year medical students.

Lipsitt, D.R. (1980). Psychiatry and medicine: Partners in primary care. *Resident & Staff Physician, 26,* 99–108.

Lipsitt, D.R. (1981). Psychiatry. In E. Bernstein (Ed.). *Medical and Health Annual.* (pp. 291–295). Chicago, IL: Encyclopedia Britannica.

Lipsitt, D.R. (1983). The influence of dualistic thinking on the role of psychiatry in medicine. In J.R. Lopez-Ibor, J. Saiz, & J.M. Lopez-Ibor (Eds.). *General Hospital Psychiatry.* (pp. 18–24). Amsterdam: Excerpta Medica.

Lipsitt, D.R. (1992). Challenges of somatization: Diagnostic, therapeutic and economic. *Psychiatric Medicine, 10,* 1–12.

McKegney, F.P., & Beckhardt, R.M. (1982). Evaluative research in consultation-liaison psychiatry. *General Hospital Psychiatry, 4,* 197–218.

Menninger, K.A. (1924). The place of the psychiatric department in the general hospital. *Modern Hospital, 23,* 1–4.

Menninger, W.C. (1945). Psychosomatic medicine on general medical wards. *Bulletin United States Army Medical Department, 4,* 545–550.

Menninger, W.C. (1947). Psychosomatic medicine: Somatization reactions. *Psychosomatic Medicine, 9,* 92–97.

Menninger, W.C. (1948a). *Psychiatry in a Troubled World: Yesterday's War and Today's Challenge.* New York, NY: Macmillan.

Menninger, W.C. (1948b). *Psychiatry: Its Evolution and Present Status.* Ithaca, NY: Cornell University Press.

Mosher, J.M. (1900). The insane in general hospitals. *American Journal of Insanity, 57,* 325–329.

Mosher, J.M. (1909). A consideration of the need of better provision for the treatment of mental disease in its early stage. *American Journal of Insanity, 65,* 499–508.

Nemiah, J.C., Freyberger, H., & Sifneos, P.E. (1976). Alexithymia: A view of the psychosomatic process. In O.W. Hill (Ed.). *Modern Trends in Psychosomatic Medicine-3.* (pp. 430–439). London, UK: Butterworths.

Oken, D. (1983). Liaison psychiatry (Liaison medicine). *Advances in Psychosomatic Medicine, 11,* 23–51.

Parkes, C.M. (1972). *Bereavement.* New York, NY: International Universities Press.

Pasnau, R.O. (1982). Consultation-liaison psychiatry at the crossroads: In search of a definition for the 1980s. *Hospital & Community Psychiatry, 33,* 989–995.

Perez-Stable, E.J., Miranda, J., Munoz, R.F., & Ying, Y.W. (1990). Depression in medical outpatients: Underrecognition and misdiagnosis. *Archives of Internal Medicine, 150,* 1083–1088.

Pincus, H.A., Lyons, J.S., & Larson, D.B. (1991). The benefits of consultation-liaison psychiatry. In F.K. Judd, G.D. Burrows, & D.R. Lipsitt (Eds.). *Handbook of Studies on General Hospital Psychiatry.* (pp. 43–52). Amsterdam: Elsevier.

Pratt, G.K. (1926). Psychiatric departments in general hospitals. *American Journal of Psychiatry, 82,* 403–410.

Public Law 94–484. (1976). Health Professions Education Assistance Act. 94th Congress, 2nd session, 12 October 1976.

Rahe, R.H. (1977). Epidemiology studies of life change and illness. In Z.J. Lipowski, D.R. Lipsitt, & P.C. Whybrow (Eds.). *Psychosomatic Medicine: Current Trends and Clinical Applications.* (pp. 411–420). New York, NY: Oxford.

Reiser, M.F. (1974). Changing theoretical concepts in psychosomatic medicine. In S. Arieti (Ed.). *American Handbook of Psychiatry.* (Vol. 4, 2nd edition, pp. 477–500). New York, NY: Grune & Stratton.

Reiser, M.F. (1988). Are psychiatric educators "losing the mind"? *American Journal of Psychiatry, 145,* 148–153.

Reiser, M.F. (1989). The future of psychoanalysis in academic psychiatry: Plain talk. *Psychoanalytic Quarterly, 58,* 185–209.

Romano, J. (1970). The elimination of the internship: An act of regression. *American Journal of Psychiatry, 126,* 1565–1575.

Rome, H.P. (1965). The psychotherapies: The sociology of psychiatric practice in a general hospital. In M.R. Kaufman (Ed.). *The Psychiatric Unit in a General Hospital: Its Current and Future Role.* (pp. 177–192). New York, NY: International Universities Press.

Rush, B. (1812). *Medical Inquiries and Observations on the "Diseases of the Mind."* Birmingham, AL: Gryphon Editions, 1988.

Sabshin, M. (1989). Commentary. In *Proceedings of the Second National Conference on Consultation-Liaison Psychiatry.* Augusta, MI: Brook Lodge, June 22–24.

Sabshin, M. (1990). Turning points in twentieth-century American psychiatry. *American Journal of Psychiatry, 147,* 1267–1274.

Schmale, A.H. (1972). Giving up as a final common pathway to changes in health. *Advances in Psychosomatic Medicine, 8,* 21–40.

Schubert, D.S.P., & McKegney, F.P. (1976). Psychiatric consultation education: 1976. *Archives of General Psychiatry, 33,* 1271–1273.

Schulberg, H.C. (1963). Psychiatric units in general hospitals: Boon or bane? *American Journal of Psychiatry, 120,* 30–36.

Schwab, J.J. (1968). *Handbook of Psychiatric Consultation.* New York, NY: Appleton-Century-Crofts.

Schwab, J.J. (1989). Consultation-liaison psychiatry: A historical overview. *Psychosomatics, 30,* 245–254.

Selye, H. (1966). *The Stress of Life.* New York, NY: McGraw-Hill.

Small, S.M. (1965). Intradepartmental education for attending psychiatric staff. In M.R. Kaufman (Ed.). *The Psychiatric Unit in a General Hospital: Its Current and Future Role.* (pp. 342–349). New York, NY: International Universities Press.

Solomon, H.C. (1947). Incidence of combat fatigue. *Archives of Neurology and Psychiatry, 57,* 332–341.

Solomon, H.C. (1958). The American Psychiatric Association in relation to American psychiatry. *American Journal of Psychiatry, 115,* 1–9.

Sontag, L.W. (1948). Determinants of predisposition to psychosomatic dysfunction and disease: Problem of proneness to psychosomatic disorder. In H.F. Dunbar (Ed.). *Synopsis of Psychosomatic Diagnosis and Treatment.* (pp. 38–66). New York, NY: Mosby.

Spiegel, H. (1944). Preventive psychiatry with combat troops. *American Journal of Psychiatry, 101,* 310–315.

Spitz, R.A. (1944). Psychosomatic principles and methods and their clinical application. *Medical Clinics of North America, 28,* 553–564.

Starr, P. (1982). *The Social Transformation of American Medicine.* New York, NY: Basic Books.

Summergrad, P., & Hackett, T.P. (1987). Alan Gregg and the rise of general hospital psychiatry. *General Hospital Psychiatry, 9,* 439–445.

Szasz, T. (1961). *The Myth of Mental Illness.* New York, NY: Harper and Row.

Taylor, G.J. (1987). *Psychosomatic Medicine and Contemporary Psychoanalysis.* Madison, CT: International Universities Press.

Tilley, D.H., & Silverman, J.J. (1982). A survey of consultation-liaison psychiatry program characteristics and functions. *General Hospital Psychiatry, 4,* 265–270.

Wallen, J., Pincus, H.A., Goldman, H.H., & Marcus, S.E. (1987). Psychiatric consultations in short-term general hospitals. *Archives of General Psychiatry, 44,* 163–168.

Weiner, H. (1977). The psychobiology of human disease: An overview. In G. Usdin (Ed.). *Psychiatric Medicine.* (pp. 3–72). New York, NY: Brunner/Mazel.

Weiner, H., Thaler, M., Reiser, M.F., & Mirsky, I.A. (1957). Etiology of duodenal ulcer. *Psychosomatic Medicine, 19,* 1–10.

White, W.A. (1936). The influence of psychiatric thinking on general medicine. *Mental Hygiene, 20,* 189–204.

Winnicott, D.W. (1966). Psycho-somatic illness in its positive and negative aspects. *International Journal of Psychoanalysis, 47,* 510–516.

Witmer, H.L. (1947). *Teaching Psychotherapeutic Medicine.* New York, NY: Commonwealth Fund.

Wittkower, E. (1960). Twenty years of North American psychosomatic medicine. *Psychosomatic Medicine, 22,* 309–316.

Wolff, H. (1950). Life stress and bodily disease: A formulation. In H.G. Wolff, S. Wolf, Jr., & C.E. Hare (Eds.). *Life Stress and Bodily Disease.* Baltimore, MD: Williams & Wilkins.

SECTION I

Seeds and Roots

Preamble: *We are certainly not the first to say that history is relevant! The quote of Santayana that those who cannot remember the past are condemned to repeat it is almost hackneyed in its familiarity. If some parts of history can be discarded, others are worthy of repetition and retention, if only to appreciate where we have come from and upon whose shoulders we have built contemporary knowledge and thought. Many ideas and beliefs of the past are silently embedded in today's practices. To have familiarity with them broadens our scope and appreciation of the world around us. To that end, we survey the many contributions to the foundation of consultation-liaison (C-L) psychiatry, looking, like Janus, both forward and back.*

Depending on whom one reads, the origins of consultation-liaison are variously evolved from psychosomatic medicine, general hospital psychiatry, physiology, or epidemiology, or, like Topsy, "just growed."[1] *This section takes a Topsy-like position, assuming that the discipline grew from an indeterminate garden of seeds and—as exclaimed by the referee when asked about baseball pitches, "it ain't nothin' 'til I calls it"—only became "C-L psychiatry" when it was named. The chapters of this section explore roots in philosophy, physiology, psychoanalysis, psychosomatic medicine, and epidemiology.*

Each of these "seeds" enters the consultation process without announcement. This section is capped with a chapter on the consultation.

Note

1 Topsy was the young slave girl of the nineteenth-century *Uncle Tom's Cabin*, who, when asked where she came from, said, "I s'pect I growed. Don't think nobody never made me."

1

REMNANTS OF PHILOSOPHY
The Vexing Mind-Body Problem

And how far is it from the point where we find ourselves today back to the late eigh-
teenth century, when the hope that mankind could improve and learn was inscribed in
handsomely formed letters in our philosophical firmament?

—Sebald, 2004, p. 112

Few psychiatrists would fancy themselves philosophers, yet every endeavor aimed at melding perturbations of the mind with expressions of bodily distress pays homage to philosophy and to philosophers who have made our task virtually automatic. Philosophic reflections are perhaps the last thing on the consultation-liaison psychiatrist's mind when consulting at the bedside, but philosophy is in his or her DNA. And Karl Jaspers, psychiatrist-philosopher, has said that "[If a psychiatrist] thinks he can exclude philosophy . . . he will eventually be defeated by it in some obscure form or another" (Jaspers, 1963, p. 770).

Why would a C-L psychiatrist be concerned about the place of philosophy in the history of C-L psychiatry? Haven't we gone far beyond that? Aren't the ancient philosophers dust? Because we are specialists who deal with mind-body problems on a regular basis, it is enlightening to know about the controversies that surrounded this problem in the past, to understand why solutions are not readily forthcoming, and to have a greater sense of the wider world than merely our own. Fundamentally, all philosophy proposes that we all grow up with both a worldview (*weltanschauung*) and a view of ourselves (*dasein*).

Ghaemi (2003), a contemporary psychiatrist attracted to pluralism as a useful concept in psychiatry, thinks of philosophy as more-or-less simply "thinking hard," a shared function of both scientists and philosophers. Similarly, William James defined it as "an unusually stubborn effort to think clearly" (Fulford,

Stanghellini & Broome, 2004). In his book *The Concepts of Psychiatry: A Pluralistic Approach to the Mind and Mental Illness*, Ghaemi (2003) takes a broad sweep of nineteenth- and twentieth-century philosophers whose ideas articulate with today's psychiatric practitioners, beginning with the salient quote of Sir Aubrey Lewis: "The psychiatrist then is confronted, whether he likes it or not, with many of the central issues of philosophy" (p. 1). In this, Jaspers and Lewis concur (Angel, 2003).

Unless the C-L psychiatrist has made a purposeful study of philosophy, he or she is likely to draw a blank on philosophers' names, except for that of Rene Descartes and his dualistic formulations. Most of these great thinkers lived in a monistic (if not monastic) world wherein they addressed the difficult big questions of life and civilization; physicians practiced a "holistic" medicine. Descartes shattered that world with the split enduring to today as "Cartesian dualism," virtually divorced from the man who initiated it. He said we consisted of two parts, the thinking mind (*res cogitans*) and the mechanical body (*res extensa*). In our industrialized and technologized world, the notion of human as machine, with reparable or replacement parts, is too seductive to abandon. So, Descartes's (1637) ideas seem to have endured longer than even more sage utterances through the ages. And while controversy continues to swirl around the "mind-body" question, significant doubts of their relationship no longer persist as philosophers consider repercussions.

To be curious and to search for answers are, in essence, the preconditions that make everyone a philosopher. Virtually all philosophies begin with questions about the relation of mind and body and of both to the surrounding world (Denys, 2007). Thus, it is no surprise that psychiatrists would find philosophy and psychiatry most companionable (see e.g., Ghaemi, 2003; Havens, 1993; Jaspers, 1963; Hundert, 1991; Fulford, 2004; Kendler, 2005). According to Wallace, "it is difficult to imagine a more perennially vexing topic to philosophers, scientists, and physicians than the mind-body problem" (1988, p. 4). Those wedded to a "scientific life" and "practicality" are apt to disparage the work of professional thinkers in philosophy as "metaphysics" or "armchair psychologizing" or "only philosophy."

Perhaps to counteract negative attitudes toward philosophers, the Scottish religious philosopher David Hume (1738) said, "Generally speaking, the errors in religion are dangerous; those in philosophy only ridiculous" (Bk 1, pt 4, sect 7). And the American satirist Ambrose Bierce (1906), in *The Devil's Dictionary*, defines philosophy dismissively as "a route of many roads leading from nowhere to nothing." More optimistically, Briquet, in his treatise on hysteria, speaks of philosophy as that "which most often is nothing other than the establishment in scientific form of the reigning traditions and ideas of the age" (Briquet, 1859, p. 132).

If one is to ponder, observe, and understand mind-body relations—essentially where it all began when the curious wanted to understand human nature and how humans behaved, thought and felt—one cannot ignore the philosophical underpinnings of our work (Kendler, 2005). Philosophers and metaphysicists have rendered the building blocks on which contemporary thinking of mind-body interaction rests; thus, they are the scaffold upon which our psychological and psychiatric theories are built. Indeed much of what we know of homeostasis, Claude Bernard's *milieu interieur*, or physiology derives from physicians who were also philosophers of their day, the polymaths among them also being mathematicians, poets, physicists, and theologians.

The brief panoramic view I take here is a bit like standing on a cliff overlooking the Grand Canyon. We admire and exult in the beauty of the moment but may not comprehend the evolving transformations that have brought us this spectacle. As a small speck on an almost incomprehensible landscape, we can only attempt to grasp what it is, not especially how it has become. We can settle for an instant photo that fixes the moment in our perception. To know more, we will need to exert effort and diligence, to "think hard." For the interested reader of how philosophy may influence the practice of psychiatry, no better example exists than that of Yalom, writing of Heidegger, Sartre, Boss, Laing, and Rollo May as they influence the practice of existential psychotherapy (Yalom, 1980).

Yalom focuses his existentialism on the four "givens" of the human condition: freedom, isolation, meaninglessness, and mortality, with one or all giving rise to any other. He expounds on the significance in life of a search for meaning, quoting psychologist Viktor Frankl, a holocaust survivor.

Personal Philosophy

Although we may not name it as such, we all carry our personal philosophy into the work we profess. Contemplation of one's being and surround was rampant in "prescientific" ages. When facts of life are not known, there is much room for controversy or, if you will, philosophizing. Psychiatry, a discipline shrouded in much uncertainty, provides great latitude for philosophical beliefs. Beyond mind-body deliberations, one can have a philosophy about anxiety, about depression, about the relationship of the physician to his or her patient. The fact that life does not fit snugly into scientific or diagnostic paradigms is likely what prompted both Jaspers and Freud to switch interests in their pursuit of answers.

Wittgenstein, a contemporary philosopher, has written that one's "narrative" encompasses reason, imagination, and meaning and that the way these unite in one's experience constitutes one's unique "personal narrative" or philosophy (Wallang, 2010).

For example, my own philosophy of patient care is that I am unable to assume responsibility for all that patients do. If I see patients once or twice a week or even more, I cannot possibly know what they do the other many hours they are not in my office. As a C-L psychiatrist, I subscribe to an attitudinal philosophy of considered risk taking in how much latitude to allow patients (and myself) free will in decision making about medication taking, hospital admission/discharge, or participation in psychotherapeutic activity. This is my "philosophy" of treatment.

Such a philosophy embraces a broad approach to the act of suicide and substantially modifies "rescue fantasies" inculcated in medical training. I can "take care" of patients when they are with me but not when they are independently functioning. I can be caring, concerned, and professionally responsible, but I cannot prevent them from getting sick, doing harm to themselves, or even killing themselves.

Others may have similar or different personal philosophies, subscribe to oriental ideas about life, or be influenced by religious percepts about human behavior—all philosophies by which individuals construct their personal or professional lives. Some psychiatrists have personal philosophies that appear "out of the mainstream" of contemporary theory and practice, so that they may be labeled "strange" or "idiosyncratic." The "philosophic" notion of Thomas Szasz (1961), for example, that mental illness is but a myth is such a case; his position on this important issue clearly affects how he treats patients and mental function.

Knowing something of how others have accomplished theirs adds power to the creation of our own personal philosophy. Exploring the landscape of philosophy in its relation to C-L psychiatry would require great diligence by one steeped in the history and epistemology of philosophical thinking. This brief review of selected philosophical musings intends only to help establish the fact that by standing on the shoulders of many who came before us, we may be able to see further than they did over 2000 years ago. It is exhilarating as well as humbling to see how much thinking of our forebears resembles our own, though modified and expressed in different language and societal coloration, and to accept philosophy as a basic foundation of C-L psychiatry (Kendler, 2005).

Our Forebears

The essential occupation of philosophers forever has been contemplating the large mysteries of existence. Since at least the 3rd century AD, philosophers were the alchemists of the day, with the professional search for the philosopher's stone, that with which base metals would be turned to gold. In contemporary times, the universal quest for a way to assure happiness, health, and wealth is perpetuated through such meanderings as those of a Harry Potter in search of the sorcerer's or philosopher's stone. The enduring wish to find the "elixir of life" is only slightly disguised in today's voluminous consumption of supplements or "programs" promising "miracle cures" or at least improved health.

Both philosophy and psychology have long believed that humans' emotions, thoughts, and behavior somehow originate in the head (brain). Primitive evidence is implied in ancient remnants of trephined skulls. Contemporary surgery may find holes in the skull useful for reduction of pressure on the brain, but providing egress for demonic spirits was the more likely rationale thousands of years ago.

Philosophical Roots

Enter the philosophers. Before much was known about anatomy, physiology, or chemistry, there were Socrates, Plato, Aristotle, Democritus, Sophocles, Hippocrates, Luke, Galen, Paracelsus, and Descartes, to allude to only a few who struggled with the complexities of life, especially of the mind/soul and body.

Regarding science and philosophy, Macklin (1978) has succinctly stated, "The methodology and evidential support adduced may differ in philosophical and scientific theories, but there is nevertheless an overlap in the two domains. . . . The difference between these two approaches to understanding man is largely a matter of emphasis" (p. 86). For example, Freud's psychodynamic theory of development echoes Plato's conception of how reason and passion interact to create personality, although the two thinkers are separated by over 2000 years. Macklin elaborates:

> The arguments put forth in favor of one or another theoretical system are, at bottom, philosophical. Whether the proponents of these arguments identify their field of research as psychology, psychiatry, or philosophy, when engaged in this sort of metatheoretical dispute they are taking a philosophical stance on the issue.
>
> *(p. 99)*

The cogitations and theorizing of earliest thinkers constitute the bedrock of much of civilization. Virtually all great ideas can be traced historically to the dialectics of great philosophers. Cicero (Taylor & Hunt, 1918) in the first century BC said, "Philosophy is the cultivation of the mental faculties; it roots out vices and prepares the mind to receive proper seed" (*Tusculanae disputationes, Bk. II, 5*) (p. 597). Similar descriptions are attributed to Socrates, Plato, and Aristotle, Greek philosophers of the fourth and fifth centuries BC. Montaigne (1579–1580) writes that "it is philosophy that teaches us to live. . . . [T]here is a lesson in it for childhood as well as for the other ages" (p. 120). Perhaps it was fortunate that early philosophers did not have access to computers and other captivating and distracting technologies, allowing ample time merely to think and write. Of the many written works, some may be thought of as merely decorative, as Sebald (2004, p. 112), a contemporary German writer and academic, has implied in questioning whether life has improved over hundreds of years.

It cannot be the purpose here to plumb all the teachings of early philosophers whose ideas have application to the foundations of C-L psychiatry. But a taste of a few salient philosophical contributions will hopefully make the point of their foundational relevance. In a very general way, we can say that the very intent and purpose of philosophers was to delve into and to understand the human spirit, to grasp what is good and evil, to comprehend pain and pleasure and joy and sadness, to contemplate how mind (soul) and body relate one to another and how the individual relates to the external world (society)—all elements of the C-L psychiatrist's task consulting each individual patient in a biopsychosocial frame-work! Ascertaining "what really matters" in patients' personal narratives is perhaps as close to philosophical inquiry as any assessment can be. In a minimalist sense, philosophy is the attempt to bring order out of chaos, to maximize certainty in the presence of uncertainty, whether in the universe or in personal conflict—in short, etymologically "a love of knowledge."

The "Big Three"

Although there were philosophers before him, we can begin with Socrates, the elder of "the big three" of Greek philosophers, whose teaching method has been well known to us as the "Socratic method," with its obvious relevance to good interviewing technique: resist leading the patient, avoid too many direct questions, and let the patients speak for themselves, to find answers within the recesses of their own thoughts, ideas, distortions, conflicts. The "Socratic method" enters our lexicon as a respectful way to elicit an individual's internal resources, so useful in evoking relevant history, thoughts, and feelings from patients.

Socrates urged philosophical thinkers to examine themselves, to know their own minds, beliefs, dogmas, and axioms, all embedded in this famous quote: "The unexamined life is not worth living." Here is unquestionable wisdom for physicians who would understand their own influence on the patient, later elaborated by Freud in his recognition of the nature of countertransference.

From Socrates' student Plato comes emphasis on the utility of dialogue, the meaningful exchange of information, feelings, and thoughts. And Plato's student Aristotle in turn bequeaths us an appreciation that ethics, logic, and rational behavior based on social, emotional, and biological "skills" can achieve "the good life," perhaps an ancient intimation of Freud's "pleasure principle" or the biopsychosocial model of adaptation. While these thinkers certainly did not get everything right, they delivered a major boost to all that followed them.

Aristotle spent many waking hours working on "definitions," searching for the "universals" in life, perhaps the precursor to "classification," efforts to systematize existing knowledge to enhance understanding and especially meaningful communication. Aristotle worked alone, while the editors of the *Diagnostic and Statistical Manual of Mental Health* (American Psychiatric Association) required armies of experts to devise "definitions" of mental disorders, considered by some still to be based more on philosophy than on science.

As recent (!) as 1864, Ernest Renan had written,

> Socrates gave philosophy to mankind, and Aristotle gave it science. There was philosophy before Socrates, and science before Aristotle, and since Socrates and since Aristotle, philosophy and science have made immense advances. But all has been built upon the foundation which they laid.
>
> *(Durant, 1953, p. 62)*

Such proclamations are similarly made today and undoubtedly will continue throughout humankind, even as things forever evolve and change.

The philosophical aspects of "logic" and "truth" enter the picture, as well as "art." One can generalize and simplify that all who endeavor to discover the "life worth living" are indulging in philosophy, no matter the approach taken.

The clinical endeavors of the consulting psychiatrist are routinely obliged to address interdependent matters of mind and body. Most likely, this occurs mindlessly, without conscious thought of the remnants of Rene Descartes's philosophic legacy and how they constitute the dualistic challenges of our profession. Sigmund Freud was no less drawn to the enigma of mind-body relationships, but he insisted that his was a "scientific" rather than philosophical route to psychoanalysis.

Freud the "Philosopher"

In spite of Freud's disclaimer that psychoanalysis was little influenced by philosophy, one cannot escape the educational experience and influence of teachers who ultimately influence one's values, identity (self, ego), and system of beliefs. This social context contributed to both the *weltanschauung* and the *dasein* of Freud (1964). The story of Freud's education is revelatory in that regard, suggesting a strong but later minimized interest in philosophy. While Freud did not consider himself a philosopher, he has been cast in that role by serious scholars: Herbert Marcuse (1955), *Eros and Civilization*; Norman O. Brown (1959), *Life Against Death*; Philip Rieff (1959), *Freud: The Mind of the Moralist*; Joel Kovel (1991), *History and Spirit: An Inquiry Into the Philosophy of Liberation*; Paul Ricouer (1965), *Freud and Philosophy: An Essay on Interpretation*; Alfred Tauber (2010), *Freud, the Reluctant Philosopher*.

Freud (1964) defended himself against those who would label him philosopher, with the following comment in the *New Introductory Lectures on Psycho-Analysis* (Lecture xxxv):

> Philosophy is not opposed to science, it behaves itself as if it were a science, and to a certain extent it makes use of the same methods; that it can produce a complete and coherent picture of the universe. Its methodological error lies in the fact that it over-estimates the epistemological value of our logical operations . . . but philosophy has no immediate influence on the great majority of mankind; it interests only a small number even of the thin upper stratum of intellectuals, while all the rest find it beyond them.
>
> *(p. 166)*

Perhaps, to make psychoanalysis uniquely his own, Freud had to renounce philosophy's influence, as he did religion, psychiatry, and ultimately medicine.

Even before Freud's birth, the teachings of the German philosopher-psychologist Johann Herbart had been part of all classical education in Vienna. Furthermore, all of Viennese intellectual education essentially embraced then current *Naturphiloso-phie*. A "pantheistic monism" stated that the conscious life of the mind was simply the expression of a more unconscious turbulence of all the forces of Nature. During Freud's schooling, he most certainly was aware of Herbart's ideas about the unconscious and his speculation that "ideas that were once in consciousness and for any reason have been repressed (*verdrangt*) out of it are not lost, but in certain circumstances may return" (Jones, 1953, p. 374). These ideas were "in the air" of the times, as it were.

Freud's biographer, Jones (1953, p. 375), writes that the ideas of Freud's teacher, Theodor Meynert, espoused concepts of mental function that were clearly analo-gous to those of Herbart, especially in the belief of inseparability of mind and body. Meynert also spoke of ways in which affect could "attack" or "defend" one's being as well as constitute a buildup of nervous excitation that seeks expres-sion, with references to an "unpleasure principle" (p. 375).

During his medical school experience, Freud spent more time in nonrequired courses on philosophy than in aspects of medicine he found unappealing. As an 18-year-old medical student, Freud familiarized himself with a book by Franz Brentano, *Psychology From an Empirical Standpoint*, published in 1874. During medical school, as recounted by Jones, "[h]e admitted himself that he pursued in only a negligent fashion the studies proper to the medical career itself and seized every opportunity to *dally in those that interested him* as well as to *forage in neighbor-ing fields*" (italics added—au.) (p. 36). In the first two years of medical school, he attended philosophy lectures and seminars on a regular basis, several on Aristotle by Prof. Brentano, whom he characterized as a great thinker and philosopher.

Like many adolescents facing developmental quandary, as an 18-year-old medical student Freud appears to have been contemplating the existence of God (Rizzuto, 1998). Writing to a friend, Eduard Silberstein, in 1875, he expressed his own surprise at how, as a Jewish atheist, he had been captivated by this inspir-ing theological lecturer and signed up for two philosophy courses, one of which, on the existence of God, he thought his friend would be amazed to hear. To Silberstein, he wrote:

> Concerning this remarkable man (he is a believer, a teleologist [!] and a Darwinist, and damned intelligent, even brilliant), who in many ways satis-fies the requirements of the ideal. I will have much to tell you in person. But I can give you this piece of news now: under Brentano's influence especially (which has had a maturing effect), I have made a decision to sit for the doc-torate in philosophy and will study philosophy and zoology.
>
> *(Brentano, in de Mojella, 2005, p. 221)*

Freud's biographers, noting his intended change of career path, have remarked that the only time this "atheistic Jew" seemed to have a momentary metaphysi-cal hesitation was in his meeting with Brentano, the Catholic teacher/theologian

(Rizzuto, 1998, p. 151). Again, writing to friend Silberstein, he described the experience as follows:

> Ever since Brentano imposed his God on me with ridiculous facility, through his arguments, I fear being seduced one of these days by proofs in favor of spiritualism, homeopathy, Louise Lateau [a stigmatic—au.], etc. . . . It's a fact that his God is nothing but a logical principle and that I have accepted it as such. Yet, we proceed down a slippery slope once we acknowledge the concept of God. It remains to be seen at which point we stumble. Moreover, his God is very strange. . . . It is impossible to refute Brentano before hearing him out, studying him, exploring his thought. Confronted with such a rigorous dialectician, we must strengthen our intellect by addressing his arguments before confronting him directly.
>
> *(Brentano, in de Mojella, 2005, p. 221)*

Freud seems to have been conscious of his vulnerability to accepting the ideas of those he admired. He claims to have developed his interest to become a medical student only after hearing a lecture of Goethe's on Nature (Jones, 1953, p. 28). "In my youth," he wrote, "I felt an overpowering need to understand something of the riddles of the world in which we live and perhaps even to contribute something to their solution" (p. 28). No philosopher has uttered more salient words.

In another couple of years, Freud would mostly abandon his philosophical pursuits as he was increasingly influenced by another teacher, Ernst Brucke, to pursue work in physiology. Of this teacher, he wrote that he "settled down to physiology," under the influence of "the greatest authority who affected me more than any other in my whole life" (Jones, 1953, p. 39). Interestingly, Freud is said by Jones to have almost defiantly supported a more "physical" or "scientific" physiology. "In his enthusiasm for the rival physical physiology, he swung to the opposite extreme and became for a while a radical materialist" (p. 43).

Regarding thoughts on a conciliation of psychology and physiology, Freud agreed with Brentano that "philosophy and psychology are still young sciences, which cannot expect any support, especially from physiology" and that "it is more necessary to submit certain specific problems to more extensive research in order to achieve definite partial results" (Mijolla, 2005, p. 221).

Failing to reconcile mental processes with neurological principles in his *Project for a Scientific Psychology*, he pursued other paths, writing that "psychoanalysis hopes to discover the common ground on which the coming together of bodily and mental disturbances will become intelligible" (Jones, 1953, p. 395), as succinct a statement of the wish to solve the mind-body problem as exists anywhere!

Another instance of Freud's "brush with philosophy" occurred in a most unusual way that may serendipitously have led to his meeting Josef Breuer, a remarkable coincidence in the history of psychoanalysis. In a little-known biographical fact,

Freud was arrested in 1879, still a medical student, for absenting himself from army duty. To avert the boredom during the time, he translated a book by the British philosopher John Stuart Mill, allegedly not so much out of great interest but as a means of generating income. The editor of the volume was Theodor Gomperz, a well-connected Viennese philosopher and historian; Gomperz was in search of a replacement for an unexpectedly deceased translator and was given Freud's name by Brentano, who, speculation has it, may have been influenced by Josef Breuer, Brentano's personal physician. Although professing little interest in Mill, Freud later acknowledged his good impression of Mill's treatment of Plato's theory of reminiscence, ideas that found their way into discussions of hysteria and Freud's later *Beyond the Pleasure Principle.* He also acknowledged sympathy for Mill's ideas about politics.

Freud's very career is good evidence of how things evolve and change. He was fortunate to have had, in his medical education, teachers whom he revered and who significantly influenced his professional pursuits. He had found the philosophical lectures of Brentano energizing and formative, as were those of Theodor Meynert. In his postgraduate hospital experience, Freud felt that Meynert's lectures on psychiatry and neuroanatomy were the best he experienced. Meynert was not so much considered a philosopher but was very knowledgeable about the writings of Kant, Schopenhauer, and Herbart, and Freud found much in his wisdom. Freud would eventually work in Meynert's department and psychiatric clinic, learning and practicing neurology, but eventually receding from Meynert's penumbra when the two disagreed about such things as hypnoid states, hypnosis, and the neuroses. Nevertheless, from Meynert, Freud absorbed the notion that some internal "force" imposed itself on the mind to result in emotional illness. Extrapolating into "mind-body" relations, Freud, like Leibniz and Spinoza, adopted a psychophysical parallelism that postulated that "the psychical is a process parallel to the physiological" (Jones, 1953, p. 368) and that the physical always preceded the psychical, leading unquestionably to his famous remark that "the ego is first and foremost a body ego." (Freud did not believe in a "soul," perhaps influencing his retreat from psychiatry, originally defined as "treatment of the soul.")

Philosophy, Psychology, and the C-L Psychiatrist

For the C-L psychiatrist, the distillate of eons of philosophy may come down to the relevance of "mind-body problem" (Kendler, 2001) in one's daily work. Although the mysteries of the mind's relationship to body remained clouded for thousands of years, the ensuing debate has brought us a plethora of riches that affect us in how we appraise the big philosophical questions of life, death, and civilization and how they influence mind or soul and body in their relation to each other. Whatever their vicissitudes, doubts of their relationship no longer persist, a relationship that enters the experience of every psychiatric consultation.

The C-L psychiatrist, addressing the comorbidities of everyday occurrence, constantly must ponder how mental and physical reveal themselves in each patient's presentation. As Ekstein (1970) states,

> In practice, psychosomatic uses all the tools. . . . It brings in all the disciplines. . . . Mind (emotion and intellect), *demos* (individuality and society), and brain (limbic and other systems), and body (organs), run around in a circle of cause and effect.
>
> *(p. 657)*

In a sense, the C-L psychiatrist, like philosophers of antiquity, embarks on a quest for answers in every consultation: What kind of person is this, what sort of life has he or she lived, how does he view the world, what are his fears and wishes, how does she contemplate death, how does he relate to others—especially his doctor—and what does his doctor want to know about him? In this sense, the consultant follows the philosopher Kant, who, in an abbreviated sense, considered all philosophy defined by four questions: (1) What can I know? (2) What should I do? (3) What may I hope? and (4) What is Man? (Wood, 1984). All is part of the C-L psychiatrist's context as he or she brings to the patient the skills of listener, advisor, interpreter, confidant, consultant, facilitator, supporter, mediator, pharmacologist, psychotherapist, and healer.

Healing: Life in the Balance

"Healing," as it preceded medicine, has always sought as its goal to restore the imbalance between the polarities of one's existence, a mechanism defined later as homeostasis. Before that, Hippocrates and other physicians saw disease as an imbalance of humors, a disruption of the life forces of blood, phlegm, and yellow and black bile, with disease the body's response and attempt to restore balance of paired qualities. We can thank Hippocrates, dubbed the Father of Medicine, for separating medicine from the supernatural and mysticism, preparing it for scientific advancement in centuries to come.

Psychotherapy, as part of the C-L psychiatrist's healing skills, is described by Bromberg (1959) as both art and science, embodying vestiges of psychiatry's roots in philosophy. According to Bromberg in *The Mind of Man*,

> mental turmoil required a medicine more specific than the broad beneficence of religion, the leveling tranquility of philosophy and the thinned-out benefits of political science. . . . [I]t was inevitable that a personal psychotherapy should evolve, i.e., specific technics [*sic*] which would minister to the immediate cries for mental comfort.
>
> *(pp. 7–8)*

In the final analysis, even with the help of pharmacologic agents and behavior-modifying techniques, healing depends upon belief, human response, trust, faith, intellect, the whole gamut of adaptive behaviors, and, yes, even magic—attributes that dwell more in the philosophic than scientific domain. According to Eckstein (1970), the philosopher Thales (620 BC), regarded by Socrates as the first philosopher in the Greek tradition, believed that magnets possessed a soul, evidenced by their power to move iron. C-L psychiatrists, encountering patients attempting to understand their own experiences, are familiar with such primitive beliefs and attributions of illness; patients trying to comprehend bodily distress often still cling to magical thinking. Part of the C-L psychiatrist's task is to help correct patients' distorted, anxiety-provoking concepts of illness.

"The essential mechanics" of healing, according to Bromberg (1959), "are those of penetration of the patient's feelings, thoughts and attitudes by an external influence and the patient's absorption of this influence" (p. 10), characteristics that encourage our nonpsychiatrist colleagues to accuse us of being too "soft and fuzzy," proxies for "philosophical."

Individuality Matters

Recognition of the primacy of each person's individuality is fundamental to the performance of every patient consultation. On one occasion, I was asked to see a young male architect because of depression following diagnosis of acute fulminating leukemia. Entering his room, I immediately saw a large framed reproduction of one of Warhol's famous flowers, a glorious red blossom, leaning against the wall. Asked about it, he said a friend had brought it to cheer him up. "This room is going to be my casket," he said. I commented that the picture was not easily seen on the floor at the foot of his bed. He said he was told by hospital staff that nothing could be hung on the wall. I excused myself, left briefly, and returned with a hammer and nail and began to hang the picture where it could be easily seen. "You'll be fired," he said. I said I could probably get another job, but he may not. He died a week later; I did not lose my job. For the C-L psychiatrist, philosophy, art, and science go together. Sometimes, it is the small things that matter most, even in specialty consultation (Ofri, 2014).

New Interest in Philosophy

Even with the desire to distance itself from mystical, religious, and "unscientific" philosophical roots, psychiatry has seen a recrudescence of interest in psychiatry's relation to philosophy since at least the 1980s (Parnas, Sass & Zahavi, 2008). Both a journal and an organization were formed to assess the measure of philosophy's contributions to contemporary psychiatry and psychology. The Association for the Advancement of Philosophy and Psychiatry (AAPP) was founded in 1989, and its journal *Philosophy, Psychiatry and Psychology* in 1993.

A fertile intellectual and clinical field has resulted in a number of relevant books addressing the large topic of philosophy's present kinship to psychiatry, perhaps to counteract increasing technologization with a "rehumanized" medicine. It was time for a reaffirmation of values, truth, ethics, morality, humor, linguistics, hermeneutics, metaphor, symbolism, beauty, and the vagaries of life (and death) itself. While medicine in general benefits from such attention, psychiatry and psychology have the soil for the fundamentals of philosophy to plant and grow. Consultation-liaison psychiatry, of all psychiatric endeavors, arguably has most to benefit from the musings and deliberations of philosophers.

What is philosophy after all, other than, in its simplest form, "a set of ideas about how to do something or how to live." Even without invoking the more erudite dimensions of aesthetics, ethics, truth, logic, metaphysics, linguistics, or epistemology, we can embrace the notion that our training, skills, attitudes, and beliefs in interacting with a patient are all interwoven in the personal philosophy that we bring to the situation. Thus, for example, an individualized existential "mind-body problem" for us in each encounter may simply be whether we approach a situation more from a physical or a mental point-of-view or from one that hopefully is more comprehensively "biopsychosocialspiritual," referring to feelings, the senses, empathy, and communication, attuned to language, symbolism, and meaning. What beliefs, ideas, attitudes, and convictions do we bring to each encounter? What do we think about suicide, about end-of-life care, about personal responsibility—indeed, even about hospitalization itself?

Today's psychiatric philosophers attach names like "pluralism" (Brendel, 2008; Ghaemi, 2007), "existential" (Havens, 1974), or "phenomenology" (Berrios, 1992), but all are attempts to better define and organize the thinking around each school. All acknowledge that, in psychiatry, knowing a patient includes not only the observable signs and symptoms but also more of the "inner person," the perception and experience of self. According to philosopher Martin Buber, "Men's attitudes are manifold. Some live in a strange world bounded by a path from which countless ways lead inside" (Kaufman, 1970, p. 11). I am reminded of my experience in psychoanalytic training when, after presenting detailed process notes of a very puzzling case, I eagerly awaited sage words from my supervisor explicating my therapeutic dilemma. After a brief reflective pause, she said, "Aren't people funny?"—words as reassuring as nearly any I had heard.

"There is hardly a belief of the past that does not enter, in some form, into the modern world as the object of passionate allegiance," states Randall (1940, p. 679). In a profession where language, interpretation, symbols, and fantasy abound, philosophy must inevitably enter! (Ofri, 2014).

Much more recently, the philosophic patina of centuries past may be detected in the words of Harvard's President Drew Faust (2014), extolling new opportunities for research:

> Curiosity and inquiry lift the shroud of humanity's ignorance, allowing us to glimpse deeper understandings and to ask—and answer—new questions.

The desire to understand is among humanity's most beautiful capacities, and it is the wellspring from which innovations flow.

(p. 5)

It is a philosophic banner that every psychiatric consultant could well carry in each encounter with patients.

References

Angel, K. (2003). Defining psychiatry: Aubrey Lewis's 1938 report and the Rockefeller Foundation. *Medical History Supplement, 22,* 39–56.

Berrios, G.E. (1992). Phenomenology, psychopathology and Jaspers: A conceptual history. *History of Psychiatry, 3,* 303–327.

Bierce, A.G. (1906). *The Devil's Dictionary (The Cynic's Word Book)*. London, UK: Arthur F. Bird.

Brendel, D.H. (2008). Pluralism in action. Panel report. *Journal of the Psychoanalytic Association, 56,* 253–262.

Brentano, F. (1874). Psychology from an empirical standpoint. In A. De Mijolla (Ed.). *International Dictionary of Psychoanalysis.* (2005 edition, Vol. 1). Detroit, MI: Macmillan Reference USA. (March 7 Letter to Silberstein).

Briquet, P. (1859) *Traite Clinique et Therapeutique a l'Hysteric.* Paris, FR: J. B. Bailliere.

Bromberg, W. (1959). *The Mind of Man: A History of Psychotherapy and Psychoanalysis.* New York, NY: Harper Torch Books

Brown, N.O. (1959). *Life Against Death.* Hanover, MA: Wesleyan University Press.

Cicero, M.T. (1918). *(45 B.C.)* Tusculanae disputations II. In H. Taylor & M.L.T. Hunt (Eds.). *Cicero: A Sketch of His Life and Works: A Commentary.* (2nd ed., pp. 457–603). Chicago, IL: A.C.M. McClurg & Co.

Denys, D. (2007). How new is the new philosophy of psychiatry? *Philosophy Ethics and Humanities in Medicine, 20,* 2–22.

Descartes, R. (1637). *Discourse on the Method.* D.A. Cress (Trans.). (3rd edition). Indianapolis, IN: Hackett, 1998.

Durant, W. (1953). *The Story of Philosophy.* (Cardinal edition). New York, NY: Pocket Books, Inc.

Ekstein, R. (1970). *The Body Has a Head.* New York, NY: Harper & Row.

Faust, D.F. (2014). The region of ideas and invention. *Harvard Magazine.* May–June, p. 5.

Freud, S. (1964). A philosophy of life. *New Introductory Lectures on Psycho-Analysis.* Lecture XXXV (1933). *The Standard Edition of the Complete works of Sigmund Freud.* New York, NY: W.W. Norton & Co.

Fulford, K.W., Stanghellini, G., & Broome, M. (2004). What can philosophy do for psychiatry? *World Psychiatry, 3,* 130–135.

Ghaemi, R.N. (2003). *The Concepts of Psychiatry: A Pluralistic Approach to the Mind and Mental Illness.* Baltimore, MD: Johns Hopkins University Press.

Ghaemi, R.N. (2007). Existence and pluralism: The rediscovery of Karl Jaspers. *Psychopathology, 40,* 75–82.

Havens, L.L. (1974). The existential use of the self. *American Journal of Psychiatry, 131,* 1–10.

Havens, L.L. (1993). *Approaches to the Mind.* Boston, MA: Little, Brown & Co.

Hume, D. (1738). *A Treatise of Human Nature*. Bk. 1, Part 4, sect 7. D.F. Norton & M.J. Norton (Eds.). Oxford, UK: Oxford University Press (2010).

Hundert, E.M. (1991). *Philosophy, Psychiatry and Neuroscience—Three Approaches to the Mind: A Synthetic Analysis of the Varieties of Human Experience*. New York, NY: Clarendon Press, Oxford University Press.

Jaspers, K. (1963). *General Psychopathology* (1913). J. Hoenig & M.W. Hamilton. (Trans.). Chicago, IL: University of Chicago Press.

Jones, E. (1953). *The Life and Work of Sigmund Freud, vol. 1. The Formative Years and the Great Discoveries, 1850–1900*. New York, NY: Basic Books.

Kaufman, W. (1970). *I and Thou: Martin Buber*. New York, NY: Charles Scribner's & Sons.

Kendler, K.S. (2001). A psychiatric dialogue on the mind-body problem. *American Journal of Psychiatry, 158,* 989–1000.

Kendler, K.S. (2005). Toward a philosophical structure for psychiatry. *American Journal of Psychiatry, 62,* 433–440.

Kovel, J. (1991). *History and Spirit: An Inquiry Into the Philosophy of Liberation*. Boston, MA: Beacon Press.

Macklin, R. (1978). Philosophical approaches to understanding man. In G.U. Balis, L. Wurmser, E. McDaniel, & R.G. Grenell (Eds.). *Dimensions of Behavior: The Psychiatric Foundations of Medicine* (Vol. 1, pp. 85–100). Boston, MA: Butterworth Publishers.

Marcuse, H. (1955). *Eros and Civilization: A Philosophical Inquiry into Freud*. Boston, MA: Beacon Press.

Ofri, D. (2014). The little things. *New England Journal of Medicine, 371,* 1378–1379.

Parnas, J., Sass, L.A., & Zahavi, D. (2008). Recent developments in philosophy of psychopathology. *Current Opinion in Psychiatry, 21,* 578–584.

Randall, J.H., Jr. (1940). *The Making of the Modern Mind*. Cambridge, MA: Riverside Press.

Ricouer, P. (1965). *Freud and Philosophy: An Essay on Interpretation*. New Haven, CT: Yale University Press.

Rieff, P. (1959). *Freud. The Mind of the Moralist*. Chicago, IL: University of Chicago Press.

Rizzuto, A-M. (1998). *Why Did Freud Reject God? A Psychodynamic Interpretation*. New Haven, CT: Yale University Press.

Sebald, W.G. (2004). An attempt at restitution. *New Yorker.* 20 and 27 December.

Szasz, T.S. (1961). *The Myth of Mental Illness: Foundations of a Theory of Personal Conduct*. New York, NY: Harper & Row.

Tauber, A.I. (2010). *Freud, the Reluctant Philosopher*. Princeton, NJ: Princeton University Press.

Wallace, E.R., IV. (1988). Mind-body. Monistic dual aspect interactionism. *Journal of Nervous and Mental Disease, 176,* 4–21.

Wallang, P. (2010). Wittgenstein's legacy and narrative networks: Incorporating a meaning-centred approach to consultation. *Psychiatrist, 34,* 157–161.

Wood, A.W. (1984). *Self and Nature in Kant's Philosophy*. New York, NY: Cornell University Press.

Yalom, I.D. (1980). *Existential Psychotherapy*. New York, NY: Basic Books.

2

PHYSIOLOGY

Cannon's Shot Heard Round the World

Pavlov's work threw light on the mechanisms, not on the nature of mind.
—Penfield, 1971, p. 342

Ever since humanity has been aware of reactions like blushing, sweating, blanching, diarrhea, and tremor, physiological process had been inferred, without necessarily being named. So important to psychosomatic medicine is physiology that the suggestion has been made that it be considered the basic science of the field—curious, therefore, that it is absent or barely indexed in major texts of psychosomatic medicine and C-L psychiatry (Blumenfield & Strain, 2006; Wise & Rundell, 2002). Its study has been one of great complexity and difficulty. Edward Glover's (1956) *On the Early Development of Mind* refers to the "physiological octopus" (p. 254) that ensnares the psychologist who attempts to develop measurements of mind. While physiology and psychology inevitably intersect, attempts to delineate their respective influence result in separate languages, processes, and research approaches. Efforts to understand mind must encounter consciousness and, through it, attempt to combine mental processes with bodily processes, a task that relies heavily on physiology as the connector. The slowness of progress is revealed in Glover's (1956) observation that "there is a huge gap between the two frontiers," a gap that "has not yet been fully explored" (pp. 255–256).

As scientists began abandoning philosophy for physiology in the nineteenth century, so too—under the charismatic influence of his teacher, the physiologist Ernst Brucke—did Freud immerse himself as avidly in that discipline as he had earlier in philosophy; after graduating medical school, he worked in the Brucke Physiology Institute with aspirations of one day becoming professor of physiology.

Inspired by the compulsivity of Brucke's research approach, Freud left behind his infatuation with philosophy and religious curiosity and plunged into the meticulous study of nerve structure in animals.

Some years after leaving Brucke's physiology lab (1897), Freud attempted to meld the two disciplines—psychology and physiology—using brain physiology, in a *Project for a Scientific Psychology*. Greatly discouraged, he frustratingly abandoned the effort. Ultimately, he felt, the endeavor must rely on introspection, free association, and the unconscious. Subsequently, Freud bequeathed it to others to delve more deeply into physiology as he himself confined his explorations to only matters of the mind.

Early Physiology

In the early nineteenth century, when the most sophisticated technology was the galvanometer, physiologists made little effort to comprehend the psychological processes of "mind" and seemed to content themselves with the more structural measureable aspects of the body. Nevertheless, their discoveries and writings have been of inestimable value to an understanding of mind-body relationships and, thus, of great foundational influence on C-L psychiatry. Earliest issues of the journal *Psychosomatic Medicine* carried reports almost exclusively of psychophysiological research.

The scientific attitude in the early nineteenth century may be summed up by the German physician-physiologist Johannes Peter Muller's words in his *Elements of Physiology* (1838):

> Though there appears to be something in the phenomena of living beings which cannot be explained by ordinary mechanical, physical or chemical laws, much may be so explained, and we may without fear push these explanations as far as we can, so long as we keep to the solid ground of observation and experiment.
>
> *(p. 539)*

A student of Muller's—another physician-physiologist, Emil DuBois-Raymond, who is considered the father of experimental electrophysiology—wrote in 1842:

> Brucke and I pledged a solemn oath to put into effect this truth:
> No other forces than the common physical-chemical ones are active within the organism. In those cases which cannot at the time be explained by these forces one has either to find the specific way or form of their action by means of the physical-mathematical method or to assume new forces equal in dignity to the chemical-physical forces inherent in matter, reducible to the force of attraction and repulsion.
>
> *(Jones, 1953, pp. 40–41)*

It must have been this zeitgeist, the curiosity about that "which cannot be explained by ordinary mechanical, physical or chemical laws" that challenged Freud's creative genius to at least try. Freud's departure from Brucke's oath was almost an act of betrayal of his medical roots and his idolization of Brucke. Pioneers who "dared" to contemplate the workings of the mind while studying physiology were deemed "unscientific." Such explanations, revealed in Muller's oath, could only be "pushed . . . as far as we can . . . without fear" (Muller, 1838, p. 539).

Nevertheless, other researchers constantly knocked at the door of mental processes in attempts to join physiology to psychiatry and psychology. The German school of physiology made significant contributions to the field. Hermann von Helmholz, a German physician and physicist, straddled the fields of philosophy and physiology during much of the latter half of the nineteenth century. He added significantly to an understanding of perception through his studies of vision and other aspects of sensory physiology. In some sense, he was like Freud in his curiosity to translate one discipline into another, as he tried to find empirical support for the theories of idealistic philosophers like Fichte and Kant. He proposed the principle of energy conservation based on studies of muscle metabolism.

By the early twentieth century, overtures into this field had coalesced into the special study of psychophysiology.

Ivan Pavlov

While hewing close to the line of "pure" physiology, Russians historically took a much more structural approach to physiology than did the Americans. Russian physiologists, of whom Ivan Petrovich Pavlov is the most well known, contributed lasting physiological knowledge. Turning from an investment in religious studies to a career in science and experimentation at the Institute of Experimental Medicine in Russia, Pavlov (1897/1902) established the Department of Physiology where he carried out animal experiments that would earn him the Nobel Prize in 1904. His studies of the gastric physiology of dogs (and, later, children) and the process of classical conditioning have been his most widely cited studies. He avoided but was not uninformed about psychology, and in his lesser known "Wednesday Meetings" he expounded on a variety of topics including his critical opinions of psychology (Gifford, 1981). Nevertheless, he shunned attempts to connect his studies to mental function. Although Sir Charles Sherrington, British physiologist–neurologist, extended understanding of the reflex arc by showing how it involved complex integrated neural circuits, published as the text *Integrative Action of the Nervous System* in 1906, the greater relevance to mind–body interaction would await the studies of Cannon.

Walter Bradford Cannon

Cannon was a contemporary of Pavlov, whose biographers believed both should have won the Nobel prize; although Cannon was not so recognized, his friendship with Pavlov was never knowingly sullied by the omission. In fact, Cannon had been responsible for bringing Pavlov to Boston in 1929 and visited him in Russia in 1935 during the convening of the International Physiological Congress. Acknowledging Pavlov's work in a most charitable obituary, Cannon had written:

> Rarely does a man of science have opportunity to devote himself to productive scholarship for half a century, and still more rarely does he continue his devotion if he has that opportunity. And yet, for nearly sixty years Pavlov was an outstanding productive scholar. During that long period he dedicated his talents and his timeless energy to the revelation of new and significant facts in the functioning of higher organisms. With incomparable zeal and enthusiasm, and with admirable singleness of aim, he spent his life seeking the explanation of the natural processes of living creatures. As a result of his ingenious methods and extraordinary technical skill, our knowledge of the functions of the digestive glands and the functions of the more complex processes of the nervous system has been largely transformed. For infinite time, Pavlov will remain a shining example of Russian genius.
>
> *(Yerkes, 1946, p. 137)*

It does not take a psychoanalyst to conjecture that this attribution might quite as justifiably apply to Cannon himself. Cannon's biographers have speculated that the omission of the Nobel was somehow related to his political affinities (Brown & Fee, 2002)

Cannon's Physiological "Shot Heard Round the World"

Every now and then, there comes along an individual with the breadth of ingenious vision and innovation to move knowledge and understanding ahead by quantum leaps in a path to narrowing the gap between physiology and psychology. Of all the foundations of C-L psychiatry, the bedrock may well be the heralded discoveries by Walter Bradford Cannon, a graduate of Harvard Medical School in 1900 and professor and chair of their Department of Physiology in 1906. Although known parochially for his "fight or flight" hypothesis (the responsiveness of the autonomic nervous system and physiological processes in emergency situations), his impact on medicine and especially mind-body interaction extends much further. His studies encompassed a larger field than the simple reflex arc (stimulus-response) studies of his colleague Pavlov. In fact, some authors have alluded to him as the father of psychosomatic medicine (Notes from the Editors, 1989).

Born in 1871, Cannon lived in an exciting time of science, bridging two centuries. His father was a railroad worker of some status with unfulfilled dreams of becoming a physician, and his mother was a woman of great social consciousness, whose death when young Walter was only 10 left him bereft. Like many multitalented individuals, choosing a career path was not easy, and he was influenced by others who recognized his talents and intellect. His father, of course, hoped he would become a physician. Encouraged and assisted by his teachers to apply to Harvard College, he was readily accepted on scholarship. As with many first-year students at Harvard, he felt a sense of isolation and something of a misfit but nonetheless excelled in his studies. By his third year, he was well immersed in courses in philosophy and psychology, some with William James as well as with Hugo Munsterberg, the latter said to have been the first (after James abandoned the project) to establish a psychology laboratory in the United States.

Cannon's first career-oriented step was his application to Harvard Medical School, where he got permission from the chair of the Department of Physiology to embark on a research project of his and another student's design. Their first efforts were the study of swallowing in animals, progressing the next year to children (not sure how this was achieved regarding informed consent—au.) and adults. Presentation of findings to the American Physiological Society and subsequent publication in the newly established *American Journal of Physiology* launched Cannon's career into its next phase.

Carrying over his observations from animal studies in which rage affected peristaltic movements of the stomach, he made similar observations in humans. Almost as a distraction from his research, he persuaded a professor of neurology to try using the Harvard Business School style of teaching via the "case method," an educational adventure that won much praise in the medical school, followed by publication of its success in the *Boston Medical and Surgical Journal* (subsequently renamed the *New England Journal of Medicine*), and ultimately a core component of the New Pathway curriculum inaugurated at Harvard in the 1980s. Cannon, atypically for a laboratory researcher, believed that one's most important function was as a teacher, the kind of advocacy that may have foreshadowed the consulting psychiatrist's combining of practical application (consultation) with teaching (liaison).

With Cannon's academic- and research-star rising, he was sought out in his final year of medical school by the dean to serve as instructor of zoology, to teach undergraduates in both Harvard and Radcliffe Colleges. In hopes of retaining him at Harvard following graduation, the dean simultaneously appointed him instructor in physiology. He advanced quickly up the academic ladder after toying briefly with the idea of being a medical practitioner. His reputation grew, and, when Cornell offered him a professorship (at a very young age), Harvard's Dean Eliot hastily convened a committee that counteroffered Cannon the chairmanship of the Department of Physiology. (He had also been offered the deanship at Harvard, which was withdrawn under influence of the former chair of physiology, who told Dean Eliot, "It is easier to find a good dean than a good scientist") (author unknown—au.).

Accepting the post of chair, there seemed little likelihood of turning back or elsewhere. His career path had been virtually confirmed; he would remain at Harvard for the rest of his life. He resided as a kind of "interactionist" between physiology and psychology, in contrast to William James, who was also a contemporary medical school graduate and who had eased away from physiology and medicine more exclusively into the realm of psychology.

Cannon's major discoveries derived first from his studies of animals. Like Charles Darwin, he believed that there was a continuum of biological reactions to emotional stimuli, from animals to humans. Early studies of the physiological reaction of dogs and cats to fear and rage led to his famed "fight or flight" theory. Cannon observed that under threatening situations, the adrenal gland released a substance that he called *sympathin* (adrenaline). This, in turn, activated carbohydrate metabolism with a release of sugar to provide energy, while other "nonessential" processes such as appetite and digestion were inhibited. As blood is redistributed and as pressure rises, the individual is readied to confront the emergent situation through either attack or flight.

Cannon's studies—beginning with his predoctoral work on the influence of emotion on gastric motility, to an understanding of the workings of the adrenal gland in neural transmission, as well as the basic process of homeostasis—have stood the test of time. With his discoveries, he was able to challenge the James-Lange theory of one of his mentors (James) that stated that emotions arose secondarily to bodily responses; Cannon's experiments suggested just the opposite.

Connect or Disconnect

Perhaps no aspect of physiological research captures so succinctly efforts to correlate mind and body as the James-Lange Theory of Emotion. William James, physician-psychologist (and, later, philosopher), attempting to explain emotion, posited that perception of a stimulus preceded the experience of feelings; thus, for example, encountering a fear-arousing situation, a person would first experience something like trembling before becoming aware of the emotion fear. Carl Lange, a Danish physician, working independently, had arrived at a similar conclusion, writing in 1855 [1922] in his acclaimed *On Emotions: A Psychophysiological Study* that a physiological reaction of the organism occurred before it was experienced as an emotion. As has been the case with most theories of mind-body interaction, the James-Lange theory ignited much controversy about the nature of emotion.

Not many years later, the Cannon-Bard theory proposed an opposing interpretation—that is, that experienced emotion was what triggered a physiological response. In other words, emotion is first, physiological reaction second, just the reverse of the James-Lange theory. The validity of both hypotheses was tested by Cannon's discovery that injections of adrenaline (*sympathin*) could produce the emotions of fear and anger but could also cause accelerated heart rate, increased breathing, sweating, dilated pupils, and the like without the associated emotions of fear or anger. Thus, it was demonstrated that the experience of emotion is more complex than a simple physiological reaction. As described by Gross and Barrett (2011), this complexity of emotion is "a collection of psychological states that include subjective experience, expressive behavior, and peripheral physiological responses" (p. 9). The James-Lange hypothesis would be one aspect of this complexity. The clinical observation that emotional response is not always perceived in its relationship to somatic reaction was addressed by Sifneos (1996) in his conception of "alexithymia," in patients who had "no words for feelings." The puzzlement of the disconnection, previously addressed in hysteria, persists today in clinical phenomena like "somatization" and "medically unexplained symptoms" (MUS). The perpetual reclassification of somatizing conditions has resulted in the change of somatoform disorders (DSM-IV) to simply somatic symptom disorder (DSM-5), with considerable controversial repercussion (Mayou, 2014).

The apparent "disconnect" between emotional and physical reaction has punctuated the history of psychiatry and psychology. According to Jones (1953), Freud too had suggested that emotions and thoughts preceded motor and physiological responses. Dunbar (1938) reinforces an impression that Freud's ideas stem from his adherence to a biological outlook, beginning with his interest in drives and instincts, not far removed from physiology. In fact, Freud's earliest description of neurosis was as the outcome of a conflict of drives (Dunbar, p. 33). With his interest in drives, according to Dunbar, "he brought psychology and general biology together and established the foundation for a biological psychology" (pp. 32–33). Commenting further, Dunbar stated:

> [Although] psychoanalytic theory is in accord with the general findings of biology, a gap still remains between our understanding and description of the organism from the side of anatomy and physiology on the one hand, and psychology and psychoanalysis on the other.
>
> *(p. 37)*

The idea that "chemical messengers" like adrenaline could help explain how mental and physical processes intersected with each other was not new. More than a century before Cannon's work on *sympathin*, the suggestion that *internuncii*, "the intermediate Officers between the Soul and the grosser parts of the Body," mediated communication between body parts was proposed by Bernard de Mandeville in 1711 (Lipsitt, 2001). Ernest Starling (1905), a British physiologist, named these substances "hormones," but it was Cannon who added the details to these rudimentary hypotheses that were necessary to establish a basis for future endocrine studies ("psychoneuroendocrinology" became a new domain of research interest). Reference to transduction (neurotransmitters) followed with additional studies by psychosomaticians like Herbert Weiner (1977), Robert Ader (1980), and George Solomon and Rudolf Moos (1964). Weiner's text on *Psychobiology* (1977) is encyclopedic in its coverage of the field. And the pioneering work of Schildkraut and Kety (1967) on biogenic amines has brought greater clarification to the neurochemistry of depression.

Gastrophysiology

The experiments of both Cannon and Pavlov first focused on how the gut responded to stimuli. But even before these researchers, by a quirky serendipitous route, an early introduction to gastric physiology had been announced in the mid-1800s by Dr. William Beaumont. He was lionized as the "Father of gastrophysiology" for his original crude studies of gastric processes. An army surgeon, not a physiologist, Beaumont (1838) treated a man, Alexis St. Martin, who had been accidentally shot in the stomach. Because the wound did not heal, opportunity presented itself for observation of gastric activity, which Beaumont did by inserting bits of food tied to a string into St. Martin's stomach. In this way, he established the fact that digestion was a chemical, not a mechanical process. He published his observations in the book *Experiments and Observations on the Gastric Juice, and Physiology of Digestion*. This serendipitous discovery joins the list of important discoveries that are often made by accident. Records leave little doubt that Cannon was aware of Beaumont's studies, for in 1933, almost one hundred years after Beaumont's publication, Cannon lectured to the Wayne County Medical Society on Beaumont's work. His lecture was published as "Some modern extensions of Beaumont's studies on Alexis St. Martin: thirst and hunger" (Cannon, 1933).

A more contemporary sophisticated investigation of gastric physiology is that of George Engel and associates' (Engel, Reichsman & Segal, 1956) famous Monica study. Baby Monica had been born with a constricted esophagus requiring an artificial opening to the stomach for feeding. Through this aperture, Engel and his associates at Rochester's Strong Memorial Hospital could observe changes of secretion and motility as Monica responded to affect related to separation, joy, fear, and anger. The observation that Monica's gastric secretion ceased when others withdrew extended findings of Pavlov and Cannon and supported the Rochester group's theory of conservation withdrawal; under threatening circumstances, the individual attempts to conserve resources to retain organismic homeostasis. It also supported their clinical hypothesis that individuals "give up" when they are "given up" in helplessness and hopelessness (Engel, 1968). Their physiological observations became the basis for conceptualizing many somatic diseases such as leukemia and ulcerative colitis.

All Is Balance

Approaches to combating illness and restoring health have all centered on the idea of reestablishing "balance" to what has apparently become "unbalanced," a process Cannon named "homeostasis" and Engel incorporated in his notions of "conservation." This concept reaches back even to the most primitive "theories" of the humors or to ancient philosophies like yin and yang. The concept of balance permeates the entire history of medicine, in both explanation and treatment. Every medical student and intern is familiar with the importance of acid-base balance as well as electrolyte balance. Ronald Pies (2007, p. 30) called attention to the early (1198) Maimonides' *Regimen Sanitatis* (Regimen of Health), wherein he proposes an "equilibrium theory" of health. This notion comprised a healthy "balanced" diet, periodic exercise, good climate, behavioral modification, and self-mastery, all essential for maintaining a healthy balance in life. Pies argues that Maimonides may have been one of the first to write of (but not name—au.) "psychosomatic medicine" with his view of "a healthy mind in a healthy body," an interrelatedness of mental and physical well-being. Maimonides wrote that "passions of the psyche produce changes in the body that are great, evident and manifest to all" (p. 30). Indeed, treatments by early physicians like Hippocrates and Galen sought to "balance" humors when they were thrown into disequilibrium by disease. Probably, such tenets characterized the Aesculapian system of medicine practiced in the temples around 300 BC.

Religion, advocating balance in life, evolved its percepts for combating evil with good. One might say the idea mimics the maxim of physics that every force has an equal and opposite force. The teeterboard of life is laden with ambivalences like active-passive, love-hate, hard-soft, hot-cold, and so on and so on, virtually ad infinitum. No wonder that early priest-physician healers believed, for example, that "cold" problems in health could be "cured" or at least alleviated through application of its opposite, "heat." Indeed, vestiges of such applications persist today in some approaches to assuaging muscle pain and other ailments.

Fechner, Freud, Bernard, and Cannon

In the early nineteenth century, when consideration of life's foibles took a more scientific turn, the question of balance and stability was addressed more thoughtfully. As the age of Enlightenment turned more from the physical assessment of the world toward the inner workings of the mind, a psychologist named Gustav Theodor Fechner, born at century's start, became interested in ways in which organization (of the world and other entities) contrasted with disorganization, resulting in a "law of constancy." He devised experiments to study how this relationship showed itself in physiological processes and how the sense organs reacted to input from various external stimuli, studies that built on work by a physiologist predecessor named Ernst Weber. The result was the Weber-Fechner law, stating that subjective sensation is proportional to the logarithm of the stimulus intensity.

With Fechner's work and ideas, the new field of physiological psychology was begun. The ripple effect in scientific circles was profound. Sigmund Freud, well-read during these years, was acquainted with Fechner's work and is known, by Freud's own attribution, to have incorporated some of Fechner's concepts into his own "law of stability," which stated in essence that where instability is (in the mental apparatus), there shall ego be, mediating the necessary changes to restore the person to a stable state. Ellenberger (1970) notes, "A large part of the theoretical framework of psychoanalysis would hardly have come into being without the speculations of the man whom Freud called the great Fechner" (p. 218).

In other quarters, namely France, around the mid-1800s, a physiologist named Claude Bernard had proposed similar aspects of physiologic processes, in which the internal milieu (*milieu interieur*) always tended toward adjustment or balance, the concept later amplified in Cannon's reference to homeostasis, a word that has readily entered the popular vocabulary. Bernard, considered by some as "one of the greatest of all men of science," wrote that "the stability of the internal environment is the condition for the free and independent life" (Cohen, 1957, p. iii).

Cannon and Psychosomatic Medicine

Some of the earliest psychosomatic studies, published by Franz Alexander and others in the issues of the then-new journal *Psychosomatic Medicine*, owed much to the foundational principles offered by Cannon's discoveries. Such studies had prompted Alexander (1950) to state, "The increasing knowledge of the relations of emotions to normal and disturbed body functions requires the modern physician to regard emotional conflicts as just as real and concrete as visible microorganisms" (p. 47). According to Alexander and Selesnick (1966), "The development of our knowledge about the influence of emotions upon organic processes that are not under voluntary control had to wait until an American physiologist, Walter Cannon (1871–1945), introduced a new concept derived from his ingenious investigations into the bodily effects of rage and fear" (p. 480). These studies are included in Cannon's 1929 magnum opus *Bodily Changes in Pain, Hunger, Fear, and Rage*, which may also be regarded as a "bible" for basic psychosomatic explorations. A more discursive volume, *The Wisdom of the Body*, was published later (1932), with further elaborations of the homeostatic principle by which the body maintains control over "both internal and external limitations on freedom of action," thus minimizing "risks of serious damage or death" to the individual (pp. 269–270). Cannon's hypotheses about the interaction of social (external) and biological (internal) processes antedated the so-called biopsychosocial approach to medical care espoused later by George Engel (1977) and others.

Throughout his career, Cannon remained a monist as far as mind-body relations were concerned. In his autobiographical writings, describing how subjective and objective data must be equally respected, he wrote (Yerkes, 1946):

> If we agree that we are organized as a psycho-organismic unity, we need not hesitate to use any convenient terms in mentioning any aspects of behavior or experience, for then we understand that these terms designate one aspect or the other of a living, systematic whole.
>
> *(p. 140)*

After Cannon

Much, if not most, of psychosomatic research includes psychophysiological parameters and draws on studies first performed by Cannon. Extending Cannon's discoveries of the autonomic nervous system, experimental psychologist Neal Miller and others discovered that many autonomic functions previously thought to be outside willful control were in fact quite readily affected by conscious thought. A landmark study by Schwartz, Shapiro and Tursky (1971) supported the premise of Miller and DiCara (1967) (based on rat experiments) that humans could learn to control their own heart rates through operant conditioning. According to Miller and DiCara, this phenomenon had "basic significance for both the theory of psychosomatic symptoms and the theory of neurophysiology of learning" (p. 143). This discovery introduced a whole new way of looking at treatment of bodily function, a quantum leap beyond Pavlov's conditioned "psychic reflexes." It demonstrated that "the relationship between fact and theory in creative scientific research is not nearly as straightforward as the general public has been led to believe" (Jonas, 1972, p. 30).

These physiologic discoveries led to the development of the new therapeutic field of biofeedback, in which individuals could learn to control their heartbeats, blood pressure, and somatic symptoms. Of course, antedating these scientific discoveries, the ability to control one's autonomic functions was well known to Zen Buddhist monks who were adept at controlling their breathing, blood pressure, skin sensitivity, and body heat, as recorded by Benson, Lehrman, Malhotra, Goldman, Hopkins, and Epstein (1982). The oriental "wisdom of the body" sought mental tranquility through self-control of entwined mind and body. Likewise, the ancient Japanese tea ceremony (*sado*) embodies a psychophysiological and philosophical approach to an altered state of consciousness.

Psychosomatic medicine itself owes much to oriental thought and practice. But it was not until Miller and DiCara had been able to quantify these "mysterious" abilities that essential mechanisms were identified. In more contemporary times, fervent advocates of the benefits of "mindfulness" and meditation practices have brought these techniques to the psychotherapeutic armamentarium of psychiatrists and others. Even with new discoveries of the manifold ways in which mental function related to physiology, the psychological school of behaviorism (e.g., Skinner, Watson) retained aspects of early stimulus-response (S-R) approaches to behavior.

Robert S. Woodworth, Psychology, and Psychiatry

Another psychologist of that time—Robert S. Woodworth (1921), called the Dean of American Psychology—retained a more holistic view of behavior, inserting, as it were, the O for "organism," between the S and the R of "stimulus-response" psychology. Woodworth's attention to the mediating organism (O) and mapping of S-O-R interactions was a functionalist approach to psychology, later characterized as "dynamic." Perhaps Woodworth's association with both James and Cannon at Harvard had molded his orientation to the relationship of physiology (which he considered unconscious mechanisms) and psychology (regarded as conscious behavior).

During his professional career at Columbia University, Woodworth (1921) developed methods of measurement of personality and physiology and published a popular book, *Psychology: A Study of Mental Life*. In it, he tackled the dilemma of the "mind-body problem," asking, "Where shall we class sensation?" Is it "mental" or "bodily"? he queried. "Both sciences [psychology and physiology—au.] study it." Physiology, he wrote, was "more apt to go into the detailed study of the action of the sense organs," while "psychology [was more apt] to concern itself with the classification of sensations and the use made of them for recognizing objects or for esthetic purposes." He concluded that "the line between the two sciences is far from sharp at this point" (p. 6). This difficult distinction engrosses both researchers and clinicians and is evident to the latter when consultees request consultations to distinguish between "organic" and "functional" disorders in patients on whom they consult; as with Woodworth, the distinction is often "far from sharp." Anorexia nervosa, considered by some to be the paradigmatic psychosomatic disease, is a glaring example of the complexity of disease states (Kaufman & Margolin, 1948).

Antedating Woodworth's emphasis on the O (mediating organism) of psychological study, the psychiatrist Adolf Meyer (1912), in a paper *The Value of Psychology to Psychiatry* read to a joint meeting of the American Psychological Association and the Southern Society for Philosophy and Psychology, wrote, "Psychology is the only field of experience from which we can get the proper designation and understanding . . . [of] the different integrative factors of the reactions as a whole, for a reduction to terms of an experiment of nature, and for the study of its modifiability" (Lief, 1948, p. 384). The O of muscles and glands as integral parts of our total behavior—the person, indeed, as the "self-integrator"—helps us to quantify our observations of all aspects of human behavior, the psychopathology, psychology, and physiology that are the requisite integrative forces of a "commonsense psychiatry." While the physiologist "singles out" specific processes, Meyer wrote, the psychiatrist must recognize "the action of a more or less conscious person . . . with its meaning in a personal life; more than a mere series of twitches, because it is part of a flow of function . . . our doing, our walking, and breathing, including also the action of the sense organs and the brain and our muscles and glands as integral parts of our total behavior—the person, indeed, as the self-regulator." Meyer, in his "psychobiological" psychiatry, elaborates further: "We cannot report this behavior in terms of mere sensory-neuromuscular performances, but we do it in terms of action, disposals of situations, performance of tasks; and this is something we must learn to practice, just as the work in physiology and in anatomy, on the basis of concrete material, instead of just thinking and talking" (p. 443).

Meyer's psychobiological approach is very compatible with the C-L psychiatrist's orientation, except that "thinking and talking" remain essential aspects of liaison's pedagogical function.

Dr. Stanley Cobb

Another collator of physiologic and psychiatric knowledge who contributed heavily to the foundations of C-L psychiatry was Dr. Stanley Cobb, who had been a graduate student under Adolf Meyer. Meyer himself had come to psychiatry through psychopathology and neurophysiology, incorporating these elements in his "psychobiological, commonsense psychiatry." Having first worked essentially as a neuropathologist at Boston City Hospital, Cobb was urged by Alan Gregg to move to Massachusetts General Hospital (MGH) in 1934 to establish, with Rockefeller Foundation money, a general hospital-based department of psychiatry. With his interest in mind–brain relationships, Cobb (1952) brought an impressive eclecticism to "the General," ranging from anatomy to physiology to psychoanalysis.

Cobb's (1928) interest in psychiatry emerged from his realization that a limited knowledge of anatomy and reflex physiology (a la Pavlov's conditioned reflex) was "inadequate for an understanding of the highest levels of integration" (p. 995). In this paper, he calls attention to the "void" in our understanding of mental mechanisms. He wrote, "It is here that research must be carried on for many years in order that block after block of facts may be built up to explain the observations and to support the theories now promulgated in psychiatry and in psychology" (p. 981).

Charitably acknowledging that innovators like Charcot, Freud, Janet, and Prince "are probably right," Cobb cautioned that theories often appear before proof is available to support them and that psychiatry must pass through its complex infancy before scientific "quantitative analysis" would be relevant. "One must build upward from below," he wrote, "on the basis of anatomy and physiology in order to elucidate the mechanisms of the increasing data of psychiatry" (p. 982). As part of this emerging data, Cobb refers to Cannon and his studies of endocrine and sympathetic connections that have "given the psychiatrist insight into the relationship between 'mind and body' " (p. 983). Cobb refers to the physiologic process of inhibition, as when extensor and flexor reflexes oppose one another, but he does not address the Freudian concept of repression that had already been reported in Freud's (1926) *Inhibitions, Repression and Anxiety*, rather alluding to Bernard Hart's (1916) book *Psychology of Insanity* that covers topics of "conflict," "complexes," and "repression."

Biographers have referred to Cobb's slow but positive receptivity to psychoanalysis, perhaps accounting for the omitted reference to Freud. With his characteristic caution and thoroughness, as chief of psychiatry at MGH until 1955, it would be fair to say that Cobb had constructed a sturdy "scientific" scaffold on which the C-L service could be built. When Erich Lindemann followed Cobb as chief of psychiatry in 1955, the MGH C-L service developed under the charge of Avery Weisman (a Boston psychoanalyst) and his young assistant Thomas Hackett, with contributions from several European émigré psychoanalysts. The program flourished and became an early model for similar services in the Boston community and elsewhere in the country. The seed was propagated when Ralph Kaufman and Felix Deutsch transferred from MGH to Boston's Beth Israel Hospital, establishing a consultation program continued under subsequent directorship of Grete Bibring and Ralph Kahana.

Weisman and Hackett's (1960) consultative approach achieved a psychodynamic orientation and was described in seminal articles in the C-L literature based on their experience (Hackett & Weisman, 1960a, 1960b; Weisman & Hackett, 1960). Significant papers by Kaufman (1953); Franzblau, Kairys and Kaufman (1956); and Bibring (1951, 1956) were published in the 1950s.

The Physiology of Stress

Once Cannon had broadened appreciation of the individual to more than an S-R preparation, interest was aroused in the multitude of variables that can affect individual physiologic responses. This variability in the vast repertoire of an individual's adaptive reactions led to the concept of "stress," a term Cannon had used in a general way, suggesting that it was something that might be measured (Hinkle, 1977, p. 30). Best known in the United States for his studies of stress was Hans Selye (1980); in Europe it was Lennart Levi (1984). Both addressed the balancing system of sympathetic and parasympathetic parts of the autonomous nervous system in ways that acknowledged the trend toward a view of the person as a physiologic "whole" organism.

The term "stress" was used in a variety of ways, on the one hand to refer to an internal total biological process (Kinston & Wolff, 1977; Selye, 1956) and on the other hand as any external pressure, load, stimulus, burden, or symbol ("stressors") eliciting some physiological response in the individual. Cannon (1935) had written of stress in his paper "Stresses and strains of homeostasis." The term spilled into everyday language to apply to almost any perturbed state of an individual hardship, difficulty, life situation, or social predicament. It became easier for patients to attribute their discomforts to stress than to more specific events in their lives. Lipowski (1975) eschews the term "stress" and alludes to "sensory and information inputs overload," with both overload and deprivation inducing psychophysiological repercussions.

Selye, beginning in the 1930s, had begun experimenting with the effects of "alarming" stimuli on animals, describing the stress aroused in them as a "general adaptation syndrome" (GAS). In his groundbreaking popular book *The Stress of Life* (1956), he distinguished between the normal state of being ("eustress") and a more pathological condition ("distress"). At times, the term was alluded to as "life stress," and, indeed, by the 1960s, Holmes and Rahe (1967) had constructed a "social readjustment scale" that attempted to quantify stressful life changes. The term soon found its way into the psychophysiological studies of psychosomatic medicine that attempted to establish specificity between disease and stressful stimuli, an approach that was eventually at least partially discredited.

It was the (mistaken) notion of physiological specificity that led Alexander and others to their psychosomatic studies of, for example, hypertension, peptic ulcer, asthma, and other disease states. The idea that peptic ulcer could arise in certain temperamentally predisposed individuals in high-stress environs had much appeal. Subsequent elucidation of the complexity of physiological responsiveness rendered the notion of such specificity suspect. According to Johnson (1977):

> Efforts to use physiological indices to define specific emotions, motivations and attitudes . . . have floundered due to semantic confusion on the psychological side and diffuseness and complex interaction among measures on the physiological side.
>
> *(p 260).*

Modern psychiatrists are most likely familiar with the work of Hans Selye on stress but unaware of other, even earlier, physiologists and their relevant work. One such is Walter Rudolf Hess (1924), a Swiss physician/physiologist and Nobelist (with Egas Moniz in 1949) for his work on the relation of the brain to control of internal organs. In his early research, Hess demonstrated that different parts of the brain controlled different types of responses. Thus, by stimulating the anterior part of the hypothalamus, he could affect blood pressure, respiration, hunger, thirst, micturition, and bowel function, while posterior stimulation caused marked excitement and defense-like behavior. He concluded that subcortical centers of the brain coordinated autonomic, somatic, and psychic functions and were organized through reciprocally balanced systems that he named *ergotropic* and *trophotropic* (Kiely, 1977, pp. 206–207). Ergotropic processes prepared the individual for action (not unlike Cannon's hypothesis), associated with increased muscle tone, sympathetic nervous activity, arousal, and alerting behavior, mediated through the biogenic amines norepinephrine and dopamine. The trophotropic system, on the other hand, promotes withdrawal and conservation of energy, with increased parasympathetic nervous system function, mediated largely through 5-hydroxytryptamine (serotonin) and acetylcholine. William Kiely, a director of the C-L Service at UCLA, drawing on the 1924 studies of Hess, was one of few psychiatrists who pursued research in this area. He wrote in 1977, "Neurobiological research makes increasingly clear the important modulating and regulatory influence of the component parts of these systems upon somatic sensory and motor function, visceral activity, and psychic function" (p. 207). This complex psychobiological process was further enunciated through studies of the thyroid-thalamus-pituitary axis operating, as it did, in a self-regulatory or homeostatic manner. Cannon, Binger, and Fritz (1915) had already demonstrated how chronic environmental stimuli could induce hyperthyroidism in the cat.

From studies of neuroendocrine mediating mechanisms, it became "apparent that the endocrine system constitutes a physiological mechanism of defense adapting the individual to his environment in much the same way that we conceptualize psychological mechanisms of defense" (Whybrow & Silberfarb, 1977, p. 221).

Remedicalization, Psychiatry, and Physiology

Little, if any, physiological research was accomplished in state asylums. However, to help meet the deficiency in one state, the Massachusetts legislature in 1912 founded the Boston Psychopathic Hospital ("the Psycho"), not as another custodial institution but rather as a facility for the prompt treatment and care of acute mental disorder, as well as training, teaching, and research (May, 1919, p. 21). There, with the Department of Therapeutic Research, under the directorship of Milton Greenblatt, extensive psychophysiologic research was carried out, to which hundreds of psychiatric trainees (many to later find posts as C-L psychiatrists) were exposed. With support from the Rockefeller Foundation, the department carried out metabolic and physiological studies that were published in 1934 in a volume entitled simply *Schizophrenia* (Boston Psychopathic Hospital, 1934).

As part of the Harvard residency program, psychiatrists, psychologists, psychoanalysts, and other researchers worked together to bring physiology and psychiatry closer together at "the Psycho." My own interest in psychiatry was fostered by an introductory course in electrophysiology with Greenblatt before I entered medical school.

Transition from asylums to general hospitals has permitted closer application of physiological knowledge to patient care. However, much of clinical psychiatry has tended to drift away from its physiology roots, with interest in this field remaining largely the province of psychosomatic researchers, not exclusively the domain of psychiatry. Nevertheless, recent remedicalization—aided by improved technology, neuroimaging, and enhanced psychopharmacologic studies—has included new explorations in pathophysiology and neuroscience as integral parts of psychiatry, proving what Hess's studies had only hinted at. In years past, patients with depression or anxiety were sometimes told that their disease was due to a "chemical imbalance"; this was intended, in most cases, to soften the impact of delivering a feared "psychiatric diagnosis" rather than to provide a sophisticated explanation of these disorders (see, for example, Pies at http://www.medscape.com/viewarticle/823368_2 [accessed March 2, 2015]). Current knowledge supports theories of multicausality, with increasing data from scientific studies adding considerably to our understanding of this complexity.

Beyond Fight or Flight: The New Physiology

Cannon's "fight or flight" hypotheses and concept of homeostasis did not include all of the neurohumoral awareness that now exists. Much more is now known about the neurochemistry, neurocircuitry, and physiology of anxiety and depression—as well as better-defined psychiatric diseases like schizophrenia—than was known to Freud when he abandoned his efforts to explain psychiatric disease in "scientific terms." For example, a recent issue of the *American Journal of Psychiatry* (Abdallah, Jiang, De Feyter, Fasula & Krystal, 2014; Iacono, 2014) carries articles on the neurobehavioral aspects of multidimensional psychopathology and the role of glutamate in depression. And the *New England Journal of Medicine* (Harkin, 2014) in the same month carries an article ("Muscling in on depression") describing how the metabolism of the enzyme kynurenine influences stress resilience, affecting the "pathophysiological aspects of a number of brain disorders, including depression" (p. 2333). When Freud told his Vienna Circle that they must hasten their work, lest discoveries in chemistry and physiology be at their heels, he could not have prophesied more astutely. A recent paper on translational neuroscience explanation for the pathophysiology of social anxiety disorder is in all likelihood the kind of study Freud might well have anticipated (Fox & Kalin, 2014); indeed, brain circuits involving the amygdala, hippocampus, and cortex have become decipherable only with progress in medical technology.

While Hans Selye and Franz Alexander have been referred to as the "two pillars of psychosomatics," future assessment of contributors to the field will have to "take the results of modern psychophysiology seriously into account," to comprehend, for example, how anxiety and depression affect physical conditions like cardiovascular disease, alcoholism, suicide, and perhaps even tumor growth (Kopp & Skrabski, 1989). Furthermore, the new field of psychoneuroimmunology (Excerpta Medica, 2002) has added immeasurably to our understanding of immune processes in disease, as well as to the enlarged roster of "pillars of psychosomatic medicine." Such expansion of our understanding of mental health and illness contributes a physiological component to the preventative prospects of combined psychophysiology, psychotherapy, and psychopharmacology, perhaps resulting in unwieldy terms like "psychoneuroendocrinoimmunology."

John Mason (1968) and colleagues have expanded our knowledge of psychoendocrine repercussions to stressful life circumstances by demonstrating how the pituitary-adrenal axis responds to psychological influence. These studies demonstrate how several systems can be studied concurrently rather than in isolation, thus paving the way for future "integrated" exploration. Specifically, Mason was able to show how the quotidian emotional influences of life can affect the central nervous system to exert a constant "tonicity" upon the endocrine system. In much the same fashion, previous studies demonstrated how the autonomic function affected skeletal muscular "effector systems."

Going Forward

It is a long way from the earliest galvanometer to the most modern neuroimaging technology, with which Glover's "physiological octopus" is gradually being vanquished. No longer is the line between physiology and psychology so distinct. Standing on the shoulders of important researchers like Pavlov, Cannon, Miller, Selye, and Alexander, as well as psychologists Watson, Skinner, and Woodworth, we can see further into mind-brain relationships where knowledge and language have begun to converge. Andreasen (1995) sums up:

> The process [mapping the human brain] is becoming much more sophisticated, particularly with the aid of neuroimaging techniques such as magnetic resonance imaging (MRI) and positron-emission tomography (PET), which permit in vivo study of the anatomy and physiology of the human brain in ways that were previously impossible.
>
> *(p. 131)*

Aspects of human behavior previously elusive to measurement—like those of memory, language, attention, emotion, and thought—have become more accessible through neurochemical discoveries like neurotransmitter systems (e.g., dopamine, norepinephrine, and serotonin). Another worthy attempt at integration is Eric Kandel's (2005) book, *Psychiatry, Psychoanalysis, and the New Biology of Mind.*

Hans Schaefer (1960), a German psychiatrist/physiologist has written, "There is hardly a kind of somatic disability that might not also somewhere include important psychic factors." He wondered whether attempts to "complete the arc" between psyche and soma, and psychology and physiology, were a problem "for physiologists still unborn, and for a time when psychosomatic science will have better methods than today" (p. 127). He proclaims that those who try to find correlations between psyche and soma "must hold citizenship in two realms—in the classical realm of science, and in the realm of the liberal arts (the humanities) and biographical psychosomatics" (p. 133), much as Winnicott (1966) metaphorically declared that few could "ride the two horses" (of psyche and soma). Schaefer (1960) pessimistically fears that if a synthesis of methods does not succeed, "science [would be] at risk of being thrown back on philosophy when physiochemical explanations of somatic or emotional events are not forthcoming." To some degree, "psychosomatic science is always metaphysical in so far as it attempts to transcend mere coordination of body and soul" (p. 133). The philosophers Jaspers and Dilthey have distinguished between two modes of understanding (*erklaren* and *verstehen*), useful in understanding the complementary aspects of these two kinds of knowledge (see, e.g., http://www.bu.edu/paideia/existenz/volumes/Vol.3-2Ghaemi.html [accessed March 2, 2015] [Ghaemi, 2003]).

In the context of today's incremental advancements in science and technology, Schaefer (1960) would undoubtedly have to agree that psychosomatic experiments offer us more than "a catalog of statements of the kind that under certain somatic conditions, certain psychic phenomena occur (reactions, deficiencies), whereby an enrichment of phenomenology, but no psychosomatic theory, is gained" (p. 130). What we need, wrote Schaefer,

> is a new philosophy of the state of being ill, and a new physiology of man's everyday life, two things that go hand in hand. They include the way foods agree with one; the "state of health" in the widest sense of its dependence on weather, mood, drugs, and stimulants; the problem of fatigue and psyche, interest and achievement, intelligence and a man's lot in life.
>
> *(p. 127)*

In time, we can hope that philosophy, physiology, psychology, science, and phenomenology will meld into a comprehensive wholeness of being.

While Cartesian dualism still infuses the teaching of medicine and the practice of physicians, new knowledge and understanding facilitate the transition from laboratory to bedside. There is hope on the horizon that new insights and even new "philosophies" of practice will redound to the benefit of patients. The relation of physiology to psychosomatic medicine remains of significant interest. Ever since the earliest development of instruments like the psychogalvanometer, improved technology, now encompassing great strides in computer science and imaging techniques, continues to clarify the physiology of emotion as reflected in bodily reactions. Andreasen (1995) states that, "both historically and conceptually, psychiatry grows from the soil of neurobiology" (p. 194). And we see the roots, stems, branches, and fruit grow from the seeds planted so long ago. It is a tree cultivated (and likely inhabited) by the C-L psychiatrist.

We have already begun to see progress in meeting the need now to take a multivariate look at the whole patient as he or she works, plays, and sleeps, with special emphasis on how the living organism maintains itself at optimal levels in the midst of an onslaught of exogenous and endogenous disturbances (Andreasen, 1995, p. 194).

By assessing the multiple stimulus situations (both internal and external) in a patient's life and the complex responses—influenced by factors such as personality type, coping styles, beliefs, attitudes, and intelligence—the C-L psychiatrist can assemble a "case formulation" from which diagnosis and treatment recommendations flow. No better goal can be expressed for the C-L psychiatrist, who, with each consultation, must make just such assessments.

A past half century of progress in psychobiology now solidly grounds the clinical practice of consultation-liaison psychiatry in the general hospital. The scientific base for its practice has been widened. However, the spirit of consultation-liaison psychiatry remains in its commitment to working collaboratively with nonpsychiatric caregivers about the psychiatric management of their patients (Stotland & Garrick, 1990, pp. 12–13).

References

Abdallah, C.G., Jiang, L., De Feyter, H.M., Fasula, M., & Krystal, J.H. (2014). Glutamate metabolism in major depression. *American Journal of Psychiatry, 171,* 1320–1327.

Ader, R. (1980). Presidential address—1980. Psychosomatic and psychoimmunologic research. *Psychosomatic Medicine, 42,* 307–321.

Alexander, F. (1950). *Psychosomatic Medicine.* New York, NY: W.W. Norton.

Alexander, F.G. & Selesnick, S.T. (1966). *The History of Psychiatry.* New York, NY: New American Library (Mentor).

Andreasen, N.C. (1995). The neurobiology of mental illness. In N.C. Andreasen (Ed.). *Introductory Textbook of Psychiatry.* (2nd edition, pp. 129–165). Washington, DC: American Psychiatric Publishing.

Beaumont, W. (1838). *Experiments and Observations on the Gastric Juice, and Physiology of Digestion.* Edinburgh: McLachlan & Stewart.

Benson, H., Lehrman, J.W., Malhotra, M.S., Goldman, R.F., Hopkins, J., & Epstein, M. (1982). Body temperature changes during the practice of g Tum-mo yoga. *Nature, 295,* 234–236.

Bibring, G.L. (1951). Preventive psychiatry in a general hospital. *Bulletin of World Federation of Mental Health, 3,* 224–232.

Bibring, G.L. (1956). Psychiatry and medical practice in a general hospital. *New England Journal of Medicine, 254,* 366–372.

Blumenfield, M., & Strain, J.J. (Eds.). (2006). *Psychosomatic Medicine.* Philadelphia, PA: Lippincott Williams & Wilkins.

Brown, T.M., & Fee, E. (2002). Walter Bradford Cannon: Pioneer physiologist of human emotions. *American Journal of Public Health, 92,* 1594–1595.

Cannon, W.B. (1929). *Bodily Changes in Pain, Hunger, Fear and Rage: An Account of Recent Research into the Function of Emotional Excitement.* (2nd edition). New York, NY: Appleton.

Cannon, W.B. (1932). *Wisdom of the Body.* New York, NY: W.W. Norton.

Cannon, W.B. (1933). Some modern extensions of Beaumont's studies on Alexis St. Martin: Thirst and hunger. (Beaumont Lecture) *Journal of Michigan Medical Society, 32,* 155–164.

Cannon, W.B. (1935). Stresses and strains of homeostasis. *American Journal of Medical Science, 189,* 1–14.

Cannon, W.B., Binger, C.A.L., & Fritz, R. (1915). Experimental hyperthyroidism. *American Journal of Physiology, 36,* 363–375.

Cobb, S. (1928). Physiology, psychiatry and inhibitions. *Archives of Neurology and Psychiatry, 19,* 981–996.

Cobb, S. (1952). *Foundations of Psychopathology.* Baltimore, MD: Williams & Wilkins.

Cohen, I.B. (1957). Forward. In Claude Bernard (1865) (Ed.). *An Introduction to the Study of Experimental Medicine.* (Dover edition, pp. 1–4). New York, NY: Macmillan.

Dunbar, H.F. (1938). *Emotions and Bodily Changes.* (2nd edition). New York, NY: Columbia University Press.

Ellenberger, H.F. (1970). *The Discovery of the Unconscious.* New York, NY: Basic Books.

Engel, G.L. (1968). A life-setting conducive to illness. The giving-up given-up complex. *Bulletin of Menninger Clinic, 32,* 355–365.

Engel, G.L. (1977). The need for a new medical model: A challenge for biomedicine. *Science, 196,* 129–136.

Engel, G.L., Reichsman, F., & Segal, H.L. (1956). A study of an infant with a gastric fistula. I. Behavior and the rate of total HCl acid secretion. *Psychosomatic Medicine, 18,* 374–398.

Excerpta Medica. (2002). *Psychoneuroendocrinoimmunology.* #1241 International Congress Series. Philadelphia, PA: Adelphi Group.

Fox, A.S., & Kalin, N.H. (2014). A translational, neuroscience approach to understanding the development of social anxiety disorder and its pathophysiology. *American Journal of Psychiatry, 171,* 1162–1173.

Franzblau, A.N., Kairys, D., & Kaufman, M.R. (1956). The emotional impact of ward rounds. *Journal of Mount Sinai Hospital New York, 23,* 782–803.

Freud, S. (1926). Inhibitions, repression and anxiety. In J. Strachey (Ed.). *The Standard Edition of the Complete Psychological Works of Sigmund Freud.* (Vol. 20, pp. 75–175). London, UK: Hogarth Press.

Ghaemi, S.N. (2003). *The Concepts of Psychiatry: A Pluralistic Approach to the Mind and Mental Illness.* Baltimore, MD: Johns Hopkins University Press.

Gifford, G.E., Jr. (1981). Pavlov's legacy to behavioral psychology, physiology and psychiatry: A program about Pavlov. *Journal of the History of Behavioral Science, 17,* 153–301.

Glover, E. (1956). *On the Early Development of Mind.* New York, NY: International Universities Press.

Gross, J.J., & Barrett, L.F. (2011). Emotion generation and emotion regulation. One or two depends on your point of view. *Emotion Review, 3,* 8–16.

Hackett, T.P., & Weisman, A.D. (1960a). Psychiatric management of perioperative syndromes. I. The therapeutic consultation and the effect of non-interpretive intervention. *Psychosomatic Medicine, 22,* 267–282.

Hackett, T.P., & Weisman, A.D. (1960b). Psychiatric management of perioperative syndromes. II. Psychodynamic factors in formulation and management. *Psychosomatic Medicine, 22,* 356–372.

Harkin, A. (2014). Muscling in on depression. *New England Journal of Medicine, 371,* 2333–2334.

Hart, B. (1916). *Psychology of Insanity.* Cambridge, UK: Cambridge University Press.

Hess, R. (1924). Uber die wechsel beziehungen zwischen psychischen und vegitativen functionen. *Archives of Neurology and Psychiatry, 15,* 260–264.

Hinkle, L.E., Jr. (1977). The concept of "stress" in the biological and social sciences. In Z.J. Lipowski, D.R. Lipsitt, & P.C. Whybrow (Eds.). *Psychosomatic Medicine: Current Trends and Clinical Applications.* (pp. 27–49). New York, NY: Oxford University Press.

Holmes, T.H., & Rahe, R. (1967). The social readjustment rating scale. *Journal of Psychosomatic Research, 11,* 213–218.

Iacono, W.G. (2014). Neurobehavioral aspects of multidimensional psychopathology. *American Journal of Psychiatry, 171,* 1236–1239.

Johnson, L.C. (1977). Psychophysiological research: Aims and methods. In Z.J. Lipowski, D.R. Lipsitt, & P.C. Whybrow (Eds.). *Psychosomatic Medicine: Current Trends and Clinical Applications.* (pp. 253–261). New York, NY: Oxford University Press.

Jonas, G. (1972). Visceral Learning, II. *New Yorker.* August 27, p. 30.

Jones, E. (1953). *The Life and Work of Sigmund Freud.* (Vol. 1). New York, NY: Basic Books.

Kandel, E. (2005). *Psychiatry, Psychoanalysis, and the New Biology of Mind.* Washington, DC: American Psychiatric Publishing.

Kaufman, M.R. (1953). The role of the psychiatrist in the general hospital. *Psychiatric Quarterly, 27,* 367–381.

Kaufman, M.R., & Margolin, S.G. (1948). Theory and practice of psychosomatic medicine in a general hospital. *Medical Clinics of North America, 32,* 611–616.

Kiely, W.F. (1977). From the symbolic stimulus to the physiological response: Neurophysiological mechanisms. In Z.J. Lipowski, D.R. Lipsitt, & P.C. Whybrow (Eds.). *Psychosomatic Medicine: Current Trends and Clinical Applications.* (pp. 206–218). New York, NY: Oxford University Press.

Kinston, M., & Wolff, H. (1977). Bodily communication and psychotherapy. In Z.J. Lipowski, D.R. Lipsitt, & P.C. Whybrow (Eds.). *Psychosomatic Medicine: Current Trends and Clinical Applications.* (pp. 481–487). New York, NY: Oxford University Press.

Kopp, M., & Skrabski, A. (1989). What does the legacy of Hans Selye and Franz Alexander mean today? The psychophysiological approach in medical practice. *International Journal of Psychophysiology, 8,* 99–105.

Lange, C. (1885 [1922]). On emotions: A psychophysiological study. In C.G. Lange & W. James (Eds.). *The Emotion.* (pp. 33–90). Baltimore, MD: Williams & Wilkins.

Levi, L. (1984). Work, stress and health. *Scandinavian Journal of Work and Environmental Health, 10,* 495–500.

Lief, A. (1948). *The Commonsense Psychiatry of Dr. Adolf Meyer.* New York, NY: McGraw-Hill.

Lipowski, Z.J. (1975). Sensory and information inputs overload: Behavioral effects. *Comprehensive Psychiatry, 16,* 199–221.

Lipsitt, D.R. (2001). The time has come to speak of many things. *Advances in Mind-Body Medicine, 17,* 249–256.

Mason, J. (1968). The scope of psychoendocrine research: A review of psychoendocrine research on the pituitary-adrenal cortical system. *Psychosomatic Medicine, 20,* 565–575.

May, J.V. (1919). The functions of the psychopathic hospital. *American Journal of Psychiatry, 76,* 21–34.

Mayou, R. (2014). Is the DSM-5 chapter on somatic symptom disorder any better than DSM-IV somatoform disorder? *British Journal of Psychiatry, 204,* 418–419.

Meyer, A. (1912). The value of psychology in psychiatry. *Journal of the American Medical Association, 58,* 911–914.

Miller, N.E., & DiCara, L. (1967). Instrumental learning of heart rate changes in curarized rats: Shaping and specificity to discriminatory stimulus. *Journal of Comprehensive Physiology and Psychology, 63,* 12–19.

Muller, P. (1838). *Elements of Physiology.* London, UK: Taylor & Walton.

Notes from the Editors. (1989). *Walter B. Cannon. Bodily Changes in Pain, Hunger, Fear and Rage: An Account of Recent Research Into the Function of Emotional Excitement.* Birmingham, AL: Gryphon Editions.

Pavlov, I. (1897/1902). *The Work of the Digestive Glands.* (Translated by W.H. Thompson). London: Charles Griffin.

Penfield, W. (1971). The neurophysiological basis of thought. In J.G. Howell (Ed.). *Modern Perspectives in World Psychiatry.* (pp. 314–347). New York, NY: Brunner/Mazel.

Pies, R. (2007). Maimonides. *Psychiatric News.* January 19, pp. 42, 30.

Schaefer, H. (1960). Physiology and psychosomatic medicine. *Archives of General Psychiatry, 3,* 123–134.

Schildkraut, J., & Kety, S. (1967). Biogenic amines and emotion. *Science, 156,* 21–37.

Schwartz, D., Shapiro, G.E., & Tursky, B. (1971). Learned control of cardiovascular integration in man through operant conditioning. *Psychosomatic Medicine, 33,* 57–62.

Scott, C.M. (1935) *Schizophrenia; Statistical Studies from the Boston Psychopathic Hospital,* 1925–1934. Boston Psychopathic Hospital Clinical Service and Laboratories. Boston, MA: Massachusetts Society for Mental Hygiene.

Selye, H. (1956). *The Stress of Life.* New York, NY: McGraw-Hill.

Selye, H. (1980). Stress and holistic medicine. *Family and Community Health, 3,* 85–88.

Sifneos, P.E. (1996). Alexithymia: Past and present. *American Journal of Psychiatry, 153*(7 Suppl), 137–142.

Solomon, G.F., & Moos, R.H. (1964). Emotions, immunity, and disease: A speculative theoretical integration. *Archives of General Psychiatry, 11,* 657–674.

Starling, E. (1905). The Croonian Lectures: I. On the chemical correlation of the functions of the body. *Lancet, 166,* 339–341.

Stotland, N., & Garrick, T. (1990). *Manual of Psychiatric Consultation.* Washington, DC: American Psychiatric Press.

Weiner, H. (1977). *Psychobiology and Human Disease.* New York, NY: Elsevier, 1977

Weisman, A.D., & Hackett, T.P. (1960). Organization and function of a psychiatric consultation service. *International Record of Medicine, 173,* 306–311.

Whybrow, P.C., & Silberfarb, P.M. (1977). Neuroendocrine mediating mechanisms: From the symbolic stimulus to the physiological response. In Z.J. Lipowski, D.R. Lipsitt, & P.C. Whybrow. *Psychosomatic Medicine: Current Trends and Clinical Applications.* (pp. 219–227). New York, NY: Oxford University Press.

Winnicott, D. (1966). Psycho-somatic illness in its positive and negative aspects. *International Journal of Psychoanalysis, 47,* 510–516.

Wise, M.G., & Rundell, J.R. (Eds.). (2002). *Textbook of Consultation-Liaison Psychiatry: Psychiatry in the Medically Ill.* Washington, DC: American Psychiatric Press.

Woodworth, R.S. (1921). *Psychology: A Study of Mental Life.* New York, NY: Henry Holt & Co.

Yerkes, R.M. (1946). Walter Bradford Cannon 1871–1945. *Psychological Review, 53,* 137–146.

3

PSYCHOANALYSIS

The Mysterious Leap

*In the beginning, psychoanalysis, like many other cultural movements, encountered
numerous obstacles to its acceptance in the land of its origin.*
—*Rosenzweig, 1994, p. 3*

The evolving field of consultation-liaison psychiatry has been a major force in
medicine, essentially self-appointed to try to close or at least to minimize the
existent gap between mental and physical (Lipsitt, 2006). The early foundational
contribution of psychoanalysis to psychosomatic medicine and consultation-
liaison (C-L) psychiatry has been virtually obscured by subsequent events but
remains vital to this day. It may be likened to a booster cable for automotive purposes without which the engine cannot start; once started, the cable is released,
but the engine continues powered up. In this metaphoric sense, psychoanalysis was the booster cable of psychosomatic medicine, with psychoanalytic roots
often forgotten, like a detached cable. Transition over the years from a mostly
"dynamic" to a "biological" orientation in psychiatry has drawn attention away
from psychoanalytic ideas, even as those concepts are integrally embedded in C-L
psychiatry. Furthermore, repeated cautionary warnings by seasoned C-L practitioners to avoid use of psychoanalytic jargon has perhaps diminished interest in the
psychoanalytic lexicon and its concepts.

This chapter reviews the history of hysteria and salient psychoanalytic elaborations as they have catalyzed developments in C-L psychiatry and psychosomatic
medicine. Before Freud discovered how the unconscious could convert intrapsychic conflict into physical symptoms, hysteria was attributed for centuries to
bizarre explanations and often even more bizarre "treatment." Freud's understanding of the condition was, in brief, the origin of psychoanalysis. It is thereby of

major consequence to the emergence of C-L psychiatry and psychosomatic medicine and will be a focus of this chapter.

Vibrant Vienna

At the turn of the century (nineteenth through the twentieth), Vienna was an incubator of genius, a cauldron of creative energy. A young neurologist struggled to grow his practice in order to support his family, while artists, writers, politicians, musicians, and other creative people rose to prominence in a turbulent culture. In a sense, Freud was an early neuropsychiatric consultant, asked to consult on patients with problems elusive of physical diagnosis, cases that might today be assigned the designation of medically unexplained symptoms (MUS).

All progressive ideas evolve almost imperceptibly, encounter opposition and obstacles when they emerge, then capture public interest and acclaim before reaching their full expression and embrace success or failure. Psychoanalysis was such a phenomenon, ultimately to infuse an entire culture in all its dimensions with its revelatory insights. Medicine and psychiatry likewise followed a similar course.

Dualisms

In general terms, dating back to ancient times, all knowledge evolved as a way to explain distinctions between the physical and nonphysical world. The entire history of ideas is punctuated with dualistic thinking of one sort or another, contrasting world against nonworld, physical against spiritual, right against wrong, good against evil, sin against virtue, internal against external, life against death, almost infinitely. Descartes spent a lifetime contemplating the "problem."

The enduring religious belief in a separate soul has attracted philosophers, theologians, and psychologists throughout the ages, searching for comprehension of the living being, developing theories of behavior to account for and integrate seemingly disparate, contrary forces. With Freud, too, his psychoanalytic theories were founded on the dualities of Eros vs. Thanatos; libidinal vs. physical energy; and psychology vs. biology.

In a sense, the history of medicine, psychology, and psychiatry may attribute to Freud the dominion over what has come to be known as "the mind-body controversy." The quandary of this dualism has dogged psychiatry's relationship to the rest of medicine for eons. The dilemma has given rise to designations of not just two medicines, biological (i.e., biomedicine) and psychological (i.e., biopsychosocial), but also two psychiatries ("functional" and "organic") (Luhrmann, 2000). In the 1950s and 1960s, Hollingshead and Redlich (1958) referred to the "organicists" and "dynamicists" in psychiatry, while others subsequently referred to "dynamically oriented" and "pharmacologically oriented disciplines." Tensions between the two sometimes rivaled those of political opponents. When I and other analytically oriented psychiatrists worked in the Public Health Service at a research center in Washington overseen by a British-trained psychiatrist, he held us in great disdain and kept file cards of our interests and training, boldly underscoring "typical psychodynamicist."

Hysteria: A Place to Start

When one speaks of the foundations of psychiatry and its ancillary specialty of C-L practice, hysteria is a good place to start; it is where psychoanalysis itself began (Nemiah, 1967). What has taken over 2000 years to understand is today easily recognized when one is said to be behaving "hysterically." In one sense, the hysteric is someone who appears out of control of her or his emotions. A not-so-mysterious leap in the development of the field occurred when Freud made his monumental discoveries about the mind-body workings of the unconscious and how others could now intervene in therapeutic ways with processes of the mind previously unknown.

Unthinkable as it may be that anyone in the twenty-first century would doubt the connection between the mind and the body, in modern medical practice we see evidence that such dichotomous thinking persists: in the tendency to treat people in parts; in the practice of treating disease in "either-or" terms as "functional" or "organic"; and in the superspecialization of medicine inaugurated by the Flexner Report of 1910. While the existence of both physical and emotional expression was clearly recognized from ancient times, greater understanding of how they interacted can be properly said to have begun with Sigmund Freud, although he was not the first to be captivated by its mystery.

A Brief History of Hysteria

Hysteria's history is therefore relevant to the foundations of C-L psychiatry. Hysteria had been described in earliest medical texts and laypersons' health publications. As noted by Nemiah (1967), "[H]ysterical symptoms had been known for centuries, although the explanation of them had varied through the ages in a series of shifting theoretical concepts that mirrors the intellectual history of mankind" (p. 871). Earliest references to hysteria have been recorded in Egyptian papyrus around 1900 BC but came into greater prominence from the time of Hippocrates, whose observations evolved into the "wandering uterus" theory. Galen and others also grappled with attempts to understand the multitudinous complaints of "hysterics" and "hypochondriacs." Its colorful, imaginative, and outlandish explanations can be reviewed in many good texts (see, for example, Bollas, 2000; Gilman, King, Porter, Rousseau & Schowalter, 1993; Micklem, 1996; Veith, 1965).

By the mid-seventeenth century, Thomas Willis (1681 [2008]) (Veith, 1965, p. 129), regarded by some as the father of neurology, had designated both hysteria and hypochondriasis as disorders of the brain, while Thomas Sydenham (1682

[2008]) (Veith, 1965, p. 140), continuing to speak of "animal spirits," around the same time may have been the first to suggest that both physical and psychological factors contributed to the disorder. By the beginning of the eighteenth century, a thoughtfully reasoned *Treatise of the Hypochondriack and Hysterick Passions* was published by Bernard de Mandeville (1711[1976]). The uneasiness with naming of these "passions" is revealed in de Mandeville's description of how hypotheses evolve:

> The real knowledge we have of Nature beyond the Ancients . . . would, I believe, upon strict Examination not amount to much; but as to the Explication of her Operations, that often changes with the times, and looking back you may all along observe a fashion in Philosophizing. . . . No Hypothesis ever became famous before it had pleased a great part of the learned World, and ever since *Paradise* Mankind has had the same strength of Thought: the rest depends all upon Experience; wherefore as long as that encreases, and our fickleness continues, it is impossible that ever a System or Opinion should be generally received, or last forever.
>
> *(p. 113; all spellings and punctuation are preserved from the original—au.)*

Clearly, the term "hysteria" had "pleased a great part of the learned World." Regarding the durability of labels, de Mandeville's comment is applicable:

> An Hypothesis when once it is established a little time becomes like a Sovereign, and receives the same homage and respect from its Vassals, as if it was Truth itself.
>
> *(p. 114)*

George Cheyne (1671–1743), the Scottish physician-philosopher-mathematician practicing in Bath, dubbed the mystifying conditions as the English Malady in a book titled *The English Malady; or, A Treatise of Nervous Diseases of All Kinds, as Spleen, Vapours, Lowness of Spirits, Hypochondriacal and Hysterical Distempers* (Cheyne, 1733).

Gradually, as de Mandeville described, the concept of hysteria, based on experience and observation, has swung, pendulum-like, from near obscurity on some occasions to resurrection of high clinical interest at others. Indeed, as underscored by Edward Shorter (1997) in *A History of Psychiatry*, "diagnostic" labels for commonly observed (but unclear) ailments may be determined as much by social attitudes as by any other empirical or observational data. Thus, from clinicians' reports we have seen aspects of hysteria acquire terms accepted by the "learned world" such as "spinal irritation," "inflammation," "English malady," "neurasthenia," "soldier's heart," "shell shock," and others. The history of medicine is populated with what Shorter (1997) calls "weasel words," applied when organic explanations for disease cannot be discovered (p. 129).

By the nineteenth century, Jean-Martin Charcot was actively engaged in the new science of neurology. Turning from studies of diseases like multiple sclerosis, Charcot's interest in hysteria became a subject of study for the rest of his career. Following a visit to Charcot's clinic in 1886, Freud (1893[1959]) became fascinated by the ailment and on return to Vienna began his "treatment" of hysterics with hypnosis as practiced at the Salpetriere.

Thus, from earliest descriptions of "womb migration" and "seminal retention" as explanations for hysteria in Hippocrates's and Galen's days, every century since has captured the imaginations and speculations of philosophers, theologians, psychologists, and others. Its durability in medical language is nothing short of amazing, surviving even those periods of temporary opacity as, for example, when the Church focused on exorcism or when "serious researchers" identified neurological or physical "explanations."

The "excitability" of hysteria was thought to be confirmed by the finding that irritability of muscle fibers could be evoked with light stimulation, suggesting that all organic tissue was capable of either too much or too little excitability, likely leading to disease. This hypothesis had appealed to neurologists of the eighteenth century who extended the theory of abnormal excitability to the entire nervous system via reflex arcs, an attribute retained in the stereotypic characterization of "hysterical" people (especially women) as flamboyant, animated, demonstrative, easily aroused. Finding areas of easy irritation on suspected hysterics led to a clinical search for "tender points" (much like the diagnosis of fibromyalgia today) and for hysteriogenic zones as described by Charcot.

Persisting into the nineteenth century, this "irritability" theory persuaded physicians to prescribe such disparate "treatments" for "sensitivity to the genitalia" as soothing baths and surgical removal of the ovaries, uterus, or clitoris (a procedure sadly practiced in some regions of the world even today).

Briquet's Disease

The first to attempt quantification of the symptoms of this prevalent but elusive disease was the French physician Pierre Briquet (1859) at the Charite Hospital in Paris in the mid-1800s. His studies "established" a hereditary factor in hysteria, although critics considered the etiology to be nurture as much as nature. This attribution to "constitutional factors" unfortunately gave rise to such terms as "constitutional inferior," "poor protoplasm," "genetic weakness," or "constitutional weakness." Even Janet (1907), credited with advancing ideas about hysteria, referred to "cerebral impotence" before advancing to concepts of psychasthenia and dissociative reactions. There followed labels of "chronic nervous exhaustion" (not unlike chronic fatigue syndrome of today) and neurasthenia. All such terms perpetuated the stigma, bias, and negative attitudes of physicians and the public toward patients who were called "hysterics," "hypochondriacs," and "psychosomatic." Perhaps later designation as "somatoform" and "medically unexplained symptoms" softened the prejudice somewhat, although patients with mystifying ailments continue to draw the ire of most physicians.

Even Briquet expressed unease with the profusion of names assigned to hysteriform syndromes: "The names under which the disorder has been known are numerous; they can be divided into two kinds: the first kind, which refer to the womb, the presumed cause of the disease, such as *strangulatus*, suffocation, *praefocatio uteri*, womb's ill, mother's ill, metronervia, *etioangiovaric neuropallia*, are, to my thinking, the result of an error. The others, employed by the authors who place the disease either in the economy as a whole, or in the nervous system, such as vapors, bad nerves, Georget's spasmodic encephalitis, Brachet's neurospasmia, M. Girard's acute cerebropneumogastric neuropathy, are too general and do not characterize hysteria" (Cousin, Garrabe & Morozov, 2008, pp. 136–137). Out of this miasma of terminology, Briquet (1859) pronounced: "I will therefore adopt the term *hysteria*, because it was the first to be employed, because it is the one most generally used, because it is known to all, and finally because I hope that with time it will have lost its etymological value and will become simply a proper noun, like *gold, iron, lead*" (*sic*; p. 137; italics original). Today, with the same frustration, practitioners continue the search for the most proper descriptor of multisymptom somatizers (Guze, 1967).

The British psychiatrist Slater (1961), cautioning against misapplication of the term "hysteria," showed, in a longitudinal study, that many patients so-named turned out to have identifiable organic neurological or diagnosable psychiatric disease, and Slater warned physicians not to jump too quickly to dismiss patients as having hysteria. With intentions to put hysteria back on a "scientific" basis, Guze and Perley (1963) at Washington University in Saint Louis urged a return to the designation Briquet's syndrome, counting symptoms. This effort was not only cumbersome but also only sporadically appreciated and subsequently over-shadowed by more psychodynamic factors, an offshoot of the ascendancy of psychoanalysis during the early twentieth century.

By the end of the nineteenth century, increasingly fanciful etiologic theories were still being proposed. Freud's very close friend Fliess had subscribed to a "theory" floated by a German physician that hysteria could be related to inflammation of the nasal mucosa. Surprisingly, he was able to persuade Freud of such a hypothesis, with recommendation of cocaine or cauterization as treatment. Freud actually experimented with such treatment on himself and his patients (Jones, 1953, pp. 78–97), with decidedly poor consequences.

An American Disease

With the approach of the twentieth century, "hysteria" was a thoroughly embraced American disease, referred to as "nervous exhaustion" or as "neurasthenia," a term previously devised by an American neurologist, George Beard (1869). Not to be outdone by the British, he also termed it "American nervousness." According to Beard, "[I]f a patient complains of general malaise, debility of all the functions, poor appetite, abiding weakness in the back and spine, fugitive neurologic pains, hysteria, insomnia, hypochondriasis, disinclination for consecutive mental labor, severe and weakening attacks of sick headache, and other analogous symptoms, and at the same time gives no evidence of anemia or of any organic disease, we have reason to suspect . . . that we are dealing with a typical case of neurasthenia" (p. 218).

This catchall diagnosis seemed to fulfill a great need to account for multitudinous unexplained symptoms, with Beard stating that this syndrome was "the most frequent, most interesting, and most neglected nervous disease of modern times" (Bunker, 1944, pp. 213–214).

Thoroughly embraced as a virtual emblem of social class, it was accepted as *physical* evidence of *stress* or *overwork*, not one of *psychological weakness*. Its popularity was far-flung and exists in continual use today in preference to psychiatric terminology by countries such as China. Early in his career, Freud took issue with Beard's overinclusiveness of symptoms, narrowing the definition of the neuroses to "the injurious influence of culture [that] reduces itself in all essentials to the undue suppression of the sexual life in civilized peoples (or classes) as a result of the 'civilized' sexual morality which prevails among them" (Bunker, 1944, p. 215), a concept appropriated from the little-known and rarely referenced A. J. Ingersoll, later identified by Freud's biographer A. A. Brill as "the first American physician to my knowledge who stressed the sexual factors in the neuroses" (Bunker, 1944, p. 215).

Freud Begins to Set the Record Straight

Freud's delving into sexuality and the unconscious startled his universe. His impact might never have occurred had it not been for certain serendipitous events throughout his career. While he was clearly a man of considerable ambition and intellectual acuity from an early age, a lesser individual might not have survived the calumny and opposition he encountered in his own country. In his words, the turning point in his life, his career, and his fame came with the invitation from G. Stanley Hall, then dean of Clark University in Worcester, Massachusetts, to participate as a lecturer in the twentieth-year celebration of the university. Following a few negotiations, he eagerly accepted what was to become the realization of an "incredible daydream" (Rosenzweig, 1994, p. 34).

In his later autobiographical account, Freud wrote, "In Europe I felt I was despised: but over there [America] I found myself received by the foremost of men as an equal" (Rosenzweig, 1994, p. 13). This recognition by the foremost scholars of psychology, philosophy, biology, and other sciences from America as well as invitees from other countries to Hall's "party" launched this 53-year-old physician and his psychoanalysis on its epochal trajectory.

While some attendees of the Clark meeting had opposing ideas of personality development from those of Freud, there were nonetheless others who became ardent advocates and friends. James Jackson Putnam was one such celebrant, and attendance at Freud's lecture by medical student Alan Gregg would be pivotal for the establishment of C-L psychiatry (see chapter on benefactors). Also attending was Adolf Meyer, who saw much in Freud's theories that he modified in his own psychobiological approach to patients.

The serendipitous route through which Freud came to the study of hysteria is not so linear as is usually recounted. Ambition not to be discounted, the young Freud, a medical student in his 20s, was not hell-bent on trying to grasp how mental processes were converted to physical embellishments; he had begun his career dissecting eels. He was much more attuned to finding ways to earn a living, expecting to enter practice "of some specialty," to be decided.

As was the cultural orientation of his time, Freud desired assurance of a proper "living" before he would marry his fiancée, Martha Bernays. Freud had come from a very impecunious background, and the need to earn money with a prospect of having to support a family became a very compelling incentive for his change of direction. Nonetheless, it was fortunate for science and the world that his wide-ranging curiosity from the nerve cells of eels to a profound interest in philosophy conflated to result in the "discovery" of psychoanalysis.

This "distraction" drew him away from his preferred laboratory research in cellular physiology, with abandonment of thoughts of one day assuming the chairmanship of physiology in the university. On completion of his medical studies in 1882, and with his mentor Brucke's urging, he began routing around for ways to assure a livelihood. To acquire the necessary skills and knowledge of a medical practitioner required a return to training in the general hospital, thoughts of which repelled him. He took turns at dermatology, ophthalmology, even psychiatry, almost mirroring the modern "rotating internship." In a later self-deprecating description of his ambivalence for medicine, he wrote, "During my first three years at the University I was compelled to make the discovery that the peculiarities and limitations of my gifts denied me all success in many of the departments of science into which my youthful eagerness had plunged me" (Jones, 1953, p. 38).

Of his own idiosyncrasy, he quoted Mephistopheles' warning: "It is vain that you range round from science to science; each man learns only what he can" (Jones, 1953, p. 39). He expressed deep regret at having to leave the laboratory for the "real world." I recall a quote in which he stated, "Men cannot remain children forever; they must in the end go out into 'hostile life'" (Freud, 1927, p. 49).

As mentioned, part of Freud's preparation for practice was a trip to Paris to learn from the great Charcot at Salpetriere how to treat neurotics. There, Freud had his first contact with hysterical patients. Observation of patients in Charcot's clinic and later collaboration with Josef Breuer (14 years Freud's senior) on a most influential book on hysteria catalyzed a universe of new mental research and treatment. Charcot adhered to organic, neurological, or heritable explanations and was allegedly uninterested in Freud's psychological speculations about the condition.

In time, curiosity about the way neurology might explain how certain somatic ailments could be generated without revealing the physical route by which they occurred prompted Freud as a neurologist to grapple with the dilemma. This step initiated explorations into an understanding of the "mysterious leap" of the mind to the body (Deutsch, 1959). At first, Freud attempted to solve the riddle through neurological knowledge, a famously quoted effort that resulted in the subsequently aborted *Project for a Scientific Psychology* (1895) when he was unable to translate psychological events into physiological or neurological processes. This frustrating application of known physiology launched Freud's journey into unknown territories, ultimately to astound the psychological world.

In *Studies on Hysteria*, Breuer and Freud (1895) credit Charcot with "[giving] us a schematic description of the 'major' hysterical attack, according to which four phases can be distinguished in a complete attack: 1) the epileptoid phase; 2) the phase of large movements; 3) the phase of '*attitudes passionelles*' (the hallucinatory phase); and 4) the phase of terminal delirium" (p. 13).

All phases need not be present in each case, and Breuer and Freud expressed their primary interest in the third phase. With Freud's remarkable curiosity and imagination, attention to physical energy switched to psychical energy, interest in dream production, and consequences of libido expression. Vicissitudes of the "pain-pleasure principle" and foibles of the "unconscious" supplanted reference to "neural excitation."

Freud was finally on his way to discovering "the mysterious leap from the mind to the body," an expression he used in his *General Introduction to Psychoanalysis* (Freud, 1916–1917 [1920], p. 229). The frustration experienced in his struggles with the "Project" must have stayed with him throughout his career, for he frequently alluded to the difficulties of integrating the languages of the body (physiology) and the psyche (psychology). He was, after all, trained in the mostly precise science of neurology, neuropathology, and neuroanatomy. As a physician, he was aware that individuals were just "undivided" beings from birth, calling forth a monist approach to the living person. On the other hand, he was heir to the dualism in medicine propounded by Descartes and others in their efforts to understand how body and mind interacted, a dilemma faced by every physician before and since. There emerged separate languages, the physiological/biological and the psychological/emotional.

Ultimately, Freud did not really believe there was such a thing as a "leap" from mind to body (or the reverse), since all processes were mediated through a central nervous system, various organs of the body, endocrine hormones, and the circulatory system. No bodily functions occurred without psychological representation, and no psychological events occurred without bodily accompaniments, a later fact incorporated in the word "psychosomatic" (or its reverse "somatopsychic"), still believed by many to be an inadequate descriptor of what takes place in the human organism, although somewhat further enhanced by Claude Bernard's and Walter Cannon's concepts of *milieu interieur* and homeostasis.

Freud had predicted that, one day, science would possess the capacity to explain all "unexplainable" perturbations of the individual through a single (monist) language that can help close the persistent gap of dualism, facilitated in the future by study of psychoneuroendocrinology and neurotransmitters and their relation to psychiatric disease. However, descriptions of famous cases in the history of psychoanalysis reveal Freud's use of concepts extant in his practice of the time.

Anna O

Perhaps the most famous case of "hysterical neurosis" studied by Freud and shared with his older colleague Josef Breuer was Anna O, her true identity revealed in the 1950s to be Bertha Pappenheim by one of Freud's biographers. Bertha's "condition" began first with an unremitting cough, then paralysis of several extremities, and inability to use her hand for writing or her eyes for reading. She also manifested a degree of aphonia. She was described as an attractive, intelligent, winsome, and previously vivacious young woman, and perhaps her features are what gave rise to later descriptions of such patients as "hysteroid" in character or possessing "hysterical personality." Although Breuer was an internist rather than psychiatrist, he treated Bertha with hypnosis and what later was described by the patient as "the talking cure." Breuer had actually treated Bertha for several years, eventually withdrawing from the case when she developed a "phantom pregnancy" out of what were assumed to be complex transference/countertransference complications with Breuer.

Freud actually never saw Bertha, although she was friendly with Freud's fiancée, Martha Bernays. But he discussed her fully with Breuer and ultimately claimed that it was his familiarity with the case that gave rise to his appreciation of the role of the unconscious in the development of "unexplained" symptoms. Freud and Breuer first published an account of Anna O in a neurological journal, describing hysterical patients as "suffering from reminiscences" (Breuer & Freud, 1895 [1957], p. 221) related to "repressed memories," with symptoms arising when these memories "threaten" to emerge in awareness; these "substitutes" for the impulse were later described as "conversion reactions" or "somatic compliance" (Freud, 1905, pp. 40–42).

Katharina

Another case, that of Katharina (1895), seen only once by Freud and reported in the *Studies in Hysteria*, reads almost like a C-L consultation with its detailed inquiry of the patient's medical symptoms, elaboration of more psychological detail, and final formulation. Freud acknowledged that the case was concocted with little available data, resulting in his "jumping to conclusions" on the basis of what was believed about hysteria, repression, and denial. He recorded that "this case history [was] more as one of guessing than analysis" (Breuer & Freud, 1895 [1957], pp. 125–134). Nevertheless, it reflected the practice of C-L in those instances where time and relevance is not adequate to explore all aspects of a patient's life history; one may then address only the consultee's question and engage the patient in an interview only as deep and extensive as required as time permits to make intelligent guesses in response to the consultee's question. This case should be required reading of all C-L psychiatrists interested in bedside (medical) psychotherapy (Lipsitt, 2002).

Like so many practicing physicians who search for the best way to treat chronic ("neurotic") somatizers, Freud experienced similar frustration. However, as the only doctor in Vienna accepting these patients, he had no one to refer such patients to, so he set about searching for other means of treatment himself. Reflecting on early beginnings of psychoanalysis and recalling his experience as a novice practitioner, he reveals (1914[1959]):

> I had only unwillingly taken up the profession of medicine, but I had at that time a strong motive for helping neurotic persons or at least wishing to understand something about neurotic states. I had already devoted myself to therapy and had felt absolutely helpless after the disappointing results I had experienced with Erb's electrotherapy which was so full of detailed indications.
>
> *(Roazen, 1992, p. 66)*

Freud's search for effective treatment of "neurotics" mimicked the behavior of so many of today's primary care physicians with little psychological training for whom managing patients with chronic somatization has been a "seat-of-the-pants" affair (Lipsitt, Joseph, Meyer & Notman, 2015).

The shift to psychological and psychoanalytic investigation of so-called unexplainable symptoms can be attributed to Freud and his colleagues. Insights into the nature of hysteria would be a momentous enough contribution of psychoanalysis to C-L psychiatry, but there is much more.

Legacy of Psychoanalysis in Psychiatry

Although psychiatry now claims the province of hysteria as its area of interest and therapeutics, major contributors to our understanding of the phenomenon of conversion have all been neurologists: Charcot, Janet, and Freud. Searching for constitutional factors to explain hysteria, Charcot had strongly held to a belief in heredity as an etiologic source, as had Briquet. Extensive debate ensued. Janet clung to a suspicion of some kind of hereditary disposition while Breuer and Freud, unable to discover evidence in their patients, tended to dismiss this explanation. This hotly debated issue largely accounted for Freud's split with Charcot.

Janet spoke of "dissociative states," while Freud adhered to the concept of "conversion." Both were discovered in patients in the "hypnoid" state, so-named from revelations under hypnosis; hysteria had begun to move away from "organic" explanations to more mental or psychical etiologies, and the studies of both Janet and Freud of the "dissociative" or hypnoid states held much attraction.

The concepts of dissociation, conversion, hysteria, and hypochondriasis have, since the advent of classificatory efforts, skipped around like lost children searching for a welcoming home; they have transiently been allied with neuroses, psychophysiological disorders, conversion disorders, organic mental disorders, somatoform disorders, and personality disorders and are now collected under the rubric of somatic symptom disorder in DSM-5 (American Psychiatric Association, DSM-5, 2013). Terms used to characterize patients as having hypochondriasis or neurasthenia have virtually disappeared, although patients with elusive symptoms have become the captivating yet sometimes irksome province of psychiatry (such patients are seen almost entirely by medical practitioners who often seek the consultative guidance of psychiatrists).

Over time, the C-L psychiatrist accumulates a vast experience with so-called "somatizing" patients, since the process frequently masquerades as physical illness. In modern "ward" medicine, hysteria has gone from its irreverent meaningless designation as "supratentorial" to MUS (medically unexplained symptoms) or simply "somatization." Either way, once considered a serious disease, it is now more flippantly regarded as a "bother" to biomedically oriented house officers and attending physicians.

A Clinical Case

I once consulted on a patient admitted to the hospital with what looked like a left-sided hemiplegia for which no neurological explanation could be found. The patient was (atypically) a 54-year-old man who had recently visited his 80-year-old poststroke mother in a nursing home. He expressed great "upsetness," insisting on his inability to return to the home again. History revealed a long-standing serious hostile-dependent relationship with his mother. Treatment consisted not of traditional psychotherapy but of educating staff to control their annoyance with the man and informing him that he had "developed a mild form of what his mother had" but that it "would resolve in a few days." It was also explained to staff that he was setting up (acting out) the same hostile-dependent relationship with them that he had had with his mother. In this case, emphasis was more on "liaison" than on consultation. No attempt was made to disabuse him of the notion that he may have had a mild stroke or to persuade him of the psychological significance of his ailment. Physical therapy was advised, and, indeed, symptoms did abate in a matter of several days.

Today's clinicians say they do not see many patients with the "old-fashioned" hysterical symptoms, although an occasional "conversion" is reported. In our technologized world, perhaps people are better informed. Much can be learned about hysteria from internet resources, unlike the situation in the early twentieth century. For example, in *A Layman's Handbook of Medicine*, Dr. Richard Cabot (1916), an internist of Massachusetts General Hospital, informed his readers that hysteria was "the rarest of the five [psychoneuroses]." Cabot wrote, "It is a long time since I have seen a case of pure hysteria, the type in which one tends to have seizures, paroxysms, fits of one kind or another" (p. 226). Cabot alludes to Janet, "when he was here [in Boston]," as having told him it was "a strange kind of forgetfulness." Cabot summarizes, intending to disabuse his reader of the notion that it is "fakery," with the following: "[I]t is an enormous subject, this subject of hysteria, but . . . [it] is not 'pure cussedness' and not organic disease, but belongs in an extraordinary limbo between those two" (p. 226). Nevertheless, the residua of "hysteria" remains forever with us, if for no other reason than removal of the uterus is still referred to as a hysterectomy, not a uterectomy.

The C-L psychiatrist is accustomed to receiving requests from psychologically unsophisticated physicians to assess their "hysterical" patient, by which they typically mean that the patient has "some complaint" for which no medically identifiable (i.e., "organic") answer can be detected. The presentation of such patients is typically no different from clinical examples described centuries ago. In some cases, there is a dramatic loss of function or use of an extremity, loss of voice or even eyesight, or spasmodic partial or total body movements, sometimes convulsion-like. Less dramatic but equally "baffling" are such symptoms as repetitive cough, unremitting pain in a variety of body areas, and tic-like patterns of speech. Primitive explanations like "demonic possession" and "floating uterus" have been replaced by more recent classifications of "conversion reaction," or somatoform disorders, but clinical descriptions of patients are little changed from those of Freud's early cases.

Hysteria as a diagnosis has had remarkable if unclear durability in psychiatric nomenclature, having being designated a psychophysiologic reaction, a neurosis, a personality disorder, and somatization. The psychoanalytic accompaniments of hysteria are virtually disguised in current official classification, but their relevance to clinical activity endures. The authors of current classification did not entirely abandon their obeisance to the importance of hysteria in psychiatry, managing to retain "Histrionic Personality Disorder" in the diagnostic manual (American Psychiatric Association, DSM-5, 2013). Homage to the psychoanalytic concept of repression is only subtly suggested in symptoms that enable the individual to avoid "some noxious activity." The word "hysteria" (absent from the manual's index) is hardly ever mentioned, although the diagnosis of conversion disorder remains, with emphasis on "pseudoneurological" symptomatology. Nevertheless, the whole realm of somatizing disorders including hypochondriasis and "psychogenic" or chronic pain disorder owe their heritage to the ancient concept of hysteria and are, in a sense, the "bread and butter" of the C-L psychiatrist.

Psychoanalysts and Psychosomatic Medicine

In time, curiosity about the way neurology might explain how certain somatic ailments could be generated without revealing the physical route by which they occurred is what prompted Freud, as a neurologist, to grapple with the dilemma. This step initiated explorations into an understanding of the so-called "mysterious leap" of the mind to the body, subsequently pursued by psychoanalysts, early pioneers of psychosomatic medicine. Many of these individuals had brought with them their experience, knowledge, and skill when they migrated to the United States to escape persecution in Europe. Their psychoanalytic roots had been largely in Vienna and Germany, to lesser extent in Britain and Hungary. Prominent among these pioneers were Franz Alexander, Felix and Helene Deutsch, Max Schur, Edward and Grete Bibring, Michael Balint, and others. They infused American medicine with groundbreaking ideas, especially in the practice of psychiatry in the general hospital. Grete Bibring described her interest and motivation as follows:

> As a psychoanalyst, I felt that I could provide doctors with a general framework that would permit them to deal knowledgably with all sorts of problems presented by medical patients. While the emotional conflicts and stresses posed by physical illness are universal, psychoanalysis teaches us how each individual deals with them in unique ways that are rooted in the history of his development.
>
> *(Bibring and Kahana, 1968, pp. vii–viii)*

Psychoanalyst Michael Balint (1957), with hardly a mention of psychoanalysis, brought an awareness of the important psychological factor in illness to the practicing internists who participated in his "research" groups. And his book *The Doctor, His Patient and the Illness* continues as a standard text in family medicine residencies (Lipsitt, 1999). Psychoanalysts like Michael Balint, Max Schur, Felix Deutsch, and Sandor Ferenczi, having come from general medical practice, seized on the relevance of Freud's discoveries to that endeavor.

The first American to apply psychoanalytic principles to general hospital medicine was probably James Jackson Putnam (1895), a Harvard neurologist, so taken with Freud's ideas that he endeavored to "spread the word," first by negotiating Freud's first (and only) visit to the United States in 1909 and then helping to found the first American psychoanalytic institute for the training of other physicians (and allied clinicians).

Jackson's attempts to apply these "strange" ideas in consultation to the medical and surgical patients of Massachusetts General Hospital were met with thinly veiled suspicion, doubt, and resistance and the naming of his small office as the *cloaca maximus* by the hospital's chief of medicine (Hackett & Cassem, 1978, pp. 2–3). Nonetheless, Hackett wrote that Jackson was the first to provide an "organized interest in the mental life of patients" at the hospital (Hackett, 1978, p. 3).

American psychoanalysts like Flanders Dunbar, Morton Reiser, Milton Rosenbaum, Herbert Weiner, Roy Grinker, Smith Ely Jelliffe, Maurice Levine, Peter Knapp, Cecil Mushatt, George Engel, Stanley Cobb, M. Ralph Kaufman, David Hawkins, Sidney Margolin, Eugene Meyer, Myer Mendelson, and others, with their positions in general hospitals, all impressed upon their medical colleagues the value of a psychodynamic orientation toward the care of medical and surgical patients. The achievements of these psychoanalysts, as they brought their psychoanalytic/psychosomatic teaching and research to the general hospital, may be called the handmaidens of C-L psychiatry.

Interactions of psychoanalysts with colleagues in medical settings has exposed medical practice to an awareness of psychoanalytic concepts like transference and countertransference; implications of conflict as a source of illness; intrapsychic stress; repression, defense mechanisms, symptom and organ symbolism, and unconscious processes; understanding psychoanalysis as a developmental psychology that emphasizes the relevance of detailed history taking and the interviewing process (e.g., Deutsch's [1958] "associative anamnesis"); an understanding of the role of trauma in subsequent disease expression; and concepts of self- and body-image.

Psychoanalytic studies have elucidated the impact of mother-child bonding, family dynamics, attachment, separation, loss, bereavement, dependence, and independence on eventual character structure and symptom manifestation. The relevance of personality style to medical treatment and hospitalization has been brilliantly demonstrated by Ralph Kahana and Grete Bibring (1964). Acknowledgement of affect (emotion) and its coloration of symptoms by fear, sadness, anxiety, distortion, and fantasy inform the consultant's assessment of a patient's "presentation." The very elements of psychotherapy have derived from in-depth psychoanalytic treatment and clarified indications for and distinctions between brief, interpersonal, supportive, cognitive, suppressive, and expressive therapies and how to select on the basis of "ego-strength" and other personality factors (Bibring, E., 1954; Lipsitt, 2002). These concepts have all sharpened the physician's understanding of his or her relationship to patients and their treatment.

Both Freud and psychoanalysis gradually drifted away from medical roots, especially as the new "science" found ever widening application beyond medicine and as the requirement of the medical degree for analytic training was abandoned. Nonetheless, Kaufman states in his paper "Psychoanalysis in medicine," "the most intimate relationship [of psychoanalysis in medical settings] has been as a medical discipline originating with Freud's immense desire for therapeutic procedures which might prove efficacious in the treatment of the neuroses" (Kaufman, 1951, p. 11).

Freud (1953[1924]) himself, in an autobiographical note, stated, "The obsessional neurosis and hysteria are the two forms of neurotic disease upon the study of which psychoanalysis was first built up, and in the treatment of which also our therapy celebrates its triumphs" (p. 269).

Among those triumphs, both psychosomatic medicine and C-L psychiatry are indebted to psychoanalysis for the germinating seeds of their respective specialties. For the C-L psychiatrist, psychoanalysis has bequeathed a rich heritage.

References

American Psychiatric Association. (2013). *Diagnostic and Statistical Manual of Mental Disorders.* (5th edition.) DSM-5, Washington, DC: American Psychiatric Association, Author.

Balint, M. (1957). *The Doctor, His Patient and the Illness.* New York, NY: International Universities Press.

Beard, G. (1869). Neurasthenia and nervous exhaustion. *Boston Medical and Surgical Journal, 80,* 217–221.

Bibring, E. (1954). Psychoanalysis and the dynamic psychotherapies. *Journal of the American Psychoanalytic Association, 2,* 745–770.

Bibring, G.L., & Kahana, R.J. (Eds.). (1968). *Lectures in Medical Psychology: An Introduction to the Care of Patients.* New York, NY: International Universities Press.

Bollas, C. (2000). *Hysteria.* New York, NY: Routledge.

Breuer, J., & Freud, S. (1895 [1957]). *Studies in Hysteria.* New York, NY: Basic Books.

Briquet, P. (1859). *Historical and Therapeutic Treatise on Hysteria.* Paris, FR: J.B. Bailliere.

Bunker, H.A. (1944). American psychiatric literature during the past one hundred years. In J.K. Hall, G. Zilboorg, & H.A. Bunker (Eds., with Editorial Board). *American Psychiatry 1844–1944.* (pp. 195–271). New York, NY: Columbia University Press.

Cabot, R.C. (1916). *A Layman's Handbook of Medicine.* Boston, MA: Houghton Mifflin.

Cheyne, G. (1733). *The English Malady. Or, a Treatise of Nervous Disease of All Kinds.* London: Powell (Scholars' facsimile reprint edition, 1976).

Cousin, F.-R., Garrabe, J., & Morozov, D. (2008). *Anthology of French Language Psychiatry Texts.* Hoboken, NJ: John Wiley & Sons.

De Mandeville, B. (1711). *A Treatise of the Hypochondriack and Hysterick Passions.* London, UK: Dryden Leach.

Deutsch, F. (1958). The associative anamnesis and sector therapy as a psychoanalytically oriented approach to patients. *Psychotherapy and Psychosomatics, 6,* 289–306.

Deutsch, F. (Ed.). (1959). *On the Mysterious Leap from the Mind to the Body.* New York, NY: International Universities Press.

Freud, S. (1893[1959]). Charcot, J. In E. Jones (Ed.). *Collected Papers.* (Vol. 1, pp. 9–23). New York, NY: Basic Books.

Freud, S. (1905). Fragment of the analysis of a case of hysteria. *Standard Edition, the Collected Works of Sigmund Freud, 7,* 7–122.

Freud, S. (1914[1959]). On the history of the psychoanalytic movement. In E. Jones (Ed.). *Collected Papers.* (Vol. 1, pp. 287–359). New York, NY: Basic Books (1959).

Freud, S. (1916–1917[1920]). *General Introduction to Psychoanalysis.* New York, NY: Boni & Liveright (New York, NY: Permabooks Edition).

Freud, S. (1927). Future of an illusion. In J. Strachey (Ed.). *The Standard Edition. Complete Psychological Works of Sigmund Freud.* (Vol. 21, pp. 5–56). London, UK: Hogarth Press.

Freud, S. (1953[1924]). *A General Introduction to Psychoanalysis.* Garden City, NY: Permabooks.

Gilman, S.L., King, H., Porter, R., Rousseau, G.S., & Schowalter, E. (1993). *Hysteria Beyond Freud.* Berkeley, CA: University of California Press.

Guze, S.B. (1967). The diagnosis of hysteria. What are we trying to do? *American Journal of Psychiatry, 124,* 491–498.

Guze, S.B., & Perley, M.J. (1963). Observations on the natural history of hysteria. *American Journal of Psychiatry, 114,* 960–965.

Hackett, T.P. (1978). Beginnings: Liaison psychiatry in a general hospital. In T.P. Hackett & N.H. Cassem (Eds.). *Massachusetts General Hospital Handbook of General Hospital Psychiatry.* (pp. 1–14). St. Louis, MO: Mosby.

Hackett, T.P., & Cassem, N.H. (1978). *Massachusetts General Hospital Handbook of General Hospital Psychiatry.* St. Louis, MO: C.V. Mosby.

Hollingshead, A.B., & Redlich, F.C. (1958). *Social Class and Mental Illness: A Community Study.* Hoboken, NJ: John Wiley & Sons.

Janet, P. (1907). *The Major Symptoms of Hysteria.* New York, NY: Macmillan.

Jones, E. (1953). The cocaine episode. In E. Jones (Ed.). *The Life and Work of Sigmund Freud.* (Vol. 1, pp. 78–97). New York, NY: Basic Books.

Kahana, R.J., & Bibring, G.L. (1964). Personality types in medical management. In N.E. Zinberg, (Ed.). *Psychiatry and Medical Practice in a General Hospital.* (pp. 108–123). New York, NY: International Universities Press.

Kaufman, M.R. (1951). Psychoanalysis in medicine. *Bulletin of the American Psychoanalytic Association, 7,* 1–12.

Lipsitt, D.R. (1999). Michael Balint's group approach: The Boston Balint group. *Group, 23,* 187–201.

Lipsitt, D.R. (2002). Psychotherapy. In M.G. Wise & J.R. Rundell (Eds.). *Textbook of Consultation-Liaison Psychiatry.* (pp. 1027–1051). Washington, DC: American Psychiatric Publishing.

Lipsitt, D.R. (2006). Psychosomatic medicine: History of a "new" specialty. In M. Blumenfield & J.J. Strain (Eds.). *Psychosomatic Medicine.* Philadelphia, PA: Lippincott Williams & Wilkins.

Lipsitt, D.R., Joseph, R., Meyer, D., & Notman, M. (2015). Medically unexplained symptoms: Barriers to effective treatment when "nothing is the matter." *Harvard Review of Psychiatry, 23,* 438–448.

Luhrmann, T.M. (2000). *Of 2 Minds: The Growing Disorder in American Psychiatry.* New York, NY: Alfred A. Knopf.

Micklem, N. (1996). *The Nature of Hysteria.* New York, NY: Routledge.

Nemiah, J.C. (1967). Conversion reaction. In A.M. Freedman & H.I. Kaplan (Eds.). *Comprehensive Textbook of Psychiatry.* (pp. 870–885). Baltimore, MD: Williams & Wilkins.

Putnam, J.J. (1895). Remarks on the psychical treatment of neurasthenia. *Boston Medical and Surgical Journal, 132,* 505.

Roazen, P. (1992). Freud and His Followers. New York, NY: Da Capo Press.

Rosenzweig, S. (1994). *The Historic Expedition to America (1909): Freud, Jung, and Hall the King-maker.* St. Louis, MO: Rana House.

Shorter, E. (1997). *A History of Psychiatry.* New York, NY: John Wiley & Sons.

Slater, E. (1961). Hysteria 311. *Journal of Mental Science, 107,* 359–381.

Sydenham, T. (1682 [2008]). Dissertatio epistolaris. In *Complete Dictionary of Scientific Biography.* Retrieved from http://www.encyclopedia.com

Veith, I. (1965). *Hysteria: The History of a Disease.* Chicago, IL: University of Chicago Press.

Willis, T. (1681 [2008]). An essay on the pathology of the brain and nervous stock. In *Complete Dictionary of Scientific Biography.* Retrieved from http://www.encyclopedia.com

Major Sources:

Hall, J.K., Zilboorg, G., & Bunker, H.A. (Eds.). (1944). *American Psychiatry 1844–1944: One Hundred Years of American Psychiatry.* New York, NY: Columbia University Press.

Jones, E. (1953). *The Life and Work of Sigmund Freud.* New York, NY: Basic Books.

4
PSYCHOSOMATIC ROOTS

Above all, it [the word "psychosomatic"] appears to imply a special field of medicine; in the best of cases, merely another specialty. This is definitely erroneous and serves to destroy precisely the structure that is being evolved. There is not, there cannot be a "psychosomatic medicine" as opposed to another concept of medicine . . . all medicine, by definition, must be psychosomatic.

—Seguin, 1970, pp. 25–26

Carlos Alberto Seguin, a little-referenced psychiatrist from the University of San Marco in Lima, Peru, had been a student of Flanders Dunbar during the formative years of psychosomatic medicine. In an introductory text on the topic, Seguin (1970) chooses to refer to "the psychosomatic tendency in medicine" (p. 25) rather than "psychosomatic medicine," intending that the new discoveries and theories should apply to all of general medicine. In a wish to avoid the clinical dichotomy between one side (psyche) or the other (soma), he states that the approach that favors a tendency toward the psychological side "not only is not true theoretically but is dangerous in practice, as it emphasizes the abyss between clinicians and psychologists" (p. 27) and "serves to maintain the dichotomy we are opposing" (p. 26).

Many teachers and writers trace the beginnings of psychosomatic medicine to ancient evidence that physicians, philosophers, and others recognized relationships between body (soma) and mind (soul, psyche). But Seguin (1970), imbued with the excitement of new discoveries, prefers to dismiss such "origins" of the new approach as "pre-history." "The history of Psychosomatic Medicine," he emphatically states, "begins in our century" (p. 24).

A new orientation to medicine had grown out of a major shift in the healing arts. Physicians were gradually awaking to the pitfalls of treating individuals like "machines," fixing one body part at a time. Psychology, previously immersed in philosophy and measurement of mental faculties, was beginning to take an interest in child development and health matters. Innovation in medical technology had facilitated physiological research that had never been done before. And appreciation of the power of the unconscious, intensified by Freud and others at the turn of the twentieth century, had fostered interest in a "new biology." As the opening quote reveals, Seguin opined that psychosomatic medicine should not be considered, "in the best of cases, merely another specialty" (p. 25). The "psychosomatic tendency in medicine," as advocated by Seguin, "has as its aim the study of man as a whole, a totality, considered as such in health and in disease, and the application of the conclusions of such study to diagnosis, prognosis and treatment" (p. 28).

Whether we agree with Seguin's definition or not, we will not in this chapter trace mind-body recognition back to the Bible, the Vedas, the Arabs, or the church fathers. We will deal only briefly with some of the "pre-history" of psychosomatic medicine as it may have bearing on its relation to C-L psychiatry. Its compendious history is beyond the scope of this book and is available in many excellent texts.[1] Our interest here is in the ways C-L and psychosomatic medicine interdigitate (or not) as revealed in literature and practice.

Origins

While it is comforting to know the origin of things, most beginnings remain shrouded in mystery. A child's earliest curiosity is reflected in this question: Where do I come from? A source of some puzzlement is whether C-L psychiatry embellishes psychosomatic medicine or the reverse is true. Maybe C-L psychiatry really sprang first from psychoanalysis since it antedated organized psychosomatic medicine. Or, its origin may be from general medical practice, in an epidemiological sense, as physicians gradually became more psychologically aware.

That psychosomatic medicine and C-L psychiatry are related, there is no doubt. The way in which that relationship exists has generated controversy for decades and continues to be debated. There is fair certainty that physiology is the scientific basis of psychosomatic medicine, while psychosomatic medicine is arguably the preeminent building block of C-L psychiatry. The foundational import of psychosomatic medicine to C-L psychiatry is much fuzzier than that of philosophy, physiology, or even psychoanalysis. Greenhill, writing of the activities of the C-L psychiatrist, states that "psychosomatic medicine became reactivated in the 1970s through the growth of liaison psychiatry as a result of medical technological advances and societal pressure" (1980, p. 255).

In the most elemental terms, one could say that psychosomatic medicine grew out of interest in joining together the two major components of the human organism. Hesitancy to do that may even be reflected in the hyphen that kept the two apart in early references to *psycho-somatic* (Winnicott, 1966). Franz Alexander, an avowed sage of psychosomatic medicine, writes that "the psychological interest [in medicine] is nothing more than a revival of old pre-scientific views in a new and scientific form" (1950, p. 17). In this definition, Alexander seems to agree with Seguin.

Naming

Process usually precedes identity and only as trends become apparent are they named. Naming permits ease of communication, discussion of ideas, actions, and behaviors (Waxler, 1981). How individual writers use names gives us insight into how they think. For example, George Engel, a preeminent internist-psychosomatician of modern times, in recent writings avoids mention of "psychosomatic medicine" or, indeed, of "mind-body problems" (Engel, 1992); in expressing disappointment in medicine's failure to achieve a more integrated approach, Engel's preference is to assess the problems of medical practice in "scientific" terms. And at least one other eminent internist-psychosomatician expressed concern that C-L psychiatry might be perceived as "all there is" to psychosomatic medicine, so prominent its existence in clinical practice (Graham, 1979). Preoccupation with this dilemma of how something is to be named emerges full-blown with the overture to seek approval for specialization. Is it C-L psychiatry or psychosomatic medicine that predominates and is accreditation worthy? When the C-L psychiatrist—with empathy, understanding, and dialogue—holistically treats a patient in distress, is the psychiatrist practicing C-L psychiatry or psychosomatic medicine? One, both, or neither?

"Pre-History"

The history of psychosomatic medicine is, in some sense, the history of human-kind's fascination with relationships between mind (or soul, psyche) and body (soma). Long before such preoccupation became a compelling force in medicine, it had been the focus of philosophers, theologians, and even mathematicians, astrologers, mystics, and magicians. Efforts to explain distinctions between the material and nonmaterial worlds were essentially the font of all knowledge.

The rudiments of a "psychosomatic perception" can be said to have begun when humans first experienced simultaneous emotions or "passions" and bodily reaction. Beisser (1964) goes so far as to say that it began when Alcmaeon around 500 BC declared that the seat of highest function of sensation was in the brain, by discovering that the eye was attached to the brain. Applying this awareness to healing, Plato (428–349 BC), quoting Socrates (470–399 BC), said, "As it is not proper to cure the eyes without the head, nor the head without the body, so neither is it proper to cure the body without the soul" (Plante, 2010, p. 34). (Was headache the first psychosomatic ailment?)

Socrates had philosophized deeply over the relative dominance of body or soul as parts of the "self" (Wright & Potter, 2000). And Plato's student Aristotle, in

350 BC, observed how emotions like joy, fear, anger, and courage affected the body. We might reasonably accept that as soon as thinkers began contemplating soul (psyche) and body (soma), psychosomatic medicine was aborning, although hardly recognized as a "movement" in the United States until the late 1920s and early 1930s.

Seeds and Roots

The *seeds* of psychosomatic medicine were sown by the Greek philosophers, but the epistemological *roots* of development originated in Europe. A German physician-philosopher, Heinrich Cornelius Agrippa (1510), often denounced for his interest in magic and occultism, wrote in *Three Books of Occult Philosophy and Magic*: "[S]o great a power is there of the soul upon the body, that whichever way the soul imagines and dreams that it goes, thither doth it lead the body" (Bk. 1, pt. 4, Ch. lxiv, line 30). For the interested reader, this fascinating document contains many insights into mind-body interactions as well as cogent observations on doctor-patient relations and ways in which fantasy (conflict?) can affect disease in oneself or others.

In the 1600s, the Reformation brought with it greater separation from religion and more reliance on "rationality." According to Schwab (1985), Francis Bacon (1561–1626), alluding to newly introduced scientific experimentation, "advocated investigation of the mental faculties and of the interactions of body and mind by case studies and by study of the relationships between the individual and society" (p. 584). Schwab anoints this advocacy as "probably the first explicit scientific statement about psychosomatic medicine in English" (p. 584). Bacon proposed two kinds of "knowledges [*sic*], one of the body and one of the mind." He referred to "the sympathies and concordances between the mind and the body, which being mixed, cannot be properly assigned the sciences of either" (p. 584).

The Split

Even as there were prominent medical interests at work attempting to better understand how this "mixed" state of mind and body functioned, other forces worked diligently to establish their separability and individuality. In the early seventeenth century, Rene Descartes (1641), considered the originator of modern philosophy, proclaimed that mind and body were clearly separate aspects of human existence. This notion imposed a dualistic dimension on the practice of modern medicine, splitting it into "organic" and "functional" approaches. Less noted by subsequent writers was Descartes's (incorrect) belief that such dualistic entities transacted their relationship in the pineal gland, a process more specifically espoused by Leibniz and Spinoza as psychophysical parallelism. This notion was revisited in the late 1970s by those who supported the concept of *linguistic* parallelism (Graham, 1967;

Hogan, 1995), a way of looking at and speaking of the same object from different views as one might a coin with heads or tails.

Early in the eighteenth century, de Mandeville's (1711) treatise on the "passions" of hypochondriasis and hysteria continued to conceptualize the interconnectedness of mind and body. He questioned "whether the soul be seated in some particular part of, or is diffused through all the brain, the blood or the whole body. . . . It is a very just inference to say that we consist of a body and a soul, [but] what every moment we may feel within our selves [*sic*], we can assert only that there must be an immediate commerce between the body and the soul." How body and soul reciprocally affect one another, de Mandeville asserted, was "not easy to be determined," but he hypothesized that some particulate matter (*internuncii*) established commerce between them (de Mandeville, 1711, p. 125). The mystery of how this occurred de Mandeville left largely to future thinkerscientists. Nevertheless, he presciently anticipated contemporary neurohumoral and psychoneuroendocrine aspects of what now is known of the process of transduction, a process some decry as an essentially meaningless term to identify that which remains unknown.

Together Again?

De Mandeville was not the only one trying to put dualistic humpty-dumpty together again. By 1733, Alexander Pope poetically knew that "the proper study of mankind is [holistically—au.] man." And the poet Coleridge, around 1800, introspectively attempting to understand his own ailments through "philosophic medicine," endeavored to integrate knowledge from philosophy, physiology, psychology, and medicine (Vickers, 2004). He is reputed to have been first to use the word "psychosomatic" and may in fact have invented the word to more succinctly communicate his preoccupation with the mind's effect on the body (Bates, 1968; Nemiah, 2000). Some of his poetry is said to have drawn heavily on Joseph Priestley's *Disquisitions on Matter and Spirit* (1777) (Levere, 1981).

George Baker, a physician who attended King George III, is said by Schwab (1985) to have delivered the first lecture on psychosomatic medicine *On the Affections of the Mind and the Disease Arriving From Them* at Cambridge University in 1755, reiterating a modification of the aphorism of Plato and Socrates that "it was 'impossible for the mind to suffer without the body becoming sick also or the body to be ill without the mind being associated with it in the distemper' " (p. 584).

Some three hundred years after Descartes' early dualism, its imprint on medicine was intensified when Abraham Flexner (1910) essentially recommended that medical specialties should be more "scientifically" differentiated. Separated from its parent medicine, the "battered child" of psychiatry (Greenblatt, 1975) has forever since sought a "remedicalized" reunion with its parent, partly achieved when psychiatry moved out of asylums and into the general hospital (Lipsitt, 1981). This move enhanced opportunities for psychiatrists to provide consultation services hospital-wide but did not rely on the presence of psychiatric inpatient beds. The remedicalization of psychiatry was promoted not only by C-L psychiatry but also by the surge of psychopharmacological research and application (Lipsitt, 1981).

First Naming: Psyche Desperately Seeking Soma

Not surprising is that this age-old intuitive recognition of mind's effect upon the body and its reverse would be reflected in language throughout the centuries. But words alone are not science, nor are they theory. This evolutional aspect of "psychosomatics" did not emerge until the 1930s, when the coexistence of technology and scientific curiosity sparked enthusiastic pursuit of the *ways* in which mind and body influenced each other.

The search for connectiveness between mind, body, and brain prevailed long before psychiatry was named in 1808 by Johann Reil (1808) or had a national board (1934). Consultation-liaison psychiatry (Billings, 1939), as such, was hardly a mote in anyone's conceptual eye, but the essentials surely were there for hypothesizing a unity of action between mind and body (psyche and soma). Their companionship had been acknowledged and studied for centuries but not referred to clinically as "psychosomatic" until Johann Christian Heinroth (1818) named the relationship. Exploring melancholy and insomnia, Heinroth wrote cryptically that "as a general rule, the origin of insomnia is 'psychosomatic' [*sic*], but it is possible that every phase of life can itself provide the complete reason for insomnia"(Margetts, 1950, p. 403). He described normal and abnormal sleep processes as psychosomatic, much as had Coleridge in his nonmedical musings. But Heinroth's is considered the first *clinical* use of the term in medicine (Lipowski, 1984, p. 155).

Heinroth (1773–1843) was a prominent figure in German psychiatry, the "first university lecturer in Europe to be appointed specifically for a psychiatric subject" at Leipzig University. (www.uni-leipzig.de). He was not only a professor of psychiatry at the famed university but also appointed professor of medicine in 1819. Strongly influenced by his devotion to Christianity, he regarded mental disorders as disorders of the soul (*Seelenstorungen*), induced by the guilt engendered by sin. Nonetheless, he devised a topology of mental structure considered by some to have been the forerunner of Freud's tripartite model of id, ego, and superego. And while Freud himself never used the word "psychosomatic" in his writings, his studies greatly expanded an appreciation of the influence of such intrapsychic variables as the unconscious, suppression, and conversion that affected the expression of mental and bodily symptomatology in hysteria, conversion, or "organ neurosis," concepts that clarified how physical symptoms could be a manifestation of emotional conflict. Psychoanalysis also brought increased understanding to physician-patient relationships through descriptions of transference, countertransference, as well as defenses like denial and somatization.

Heinroth regarded his treatment method as "directly psychic," taking into account aspects of personality that extended beyond mere somatic considerations; the relevance of personality in psychotherapeutic endeavors would later be emphasized by Alexander (1950, p. 71), Dunbar (1943), and Kahana and Bibring (1967). Heinroth's textbook on disorders of the soul states, "The person is more than just the mere body, but also more than just the mere soul; it is the whole man," (Steinberg, Herrmann-Lingen & Himmerich, 2013, p. 11), a sentiment not unlike that of Plato and others many centuries earlier. His treatments included a broad spectrum of social, dietetic, and psychological interventions. Some authors regard him as not merely the inventor of the term "psychosomatic" (although it was used only once) but the virtual founder of psychosomatic medicine itself (Steinberg et al., 2013). Once named, interest grew, and such deliberations of mind-body interrelationships were destined to become an organized system of psychosomatic knowledge.

Besides Heinroth, Leipzig University famously contributed other notable figures to the history of psychiatry as well as to psychosomatic medicine: Kraepelin took his early training there during Heinroth's tenure; Gustav Fechner, the psychologist, lectured widely on the relationship of mind and body; Wilhelm Wundt established the first psychophysiology laboratory in 1884 alongside Paul Flechsig, another psychophysiological researcher and head of the hospital, both of whom attracted such famous students as Ivan Pavlov, from Russia, and James Cattell and G. Stanley Hall, both psychologists from the United States. Cattell was the originator of mental tests for measuring individual differences and the putative first professor of psychology in America, and Hall was known to have brought psychoanalysis to America by hosting Sigmund Freud in 1909 at Clark University in Worcester, Massachusetts. Flechsig is probably best known as the "hated" physician of Paul Daniel Schreber, treated twice in the Leipzig Hospital (1884–1885 and 1893–1894) before becoming a famous case of Freud (1911); Schreber's psychoanalysis contributed greatly to Freud's theories on hysteria and conversion. Leipzig joins Burgholzi and Salpetriere as hospitals prominent in the history of psychiatry.

Expanding Interest in Psychological Medicine

Even prior to Heinroth's influence, physicians were generally diagnosing and treating mental aspects of general practice in routine Hippocratic and Galenic fashion. This began to change in the early to mid-nineteenth century during a particularly robust era of interest in the psychological aspects of medicine. A Scottish naval physician named Thomas Trotter (1808) entered private practice after leaving the navy and published a book—no doubt based on general practice experience and a "psychosomatic" sensibility—*The Nervous Temperament: Being a Practical Treatise on Nervous, Bilious, Stomach and Liver Complaints*, in 1808, popular enough to have a second edition in 1809. This was the same year that Reil, anachronistically an ophthalmologist, had allegedly attached the name "psychiatry" to efforts to comprehend mind-body medicine. He wrote of the "inseparability of mind and body," seeing them as "tied together in consciousness of the self" (Schwab, 1985, p. 585). He also founded two of the first psychiatry journals and proposed "rational psychotherapy" in his *Rhapsodies on the Application of Psychological Methods of Treatment to Mental Disorders* (Schwab, 1985, p. 585).

In 1845, ten years after receiving his medical degree, Baron Ernst von Feuchtersleben, interested in education reform, produced the book *Principles of Medical Psychology*. Both Trotter and Feuchtersleben (Feuchtersleben, (1845 [1995]) were also esteemed poets, joining the list of later poets who saw the artistic and scientific compatibility of both fields of interest, joining such poet luminaries as William Carlos Williams, Getrude Stein, John Keats , Sir Ronald Ross (Lipsitt, 1956), and others (Levere, 1981).

From early speculations emerged a rich historical journey through inquiries of the interactivity of mind and body: Breuer and Freud's explanation of hysterical conversion, 1895; Morton Prince on psychotherapeutics, 1910; Joseph Dejerine's treatment of psychoneuroses, 1913; Adolf Meyer's psychobiological medicine, 1915; Pierre Janet's studies of the dissociative process, 1922. It is believed that Felix Deutsch, an internist and former student of Freud who emigrated to America in the early 1930s, was the first to coin the composite term "psychosomatic medicine," in the early 1920s, while still in Austria. He predicted that one day this appellation would stand for all of medicine. The multiplicity of namers has left somewhat ambiguous the true identity of the real "father of psychosomatic medicine."

Does the Word Mean What It Says?

Whether in asylums or general hospitals, doctors treated patients with psychological reactions to medical or surgical illness without thinking or knowing they were practicing psychosomatic medicine or even psychiatry. In fact, when Flanders Dunbar began her efforts to establish both a journal (1939) and an organization (1943) devoted to the study and care of patients with combined illness, she was a practicing physician caring for patients admitted to New York's Presbyterian Hospital. Conceivably, she was a C-L psychiatrist even before she was a "psychosomatician." An interesting anecdote is that Flanders Dunbar, the pioneer of psychosomatic work, was dubbed the "mother of holistic [not "psychosomatic"— au.] medicine," further suggesting the substitutability of designations of the field.

When the time came to append a name to what Dunbar and others did, great uncertainty prevailed. This lack of clarity perhaps foretold the future of the field as one with more frequent changes in name than any other field of medicine. In fact, when Dunbar negotiated with the Macy Foundation to establish the journal, she was not strongly wedded to the word "psychosomatics" at all. Other titles offered for consideration included: *Physiology of Emotions*; *Emotions and Bodily Changes*; *The Physiology of Emotional Expression*; *Investigative Psychophysiology*; *A Journal of*

Psychiatry and Medicine; and *Behavior Derangement Review: a Journal for Experimental, Statistical and Critical Clinical Studies* (Levenson, 1994, p. 36). The word "psycho-somatics" was saliently absent.

Franz Alexander, a strong board member of the new journal and a research pioneer, said "psychosomatic medicine is not equivalent with what is understood by the term psychiatry . . . [and] is not restricted to any field of pathology" (Levenson, 1994, p. 39), a sentiment expressed by others who wanted to retain the broader relevance of psychosomatics to all of medicine (for example, Deutsch, Dunbar, Seguin). Some believed that the word perpetuated a dualistic connotation that the founders argued against. When the society itself was initially formed, it was called The American Society for Research in Psychosomatic Problems (Levenson, 1994, p. 65), soon changed to American Psychosomatic Society. The word "psychosomatic" came to be a more-or-less shorthand way of communicating about the complex matters of mind, brain, body, physiology, psychology, psychiatry, psychoanalysis, and other related ideas and has been uncomfortably tolerated ever since.

The origin of the word "psychosomatic" should not be confused with the origins of a field of inquiry called "psychosomatic medicine." From Plato's earliest incantations that "treatment of the body cannot occur without treatment of the head," to the English psychiatrist Daniel Hack Tuke's (1873) treatise awkwardly titled *Illustrations of the Influence of the Mind Upon the Body in Health and Disease Designed to Elucidate the Action of the Imagination*, an influence of mental processes on bodily function that already had been well appreciated.

A Cornucopia of Names

In his 1979 presidential address to the American Psychosomatic Society, internist David Graham attributed the field's poor record of influence on general medicine to the confusion and profusion of words that hampered an adequate definition of the field: "functional or organic"; "somatopsychic or psychosomatic" ; "emotional, psychological, or psychiatric"; "biobehavioral or biopsychosocial"; "stress response or psychosocial." Indeed, one author (Field, 1982) writes, "This periodic fashioning of new terms and alteration in the meaning of old ones often appears confusing, even frivolous to the outside observer" (p. 1).

Allusions to "psychosomatic" phenomena have not always been confined to medical literature. Indeed, the word "psychosomatic" itself has been variously attributed to poets, novelists, and philosophers. As noted, the poet Coleridge attributed some of his best work to mentalistic phenomena—some no doubt prompted by the use of laudanum—and is said by some (Nemiah, 1961) to have first coined the term "psychosomatic" in 1796.

Others (Lipowski, 1984) have unearthed nineteenth-century use in the novel *Hard Cash* by the English writer Charles Reade, who wrote of "a psycho-physical physician, who knows the psycho-somatic relation of body and mind." More contemporaneously, the height of psychosomatic popularity is revealed in Adelaide's song in the musical *Guys and Dolls*, when she sings, "A girl could develop a cold" as a "psychosomatic" ailment. Undoubtedly, a Sherlock Holmesian historian might detect many similar quotations in nineteenth-century writings, when the culture was absorbing the new idea of psychosomatic medicine. And, on occasion, when consultees are uncertain about a reason for requesting a consultation, they will curtly ask for a "psychosomatic evaluation."

Psychosomatic Medicine Grows in America

The seeds were planted in Greece, the roots took hold in Europe, but the tree of psychosomatic medicine was cultivated in the United States, most robustly by Dunbar and her new colleagues during and following World War II Lipsitt, D.R. (2006). Around that time, psychoanalyst physicians who had studied with Freud emigrated to America, where they promptly engaged in research and clinical work in general hospitals; their clinical activities catalyzed a growing interest in the "dynamic" nature of their studies.

Previously, American psychiatry, with its European influence a la Kraepelin, had been largely descriptive, although physicians like Flanders Dunbar and Adolf Meyer fostered growing interest in more psychobiological dynamic mind-body relationships in illness. Dunbar's first edition of the impressively rich *Emotions and Bodily Changes: 1910–1933* had appeared in 1935, anticipating the journal in 1939 and the society in 1942, with Dunbar the driving force of both. The Weiss and English textbook on *Psychosomatic Medicine* soon followed in 1943, considered by some to be the first American textbook on the subject. As indicated, Dunbar was a practicing physician at New York's Presbyterian Hospital, where, most likely, she was already addressing the complex comorbid ailments of the hospital's patients, the kind so amply illustrated in her 1935 volume.

Franz Alexander, having emigrated from Germany via Boston to Chicago, had already established his Institute for Psychoanalysis in 1932 with Rockefeller Foundation support, providing a platform for early psychosomatic research. He and his psychoanalytic and psychiatric associates were instrumental in the publication of much of the earliest psychosomatic research in the United States. With meticulous research methodology, he would formulate the specificity theory of psychosomatic disorder that held sway for a couple of decades before being judged inadequate to explain mind-body relationships in disease. But Alexander's work opened the field to a burgeoning interest of physicians, psychologists, social workers, and others. By this time, "psychosomatic medicine" rose to a threshold of organizational excitement and activity.

Psychosomatic medicine was already being taught and practiced in Europe, but allegedly without the critical and organizational focus of the American movement. Georg Groddeck (1949) in Germany, for example, sometimes referred to as the "wild analyst," is said to have influenced Freud in some of his own interpretative views of symptoms and dreams. Heidelberg's professor of medicine, Vicktor von Weizsacker, applying Freud's psychoanalytic views, espoused ways in which emotions affected bodily disturbances and could be applied to community health care (Rossler, Riecher & Meise, 1994). Of course, Franz Alexander, as an émigré to the United States in the early 1930s, had brought with him much that was already known about psychosomatic medicine in Germany.

With these events, psychosomatic medicine in the United States was launched and embraced by a public that was prepared for more humanism in the world following the atrocities of a world war. Some authors have even referred to interest in this psychosomatic aspect of medicine as a reformist humanist movement against gradually increasing mechanization of medical practice.

Consultation-liaison psychiatry itself has often been characterized as a clinical endeavor to retain medicine's holistic and humanistic roots. Physicians returning from war had seen the achievements of a "dynamic" approach to battle-induced illness and were prepared to endorse a new method of treatment. Many writers over the years have hailed psychiatry and psychoanalysis as "carrying the torch for humanism" (au.) in an increasingly impersonalized medicine (Engel, 1977).

Holism and Humanism

Dubbed as it was a "reformist" movement, psychosomatic medicine was seen to hold promise for the preservation of humanism in medicine and restoration of a "holistic approach to the patient." Such treatment would absorb information from all facets of the patient's life (Schwab, 1985, pp. 225, 243) in formulating a portrait of the patient's illness, much as proposed by Adolf Meyer in his "psychobiology." Reminders of the importance of retaining the humanism in medicine confront all physicians in their training and professionalization, but this training is said by some to be readily dissipated over time. At risk of being overshadowed by technological advances and even new nomenclatures that attempt to standardize diagnosis and treatment, human interaction can readily be reduced to "case reports" and dry, homogenized caricatures of real people.

As long ago as 1927, Francis Peabody, idolized for his classic paper on the "care of the patient," cautioned students and physicians of the risks of being engulfed by the "progress of science" to the detriment of the patient. At times it would appear that science and humanism are immiscible.

Psychosomatic medicine and C-L psychiatry have traveled *pari passu* in a kind of symbiosis through the decades in more-or-less uncomfortable relationship to one another. But, since the first identifiable C-L paper of George Henry preceded in 1929 the foundation of American psychosomatic medicine (1939), it seems proper to say that C-L psychiatry did *not* spring from psychosomatic medicine but may only have been enhanced by it in later years. Whatever their relative sequential developmental histories, there is little doubt that they are related. Just how they relate will be revisited later, when the question of accreditation arises and examines their record of collaboration. Their kinship has contributed to the growth of both, while being partly responsible for the bumpiness in the road to specialization.

Note

1 Alexander, 1950; Blumenfield & Strain, 2006; Cheren, 1989; Hill, 1976; Levenson and Wulsin, 2010; Lipowski, Lipsitt & Whybrow, 1977; Seguin, 1970; Shorter, 1997; Wise, M.G., & Rundell, J.R. (Eds.). (2002).

References

Agrippa, H.C. (1510). *Three Books of Occult Philosophy and Magic*. London, UK: Moule (1651).

Alexander, F. (1950). *Psychosomatic Medicine*. New York, NY: W.W. Norton & Co.

Bates, W.J. (1968). *Coleridge*. New York, NY: Macmillan.

Beisser, A.R. (1964). The fundamental psychosomatic discovery. *American Journal of Psychiatry, 121*, 614–615.

Billings, E.G. (1939). Liaison psychiatry and intern instruction. *Journal of the Association of American Medical Colleges, 14*, 375–385.

Blumenfield, M. & Strain, J.J. (2006). Psychosomatic Medicine. Philadelphia, PA: Lippincott Williams and Wilkins.

Cheren, S. (1989). *Psychosomatic Medicine: Theory, Physiology, and Practice*. (Vol. 1). Madison, CT: International Universities Press.

DeMandeville (1976[1711]). *A Treatise on the Hypochondriack and Hysterick Passions*. New York, NY: Arno Press (Reprint).

Descartes, R. (1641). *Meditations of First Philosophy*. (Translated by J. Cottingham). Cambridge, UK: Cambridge University Press.

Dunbar, H.F. (1935). *Emotions and Bodily Changes: A Survey of Literature on Psychosomatic Interrelationships 1910–1933*. New York, NY: Columbia University Press.

Dunbar, H.F. (1943). *Psychosomatic Diagnosis*. New York, NY: P.B. Hoeber.

Engel, G.L. (1977). The need for a new medical model: A challenge for biomedicine. *Science, 196*, 129–136.

Engel, G.L. (1992). How much longer must medicine's science be bound by a seventeenth century world view? *Psychotherapy and Psychosomatics, 57*, 3–16.

Feuchtersleben, E.V. (1845 [1995]). *Principles of Medical Psychology*. New York, NY: The Classics of Psychiatry and Behavioral Sciences Library (Fine Facsimile Reprint edition).

Field, H.L. (1982). Psychosomatic illness: Semantic and theoretical evolution. In R.L. Gallon (Ed.). *The Psychosomatic Approach to Illness*. (pp. 1–15). New York, NY: Elsevier Biomedical.

Flexner, A. (1910). *Medical Education in the United States and Canada: A Report to the Carnegie Foundation for the Advancement of Teaching*. Bulletin No. 4, New York, NY: The Carnegie Foundation for the Advancement of Teaching.

Freud, S. (1911). Psychoanalytic notes on a case of an autobiographical account of a case of paranoia (dementia paranoides). In J. Strachey (Ed.). *Standard Edition of the Complete Works of Sigmund Freud*. (Vol. 12, pp. 3–82). London, UK: Hogarth Press, 1955.

Graham, D.T. (1967). Health, disease, and the mind-body problem: linguistic parallelism. *Psychosomatic Medicine, 29*, 52–71.

Graham, D.T. (1979). What place in medicine for psychosomatic medicine? *Psychosomatic Medicine, 41,* 357–367.

Greenblatt, M. (1975). Psychiatry: The battered child of medicine. *New England Journal of Medicine, 292,* 246–250.

Greenhill, M. (1980). Therapeutic intervention in liaison psychiatry. *Journal of the University of Ottawa, 5,* 255–263.

Groddeck, G. (1949). *The Book of the It.* New York, NY: Vintage Books (Random House).

Heinroth, J.C. (1818). *Lehrbuch Der Storungen Des Seelenslebens.* Leipzig: Fcw Vogel.

Hill, O.W. (Ed.). (1976). *Modern Trends in Psychosomatic Medicine 3.* London, UK: Butterworths.

Hogan, C.C. (1995). *Psychosomatics, Psychoanalysis, and Inflammatory Disease of the Colon.* Madison, CT: International Universities Press.

Kahana, R.J., & Bibring, G.L. (1967). Personality types in medical management. In N.E. Zinberg (Ed.). *Psychiatry and Medical Practice in a General Hospital.* (pp. 108–123). New York, NY: International Universities Press.

Levenson, D. (1994). *Mind, Body, and Medicine: A History of the American Psychosomatic Society.* Philadelphia, PA: Williams & Wilkins.

Levenson, J.L., & Wulsin, L. (Eds.). (2010). *The American Psychiatric Publishing Textbook of Psychosomatic Medicine: Psychiatric Care of the Medically Ill.* Washington, DC: American Psychiatric Publishing.

Levere, T.H. (1981). *Poetry Realized in Nature: Samuel Taylor Coleridge and Early Nineteenth Century Science.* Cambridge, UK: Oxford University Press.

Lipowski, Z.J. (1984). What does the word "psychosomatic" really mean? A historical and semantic inquiry. *Psychosomatic Medicine, 46,* 153–171.

Lipowski, Z.J., Lipsitt, D.R., & Whybrow, P.C. (Eds.). (1977). *Psychosomatic Medicine: Current Trends and New Applications.* New York, NY: Oxford University Press.

Lipsitt, D.R. (1956). Doctors afield: Sir Ronald Ross. *New England Journal of Medicine, 292,* 246–250.

Lipsitt, D.R. (1981). The remedicalization of psychiatry. In E. Bernstein (Ed.). *Medical and Health Annual.* (pp. 291–295). Chicago: Encyclopedia Britannica.

Lipsitt, D.R. (2006). Psychosomatic medicine: History of a "new" specialty. In M. Blumenfield & J.J. Strain (Eds.). *Psychosomatic Medicine.* Philadelphia, PA: Lippincott Williams & Wilkins.

Margetts, E.L. (1950). The early history of the word "psychosomatic." *Canadian Medical Association Journal, 73,* 402–404.

Nemiah, J.C. (1961). Introduction to Taylor, G.J. *Psychosomatic Medicine and Contemporary Psychoanalysis.* (pp. 1–10). NY: International Universities Press.

Nemiah, J.C. (2000). A psychodynamic view of psychosomatic medicine. *Psychosomatic Medicine, 62,* 299–303.

Peabody, F. (1927). The care of the patient. *Journal of the American Medical Association, 88,* 877–882.

Plante, T.G. (2010). *Contemporary Clinical Psychology.* Hoboken, NJ: Wiley.

Reil, J.C. & Hoffbauer, J. (1808) Beytrage zur Befordenung Einer Kurmethode auf Psychischen Wege. Halle, Ger: Curtische Bucchandlung.

Rossler, W., Riecher-Rossler, A., & Meise, U. (1994). Wilhelm Greisinger and the concept of community care in 19th century Germany. *Hospital & Community Psychiatry, 45,* 818–822.

Schwab, J.J. (1985). Psychosomatic medicine: Its past and present. *Psychosomatics, 26,* 583–593.

Seguin, C.A. (1970). *Introduction to Psychosomatic Medicine*. New York, NY: International Universities Press.

Shorter, E. (1997). *A History of Psychiatry: From the Era of Asylum to the Age of Prozac*. Hoboken, NJ: Wiley.

Steinberg, H., Herrmann-Lingen, C., & Himmerich, H. (2013). Johann Christian August Heinroth: Psychosomatic medicine 80 years before Freud. *Psychiatria Danubina, 25*, 11–16.

Trotter, T. (1808). *The Nervous Temperament: Being a Practical Treatise on Nervous, Bilious, Stomach and Liver Complaints*. Troy, NY: Wright, Goodenow & Stockwell.

Tuke, D.H. (1873). *Illustrations of the Influence of the Mind upon the Body in Health and Disease Designed to Elucidate the Action of the Imagination*. Philadelphia, PA: Henry C. Lea.

Vickers, N. (2004). *Coleridge and the Doctors*. New York, NY: Oxford University Press.

Waxler, N.E. (1981). The social labeling perspective on illness and medical practice. In L. Eisenberg & A. Kleinman (Eds.). *The Relevance of Social Science for Medicine*. (pp. 283–306). Boston, MA: Reidel.

Weiss, E., & English, O.S. (1943). *Psychosomatic Medicine*. Philadelphia, PA: W.B. Saunders Co.

Winnicott, D. (1966). Psycho-somatic illness in its positive and negative aspects. *International Journal of Psychoanalysis, 47*, 510–516.

Wise, M.G., & Rundell, J.R. (Eds.). (2002). *The American Psychiatric Publishing Textbook of Consultation-Liaison Psychiatry*. Washington, DC: American Psychiatric Publishing.

Wright, J.P., & Potter, P. (2000). *Psyche and Soma*. New York, NY: Oxford University Press.

5

EPIDEMIOLOGY

Neither Physiology nor Philosophy

[O]ur powerful science has not yet unearthed the causes of, or precise predispositions to, the pathogenic initial disequilibria and the cascade of consequences we recognize as symptomatic disease. Thus, with all our power, we have promises yet to deliver and miles to go.

—Freedman, 1992, p. 862

Iago Galdston (1954), a psychoanalyst and erudite writer, has suggested that interest in psychosomatic phenomena arose not so much from psychoanalysis and psychiatry but rather from epidemiological roots. While the words "psyche" and "soma" were "as ancient as the Greek tongue," no mention of "psychosomatic" appeared before the nineteenth century. Its sudden upsurge, Galdston claims, can only be accounted for "as the result of some abrupt conceptual transmutation, some sudden conversion in thinking pattern, some radical change in ideational *gestalt*" (p. 128). This occurred at the point in medical history when most acute infectious disease had been diminished, with a change of focus to a "new order of morbidity, the sick man and the ailing woman who had 'nothing the matter with them' and yet were not well" (p. 130). The need to "arrive at some suitable and competent etiological factor . . . for [these] unaccountable morbidities," led naturally to perturbations of the "psyche" (p. 130). Thus, it was, claims Galdston, an "epidemiological necessity" rather than psychoanalytic or psychiatric insight that "initiated and motivated the psychosomatic movement" (p. 130). With infectious diseases under better control in the first quarter of the twentieth century, practitioners' attention could turn to an interest in the epidemiological incidence of mind-body (psychosomatic) morbidity and mortality in their practices. Indeed, the epidemiological studies of John Schwab and associates (Schwab, Fennell & Warheit, 1974), pioneers of consultation-liaison psychiatry and social psychiatry, established a clear link between the prevalence of psychophysiological symptomatology and social change.

Credence for this intriguing idea exists in the inevitable awareness of primary care physicians (previously general practitioners) that large segments of their daily practice consist of patients whose symptoms do not readily disclose "organic" origins. While an expedient gesture is to declare "nothing the matter," the more perspicacious practitioner acknowledges a mental or "functional" component to puzzling complaints (Lipsitt, Joseph, Meyer & Notman, 2015). Figures for this observation have been fairly constant for at least a century, with anywhere from 30% to 80% of patients in doctors' offices presenting with somatized complaints of unspecified origin, the most recent iteration of labels being "medically unexplained symptoms" (MUS) (Fink, Sorensen, Engberg, Holm & Munk-Jorgensen, 1990). For general practitioners, how to integrate the mental and physical components of illness (psyche and soma of past centuries) presents a clinical challenge for which medical school has inadequately prepared them (Lipsitt et al., 2015).

Ultimate acceptance of this fact by medical practitioners, generalists, as well as specialists has clear implications for the need of assessment, diagnosis, and management by psychiatrist colleagues. Singular consultations to physicians and their patients were simply called that—that is, "consultation." With increasing frequency and the passage of years, the process of consulting evolved into a more organizational designation, called "consultation-liaison psychiatry" (Billings, 1939). Thus began an appreciation of the "integration" of health resources, both physical and psychological, looking and sounding curiously like the beginnings of "psychosomatic medicine"! Felix Deutsch (1959), an internist-become-psychoanalyst in Vienna, for a time Freud's physician, is recorded as having given the field its name in the mid-1920s, before there was evidence of "psychosomatic research."

This chapter follows this possibly fanciful idea with a brief survey of how medical practice is accustomed to dealing with patients' somatizing (or psychologizing) distress. For many physicians through the ages, these patients have been characterized as "difficult" (Lipsitt, 2003). It was not uncommon to hear demeaning references to "high-utilizers," "frequent-flyers," "problem patients," and "heartsink patients." The process inferred by Galdston's "epidemiological" hypothesis can be characterized as (1) physicians' awareness in general practice of the emotional component of illness and its somatization leads to (2) an interest in and need for psychiatric involvement that leads to (3) psychiatric consultation and "medical psychotherapy" that leads to (4) a "psychosomatic" approach and, by my own extrapolation, to psychosomatic medicine and C-L psychiatry. This chapter endeavors to follow this pathway.

General Medical Practice: The Universality of Somatization

People have experienced and complained of aches, pains, twinges, and sprains long before there was medicine, psychiatry, psychoanalysis, and psychosomatic medicine.

In fact, it was those very perturbations besides other more serious malfunctions of the body that gave rise to the various "provider" professions, originally called healers; as has been said, there were patients before there were doctors. Most puzzling to the healers were those conditions that were most "bizarre," but any variety of incantations, potions, and practices seemed to "cure" most (see, for example, Frazer, 1922).

The need to name that which is "unnameable" in medicine probably accounts for the overuse of words like hysteria, neurasthenia, functional, hypochondriasis, idiopathic, and neurotic, a process referred to by Freedman (1992) as "the game of the name" (p. 865). The experience of "not knowing," of uncertainty, of puzzlement that complexes of symptoms do not readily fit well-studied and well-known rubrics of medicine is almost certain to prompt such a flurry of specious names and a request for help from psychiatric consultants.

This trend persisted until the late 1800s when Wilhelm Stekel, a physician student of Freud, referred to bodily pain without organic findings as "somatization" (Marin & Carron, 2002, p. 250).[1] In all subsequent official nomenclatures, symptom complexes without organic findings have been referred to as "somatoform" (American Psychiatric Association, 1980).

Treatments of somatoform disorders through the ages have been as varied (and useless) as their names. The artist Daumier (1841) caricatured that most iconic of all "somatized" afflictions, hypochondriasis, treated with "white mustard, red Paraguay, Regnault paste, Clysobol, and in general all inventions for relieving unsuffering humanity." This caption for his drawing of the wretched hypochondriac proclaimed that this ailment was the "providence of the medical profession, the benediction of the drug trade," in other words "the bread and butter" of medical practice of the day.

Less than 100 years later, the revered Harvard professor/teacher Francis Peabody (1927) uttered virtually the same message; in his classic paper, *The Care of the Patient*, he wrote:

> [M]any physicians whom I have questioned agree . . . that, excluding cases of acute infection, approximately half of their patients complained of symptoms for which an adequate organic diagnosis could not be discovered. Numerically then, these patients contribute to a large group, and their fees go a long way toward spreading butter on the physician's bread.
>
> *(p. 878)*

Requests for help with these patients most often fell to the psychiatrist. And because many patients had what were considered somatizing disorders, the concept of somatization became a constant element in the history of C-L psychiatry. Classifiers for centuries have struggled with the problem of characterizing those patients whose physical complaints do not match known anatomic or physiologic paradigms. Even formalized classification has had its problems, resulting in "official" appellations like psychophysiological reaction, adjustment reaction, transient situational personality disturbance, psychological factors affecting physical condition, and somatoform disorders. The problem remains with us, and, after many iterations, it is now identified as "somatic symptom disorder" (American Psychiatric Association, 2013).

One Doctor's Experience

In April 1886, a young Viennese neurologist reluctantly entered medical practice. As the "new doc on the block," he was promptly referred those patients whose symptoms perplexed Vienna's general practitioners. Early psychoanalytic practice in all likelihood drew patients from the large reservoir of "somatizers," commonly referred to at the time as "hysterics." When their treatment with techniques like womb "fumigation" failed, patients were referred to "head doctors." It was as though "it's all in your womb" became "it's all in your head."

Freud's experience is replicated daily in the practices of today's primary care physician. Patients with puzzling nonorganic symptoms present puzzling diagnostic challenges. Efforts to understand his patients' symptoms led Freud to concepts of "conversion" and "somatic compliance," basically equivalent to today's "somatization." Perhaps the most quoted definition is that by Lipowski (1988):

> [S]omatization is the tendency to experience and communicate somatic distress and symptoms that have no pathological findings, to attribute them to physical illness, and to seek medical help for them.
>
> *(p. 1359)*

Throughout the history of humankind, individuals have experienced the symptoms of everyday life—the backaches, the headaches, the stiffness, and the shortness of breath, recognized in the past as transient and of little consequence. With continual medical progress, pharmacologic innovation, industry promotion, growing self-awareness, and stimulation through advertising and extensive cybernetic communication, symptoms once ignored have been brought to prominence (Barsky & Borus, 1995). With frequency of doctor visits, and high utilization of health care resources, somatizers threaten to glut the health care system, so that, in general medical settings, somatizing patients generate psychiatric consultation like no other circumstance.

In the extreme, we might say that C-L psychiatry and psychosomatic medicine may not have existed had there been no phenomenon of somatization, formerly called "spinal irritation," "neurasthenia," "hysteria," or similar somatoform designations. Freud's intrigue with the machinations of the unconscious very likely began with curiosity about those patients whose symptoms had "no explanation." Ernest Jones's (1953) account of the life and work of Sigmund Freud relates of him that he had to accumulate personal experience of neurotic cases before he could feel in a position to say anything new about them. Material there was in plenty, for like all neurologists, he found that his practice would consist largely of psychoneurotics who were under the impression that 'nerve specialists' could cure 'nerves' as well as disease of the spinal cord. Unlike most neurologists, however, he regarded this state of affairs not as *a humiliating nuisance* in view of their total ignorance of the subject, but as an opportunity to explore a new and fruitful field.

(pp. 228–229; italics by au.)

This receptivity to others' "rejects" would become familiar to psychiatry's future C-L practitioners.

A Need for Consultation

Medical practice, in whatever age, has had to address patients' distress in whatever form presented. Every practice has its share of patients whose symptoms do not easily lend themselves to definitive diagnosis. In early Greek medicine, Hippocrates, Galen, and other physicians did not distinguish between emotional and physical perturbations in their ministrations. But, in time, as physicians became more burdened, attending to the psychological needs of their patients became less possible or appealing. Even the Greeks had their "specialists," and patients with symptoms of doubtful origin may well have been referred, for example, to Aesculapian practitioners and their temples or others for consultation, diagnosis, and management.

One of the earliest of "problem patients" consulted on, although not seen by Freud, was the pseudonymous Anna O (see chapter 3), a patient with multiple somatic complaints "untreatable" by other physicians. She had first come to the attention of Josef Breuer, who treated her until encountering an "impasse" (Breuer & Freud, 1895, pp. 40–41). Freud's consultation began an exploration of the patient's symptoms that ultimately led to the "talking cure" and psychoanalysis. One may wonder to what extent the treatment of "problem patients," somatizers like Anna O, that "no one likes" contributed, over the centuries, to the stigma attached to the fields of psychiatry and psychoanalysis.

Although Peabody (1927), like Daumier, may have felt that these patients' fees "put bread on the table" at that time (*vide supra*), changes in practice structure, compensation, and reimburseability have rendered somatizing patients more punishing than rewarding for practicing physicians. The marginalizing of these patients has placed them visibly in the psychiatric domain, sometimes as irksome to psychiatrists as to their nonpsychiatrist colleagues (even Briquet found these patients a source of frustration). For the general physician with little interest in such matters, they represent only frustration and likely rejection. And psychiatrists, like their nonpsychiatrist colleagues, often have little relief to offer than a listening ear, often an ameliorative intervention of its own (Lipsitt et al., 2015).

Emergence of the "Liaison" Psychiatrist

Because somatizing patients, not recognizing an emotional basis for their own distress, do not typically seek psychiatric attention, they tend to populate the practices of physicians. Those who find such patients vexing and ungratifying may then seek the assistance of consulting psychiatrists. Some observers of the health care scene believe that somatization may be a greater basis of medical utilization than it was a century ago (Shorter, 1992).

The psychiatrist interested in patients who are "suitable for psychotherapy" finds these patients of little appeal, but a new breed of psychiatrist with interest in how mind-body interaction relates to baffling physical symptoms in medical settings emerged. For the C-L psychiatrist, somatizing patients represent a major concern, with questions of how internal (unconscious) emotional factors find expression in physical symptoms.

In the interests of better serving these patients, consulting psychiatrists recognize a need to familiarize referring physicians with techniques for managing and treating these patients in their practice without having to refer them to psychiatry, regarded by some as a "fool's errand," but out of which grew the need for "liaison." This interaction affords an opportunity for instructing the physician in more salubrious management, with consequent benefit to both patient and physician, as well as potential reduction in suffering, costs, excessive use of resources, and patient and physician frustration. When the diagnosis of these patients is missed or physicians dismiss them with "nothing the matter," patients are likely to become chronically ill, placing a great burden on the health care system and themselves (Lipsitt et al., 2015).

Medical literature overflows with thousands of papers on the process of somatization, imploring primary care physicians to learn how better to care for patients who manifest somatoform illness. Indeed, the resources have, for the most part, been suboptimal. The many articles advising physicians on the "management" of the "difficult" or "problem patient" are testimony to the lack of definitive diagnostic and therapeutic clarity. Much advice derives from purely anecdotal and experiential wisdom from treaters who hold strong beliefs in their own unique approaches (Lipsitt et al., 2015)

While no definitive treatment exists for most somatizing conditions, long experience of practitioners has led empirically to a number of "suggestions" for "management" and "support" of the ailing somatizer, whether diagnosed as hypochondriasis, somatization disorder, or chronic somatic disorder. Included in this compendium of "principles of management" are the following: respect the patient's symptoms and their validity; avoid the temptation to "label" in the face of uncertainty; know when to limit a workup; assign regular appointments without waiting for escalation of symptoms; explore psychological and psychosocial aspects gradually; reassure sparingly; restrain temptation to refer or write prescriptions; tolerate your own discomfort and promote a "working alliance." Variations on these basic themes are as plentiful as there are practitioners, but general adherence reportedly eases discomfort in both patient and physician.

Professional classifiers, attempting to assist practitioners and researchers, have struggled with the varieties of somatizing disorders, from somatization disorder to "abridged" somatization disorder (Escobar, Rubio-Stipec, Canino & Karno, 1989) to multisomatoform disorder (Kroenke et al., 1997). The fact that each classification introduces new names attests to the enormity and uncertainty of the task. And the commonly observed "overlap" of syndromes calls attention to the fluidity of diagnosis.

Noted by at least one cohort of researchers, "the high prevalence, serious impairment, and deterioration over the course of one year suggest the importance of developing primary care interventions to alleviate the physical burden that somatizers suffer" (Dickinson, Dickinson, deGruy, Candib, Main, Libby & Rost, 2003, p. 6).

Since the somatizing process is a fact of nature unlike TB or other controllable diseases, it will never be eliminated; the assistance of C-L psychiatrists will therefore always be relevant, to whatever extent they may be utilized. Much research will be stimulated to assess the methods of treatment, the experience of primary practitioners with these patients, and the extent to which applied therapeutics influence well-being, clinical efficacy, service utilization, and cost. Further consideration of somatization is instructive.

Theories of Somatization

The subject of somatization provides a rich context in which to ponder the interaction of psyche and soma. As a process rather than a disorder or disease, it is a valuable researchable resource, although this has evolved slowly. Specific studies have waited on technological advances such as imaging to facilitate creative investigations by C-L researchers, of which there are few (Lane, 2008).

To date, the best explanation of the process of somatization appears to be that of Max Schur (1955), Freud's one time personal physician and an eventual psychoanalyst. One might speculate that Freud's hypochondriacal tendencies were a stimulus for Schur's contemplation of this process; Freud was not reluctant to refer to his own "neurasthenia." Schur hypothesized that we are all born as undifferentiated somatizers, with access only to bodily expression to make known our needs and wants. As neurologic and emotional maturation occur in the child, language facilitates greater elaboration of need expression. Accompanying ego mastery and linguistic facility enables new forms of communication. In this developmental stage, according to Schur, gradual *de*-somatization occurs, with less reliance on the body for emotional communication. However, trauma, stress, loss, disease, or developmental failure can readily return (regress) the individual to *re*-somatized states.

Applying Schur's hypothesis, one searches for a history of early losses, deprivation, abuse, or other trauma in patients who repeatedly or chronically re-somatize in their attempts to find need fulfillment from nurturant doctors, from themselves through "self-mothering" (as seen in hypochondriasis), and through dependency on others (Lipsitt, 2001).

Other theories of somatization draw on concepts of alexithymia (Sifneos, 1996) and early attachment experience (Bowlby, 1958; Waller, Scheidt & Hartmann, 2004). Attachment theories add to an understanding of the "object hunger" of somatizing patients, a notion that helps to explain their characterization as "high utilizers" of medical resources.

Emergence of Medical Psychotherapy

Since the problem of the somatizing patient never disappears in medical practice from one century to another, recognition of the "psyche" as the distressed "organ" has fostered a search for therapies of the psyche. With new recognition of the existence of the numbers of neurotics in general practice came a natural interest in the need to develop treatments for them. Interest in medical patients with emotional distress led quite naturally to the application of various forms of psychotherapy. Psychotherapy has a long and muddled history, ranging from merely sitting quietly with a patient to a full lengthy psychoanalysis, and rudimentary forms of "psychotherapy" have existed for centuries throughout the world, but formalized psychotherapy is considered to have originated in Vienna with Freud. Freud had said that psychotherapy was "anything one does to affect an emotional response," that in medical care it was the "mental factor," the "exerting of a mental influence" over the patient, that characterized psychotherapy.

If it were easy to define psychotherapy, there would probably not be the more than 400 interventions referred to as psychotherapy. Although many psychiatrists originally chose the field of special study to prepare for a career "doing psychotherapy," changes in the medical, social, and psychological landscape began to alter what consultants found most useful at the bedside of hospitalized medical and surgical patients (Greenhill, 1980). For some, greater therapeutic valence was invested in psychopharmacology than in psychotherapy as such.

In the United States, whether through the beseeching of medical leaders, the decreased prevalence of infectious disease, the postwar turn to humanism, or protestation against increased industrialization and technology, the path toward psychotherapy seemed ineluctably to arise from growing interest in the emotions in patients' complaints. Psyche and soma were beginning to come closer together!

The Boston Roots: "Boston Group"

In Boston, where other revolutions had begun, a center of "medical psychother-apy" was arousing interest. As early as the 1890s, at the country's oldest university, Harvard's professor of medicine Robert T. Edes and neurologist James Jackson Putnam were advocating "medical psychotherapy" (Gifford, S., 1978, p. 106). George Beard (1869) had previously been administering "practical treatment" of neurasthenia, consisting largely of rest, baths, and healthy living habits, which he termed "mental therapeutics." The national popularity of "rest cures" seemed to have softened perception of "nervous disorders" as acceptable ailments for which treatment was available. Hypnosis and suggestion were techniques already being used by internists and surgeons in Boston (Gifford, G., 1978).

Edes and Putnam were joined by colleagues Walter Cannon and William James, both physicians and Harvard professors, and informally began what came to be known as the "Boston Group." Putnam was imbued with new Freudian ideas and was able to interest James's student Boris Sidis, a psychologist/psychia-trist who helped found the *Journal of Abnormal Psychology*; an internist, Joseph Pratt from Tufts Medical School, later credited with founding "group therapy"; Richard Cabot, chief of medicine at MGH; Herman Munsterburg, director of James's psychology laboratory; Josiah Royce, the philosopher friend of James; G. Stanley Hall, psychologist from Clark University who had invited Freud to Amer-ica in 1909; Edward Cowles, director of McLean Hospital; and Morton Prince, a Boston neurologist who had studied with Charcot and aroused American interest in abnormal psychology through his published account of Christine Beauchamp's multiple personalities (Prince, 1905). Adolf Meyer, then at Worcester State Hospi-tal, would make occasional visits (Hale, 1971).

William James (1895) had reviewed Breuer and Freud's (1895) work on hys-teria in the *Psychological Review*, and in that same year Edes (1895) had given an important local lecture on *The New England Invalid* (Gifford, S., 1978, p. 327). Josiah Royce, a teacher of "practical philosophy," and his close friend James had been "practicing" psychotherapy and were a strong influence on Putnam and Meyer (Hale, 1971). The visit to Clark University by Freud, Jung, and Ferenczi in 1909 created considerable excitement about the possibilities of a serious psycho-logical therapy (Rosenzweig, 1974).

Richard Cabot had pioneered the profession of social work in the general hospital, appointing Ida Cannon, Walter Cannon's sister, as chief of that service at the Massachusetts General Hospital. He may be credited with originating the notion of the "team approach" in caring for patients with mixed physical, social, and psychological problems.

This dynamic "Boston Group" of psychologists, physicians, philosophers, and researchers vigorously promoted the use of "medical psychotherapy" to address the day-to-day complaints of a troubled population (Gifford, S., 1978). According to historian Hale (1971), this small circle of diverse specialists "developed the most sophisticated and scientific psychotherapy in the English-speaking world between 1890 and 1909" (p. 11).

The Emmanuel Movement

Joseph H. Pratt (1922) had expressed a long-standing interest in the role of emotional and social events on all physical illness. At Harvard and Tufts, believing that the "common neuroses" should be treated by the internist and not the psychiatrist, he applied his "class method" of group therapy to patients with organic diseases like TB (Pratt, 1922), a technique adapted from the more religious counseling approaches of the so-called Emmanuel Movement, begun at the Emmanuel Church in Boston in 1905.

The Emmanuel Movement began with Elwood Worcester, an ordained minister and former professor of psychology and philosophy at Lehigh University, when he moved to Boston in 1904 to become rector of Emmanuel Church. Having been friendly with the neurologist S. Weir Mitchell and having studied in Europe with psychologists Wilhelm Wundt and Gustav Fechner, he felt qualified to open a clinic "for the moral and psychological treatment of nervous and psychic disorders" (Gifford, S., 1978, p. 112).

Worcester had been impressed with William James's description of the "mind cure movement," described in James's book *The Varieties of Religious Experience* (James, 1902, pp. 87–89). Although James was clearly aware of Worcester's endeavors, his involvement with them is unclear. He had already known about the studies of Breuer and Freud as early as 1894 (Gifford, S., 1978, p. 107) and was a proponent of psychotherapy. In fact, in *Varieties of Religious Experience* (1902), James wrote that the American public was *unusually receptive to the movement of medical psychotherapy* and that the "practical character of the American people" had made it possible for them to "intimately knit up" their "systematic philosophy of life" with "practical therapeutics" (Gifford, S., 1978, p. 327). Richard Cabot (1909), influenced by Janet's and James's books, published a paper, "The American type of psychotherapy." Pliny Earle (1868) had expressed interest in making "psychological medicine" a standard part of the medical curriculum and every physician's practice. Indeed, he was named the first professor of psychological medicine at the Berkshire Medical Institution in Pittsfield, Massachusetts, in 1853, reflecting the receptivity to this aspect of medical care in New England at the turn of the century. The excitement about looking at patients differently was in the air, not only at academic centers.

With support from Putnam, Cabot, Pratt, and Boston neurologist/psychoanalyst Isadore Coriat, Worcester trained lay therapists to provide care. As the clinic gained notoriety, it was criticized by the medical community. Putnam withdrew, citing inadequate medical supervision, while Cabot, Pratt, and Coriat remained as advisors. The clinic survived for 23 years, gradually focusing almost exclusively on the treatment of alcoholism and drug addiction. Although compared by some critics to Christian Science, the movement was influenced by psychology and psychoanalysis and had attracted serious interest by the medical psychotherapists in Boston.

Worcester collaborated with Coriat and McComb in 1908 to publish a book, *Religion and Medicine, the Moral Control of Nervous Disorders*, which enjoyed nine printings in its first year. Worcester had become a major devotee of Freud's work and incorporated psychoanalytic ideas into his practice (Gifford, S., 1978, p. 117). During his 1909 visit to America, Freud was informed of the Emmanuel Movement's work, but he essentially dismissed it because of its religious connection. He nevertheless admired the energy invested by the Boston Group in "medical psychotherapy," for he always advocated that all physicians should be capable of offering their patients "mental health treatment." Adolf Meyer's advocacy of "commonsense psychiatry" was a timely contributor to the fervor for treatment of mental illness. In a commemorative speech given at Bloomingdale Hospital in 1921 (where Henry and Earle worked), Meyer (Lief, 1948) said:

> Today we feel that modern psychiatry has found itself—through the discovery that, after all, the uncritical commonsense view of mind and soul is not so far remote from a critical commonsense view of the individual life and its activity, freed from the forbidding and confusing assumptions through which the concept of mind and soul has been held in bewildering awe.
>
> *(p. 1)*

Although Meyer was not a psychoanalyst, he held psychoanalysis in high regard and even cofounded one of the first psychoanalytic institutes in the United States; his simple translation of emotional aspects of illness found broad receptivity in medical audiences and common people, and many of America's early psychiatrists studied with him at Johns Hopkins.

Caring for Patients

With all the excitement about psychotherapy, physicians still needed to be urged to seek treatment for "neurotic" patients. Peabody (1927) lectured medical students at Harvard to pay more attention to those patients who were being dismissed as "having nothing the matter." And Walter Cannon, although vigorously involved in psychophysiological research, was still concerned as a physician about the care of patients with emotional problems. In a lecture to the Massachusetts Medical Society (1928), he said:

> I think we must admit that, although physicians have not infrequent occasions to observe instances of functional disturbance due to emotional excitement, there is an inclination to minimize or to slight that influence, or

even to deny that it is part of a physician's service to his patient to concern himself with such troubles.

(p. 877)

Cannon added that physicians' unwillingness to consider the importance of emotional aspects of illness was probably due to two factors: too great an interest in "pathology" and too little interest in "the psyche." He told his audience that the altered structure of some organ and the altered function of the nervous system may be causally related and may have to be *treated as a single disorder* (p. 877).

While entreaties by a "bench" scientist to a group of practicing "trench" physicians may be less than impactful, Cannon set the stage for "next steps" when he concluded his talk:

> The doctor is properly concerned with the workings of the body and their disturbances, and he should have, therefore, a natural interest in the effects of emotional stress and in the *modes of relieving it*. The field has not been well cultivated; much work still needs to be done in it.
>
> *(p. 884; emphasis by au.)*

How much influence these importunings had on further events is speculative, but concern by leading medical educators emphasized their importance.

Interest in medical psychotherapy was not confined to Boston. A textbook of psychotherapy by Dejerine and Gaukler (1913) in France was translated into English in 1913 by the New York psychoanalyst Smith Ely Jelliffe, an early psychoanalytic "psychosomaticist." It drew on the work of Emil DuBois-Raymond (*The Psychic Treatment of Nervous Disorders*, 1905) and Janet (*Psychological Automatism*, 1889) for its techniques of treatment (Gifford, S., 1978, p. 109), and it had achieved some popularity with Pratt and his colleagues. Dejerine believed that emotional training and reeducation were the essential elements in treatment and that psychosomatic symptoms were caused by suggestion and therefore could be cured by either hypnotic suggestion or "rational persuasion."

"Medical therapists" were much influenced by Janet's book *Principles of Psychotherapy* (1924), as well as his *Psychological Healing* (1925). Janet himself was reciprocally influenced by many American writers and teachers of the medical psychotherapy group, such as S. Weir Mitchell, Morton Prince, and William James, referred to in his treatise.

Dorothy Levenson's (1994) excellent history of the American Psychosomatic Society describes how Dr. Austen Fox Riggs, an internist, working at New York's Presbyterian Hospital

> became interested in that large group of patients who were sick to a degree that was out of proportion to the organic findings and in patients in whom

there was no demonstrable pathology. Riggs found that he could help [them] by encouraging them to talk freely to him about their lives.

(p. 12)

When he contracted tuberculosis, Riggs moved to western Massachusetts to recuperate and founded the well-known Austen Riggs Center for the care of "treatment-resistant" patients in 1913, providing treatment that would utilize growing interest in "psychosomatic medicine" and "therapeutic psychology" to encourage "precepts for successful living." Other clinics began offering such treatment as well. Even in Vienna, Freud's Ambulatarium or Free Clinic (Danto, 2005), using psychoanalytic methods, addressed the complaints of individuals who were not helped by traditional medical intervention.

Role of the General Hospital

If, as was being reported in medical circles, general practice consisted of large numbers of "neurotic" patients with symptoms that were being overlooked, it would be only natural to expect that many of these patients would be found in the general hospital. In fact, it was to this group that Peabody called attention in 1927. Once recognized, a need for psychiatric assistance followed. Was this not the germination of consultation-liaison psychiatry? Histories of C-L psychiatry date the beginnings of the field to Henry's paper (1929; see prologue), only one year after Cannon's stirring speech; Henry elaborated on his experience in a general hospital. This psychiatric experience led readily to recommendations for improved psychosocial care of hospitalized medical and surgical patients. And the field of psychosomatic medicine had not yet been established. By the 1930s, there was an escalating clamor for psychiatric care in general hospitals, not by beds alone (Lipsitt, 1984), but by availability of collaborative care for the many patients whose syndromes were more than simply organic. Numbers of general hospitals increased sharply for the next couple of decades, and, by the 1960s, patients discharged from these institutions with psychiatric diagnoses exceeded by far all similar data from state, county, and other psychiatric institutions. In 1964, statistics released by the American Hospital Association recorded 1,005 general hospitals in the United States that accepted psychiatric patients (*Medical Tribune*, 1964, p. 8). Only 45% of these hospitals included separate psychiatric inpatient beds. The need for psychiatric consultation was expanding.

As psychiatric services developed in general hospitals, opportunities arose for pedagogical offerings in those settings, especially in academic centers. Occasions for teaching abounded, so that avid psychiatric educators, who "knew so much more than their 'medical' colleagues," had to be cautioned to avoid "missionary zeal" or a "proselytizing" educational fervor (Lipowski, 1983, p. 337). Nonetheless, in academic settings where attending physicians, house officers, and medical students all gathered as in a small university, exposure to psychiatry was inevitable.

Described elsewhere in this book, "liaison" emerged as a shorthand way of referring to the psychiatrist's "educational" interaction with other staff members.

Reconciliation of medicine and psychiatry seemed rife, after what one writer characterized as "a long and stormy courtship, with many broken engagements, an occasional annulment, and sometimes outright divorce" (Moore, 1978, p. 413). And the recrudescence of interest in primary care (nee general practice) opened possibilities for a major role of psychiatric consultants in that endeavor, with beginnings in the general hospital.

Although many writers allude to C-L psychiatry as the "clinical arm of psychosomatic medicine," would logic not permit, as presented here, to declare that, in fact, active interest in "psychosomatic medicine" had grown out of common medical practice as it began to rely on psychiatry to assist with "problem patients"? Recognition that psyche and soma reside together in the active living patient soon fostered interest in knowing more about the phenomenon. There followed robust research investigation by people like Alexander, Dunbar, Grinker, Deutsch, and others. Alexander (1950), in *Psychosomatic Medicine*, states the progression quite clearly: "[P]sychological factors influencing physiological processes must be subjected to the same detailed and careful scrutiny as is customary in the study of physiological processes" (p. 11).

Here are echoes of Cannon! The impetus for psychosomatic research followed, as Alexander (1950) states:

> Once again, the patient as a human being with worries, fears, hopes, and despairs, as an indivisible whole and not merely the bearer of organs—a diseased liver or stomach—is *becoming the legitimate object of medical interest*. A growing psychological orientation manifests itself among physicians. This psychological interest is nothing more than a revival of old pre-scientific views in a new and scientific form.
>
> *(p. 17; emphasis by au.)*

Research followed practice! The body of C-L psychiatry had grown a head! From Hippocrates' dictum that one cannot treat the body without the "soul," to growing awareness in general practice that emotion must be acknowledged in treating somatizing patients, to the evolution of psychiatric consultation, psychotherapy, general hospital psychiatry, and liaison and psychosomatic medicine, Galdston's concept of "epidemiological necessity" seems profoundly logical! This epidemiological excursion stands as one more contribution to the foundations of C-L psychiatry.

Note

1 Although attributed to Stekel, the word was most likely coined by Stekel's translator for the German *organsprache* (organ speech), considered equivalent to Freud's "conversion" (p. 250).

References

Alexander, F. (1950). *Psychosomatic Medicine*. New York, NY: W.W. Norton.

American Psychiatric Association. (1980). *Diagnostic and Statistical Manual of Mental Disorders*. (3rd edition). Washington, DC: American Psychiatric Association, 1980.

American Psychiatric Association. (2013). *Diagnostic and Statistical Manual of Mental Disorders*. (5th edition). Washington, DC: Author.

Barsky, A.J., & Borus, J.F. (1995). Somatization and medicalization in the era of managed care. *Journal of the American Medical Association, 274*, 1931–1934.

Beard, G.M. (1869). Neurasthenia and nervous exhaustion. *Boston Medical and Surgical Journal, 3*, 217.

Billings, E.G. (1939). Liaison psychiatry and intern instruction. *Journal of the American Association of Medical Colleges, 14*, 375–385.

Bowlby, J. (1958). The nature of the child's tie to his mother. *International Journal of Psycho-Analysis, 39*, 350–373.

Breuer, J., & Freud, S. (1895). *Studies on Hysteria*. Leipzig: Deutike.

Cabot, R.C. (1909). The American type of psychotherapy. *Psychotherapy, 2*, 24–25.

Cannon, W.B. (1928). The mechanism of emotional disturbance of bodily functions. *New England Journal of Medicine, 198*, 877–884. (Annual discourse delivered before the Massachusetts Medical Society, Worcester, Massachusetts, June 1928).

Danto, E.A. (2005). *Freud's Free Clinics: Psychoanalysis and Social Justice, 1918–1938*. New York, NY: Columbia University Press.

Daumier, H. (1841). The hypochondriac. *The National Museum of Western Art*. Retrieved from http://collection.nmwa.go.jp/en/G2000–1015.html

Dejerine, J.J., & Gaukler, E. (1913). *Psychological Healing*. S.E. Jelliffe (Trans.). Philadelphia, PA: J.B. Lippincott.

Deutsch, F. (1959). *On the Mysterious Leap from the Mind to the Body: A Workshop Study on the Theory of Conversion*. New York, NY: International Universities Press.

Dickinson, W.P., Dickinson, L.M., deGruy, F.V., Candib, L.M., Main, D.S., Libby, A.M., & Rost, K. (2003). The somatization in primary care study: A tale of three diagnoses. *General Hospital Psychiatry, 25*, 1–7.

DuBois-Raymond, E. (1905). *The Psychic Treatment of Nervous Disorders: The Psychoneuroses and Their Moral Treatment*. S.E. Jelliffe & W.A. White (Trans.). New York, NY: Funk and Wagnalls.

Earle, P. (1868). Psychological medicine: Its importance as part of the medical curriculum. *American Journal of Insanity, 24*, 257–280.

Edes, R.T. (1895). The New England invalid. *Boston Medical and Surgical Journal, 133*, 53–57.

Escobar, J.J., Rubio-Stipec, M., Canino, G., & Karno, M. (1989). Somatic symptom index (SSI): A new and abridged somatization construct: Prevalence and epidemiological correlates in two large community samples. *Journal of Nervous and Mental Disease, 177*, 140–146.

Fink, P., Sorensen, L., Engberg, M., Holm, M., & Munk-Jorgensen, P. (1990). Somatization in primary care: Prevalence, health care utilization, and general practitioner recognition. *Psychosomatics, 40*, 330–338.

Frazer, J.G. (1922). *The Golden Bough: A Study in Magic and Religion*. London, UK: Macmillan Press.

Freedman, D.X. (1992). The search: Body, mind and human purpose. *American Journal of Psychiatry, 149*, 858–866.

Galdston, I. (1954). Roots of psychosomatic medicine. *Canadian Medical Association Journal,* *70,* 130–132.

Gifford, G.E., Jr. (1978). *Psychoanalysis, Psychotherapy, and the New England Medical Scene,* *1894–1944.* New York, NY: Science History Publications.

Gifford, S. (1978). Medical psychotherapy and the Emmanuel movement in Boston, 1904–1912. In G.E. Gifford, Jr. (Ed.). *Psychoanalysis, Psychotherapy, and the New England Medical Scene, 1894–1944.* (pp. 106–118). New York, NY: Science History Publications.

Greenhill, M.H. (1980). Therapeutic intervention in liaison psychiatry. *The Psychiatric Journal of the University of Ottowa, 5,* 255–263.

Hale, N.G., Jr. (Ed.). (1971). *James Jackson Putnam and Psychoanalysis.* Cambridge, MA: Harvard University Press.

Henry, G.W. (1929–1930). Some modern aspects of psychiatry in general hospital practice. *American Journal of Psychiatry, 86,* 481–499.

James, W. (1894). On the psychical mechanisms of hysterical phenomena. *Psychological Review, 1,* 199.

James, W. (1895). Review of Breuer and Freud. *Psychological Review, 1,* 199.

James, W. (1902). *The Varieties of Religious Experience: A Study in Human Nature.* New York, NY: Longmans, Green, and Co.

Janet, P. (1889). L'Automatisme Psychologique. Paris, FR: Felix Alcan.

Janet, P. (1924). *Principles of Psychotherapy.* London, UK: Allen & Unwin.

Janet, P. (1925). *Psychological Healing: A Historical and Clinical Study.* London, UK: Allen & Unwin.

Jones, E. (1953). *The Life and Work of Sigmund Freud.* (Vol. 1). New York, NY: Basic Books.

Kroenke, K., Spitzer, R.L., deGruy, F.V. 3rd, Hahn, S.R., Linzer, M., Williams, J.B., . . . Davies, M. (1997). Multisomatoform disorder: An alternative to undifferentiated somatoform disorder for the somatizing patient in primary care. *Archives of General Psychiatry, 54,* 352–358.

Lane, R. (2008). Neural substrates of implicit and explicit emotional processes: A unifying framework for psychosomatic medicine. *Psychosomatic Medicine, 70,* 213–230.

Levenson, D. (1994). *Mind, Body and Medicine: A History of the American Psychosomatic Society.* Philadelphia, PA: Williams & Wilkins.

Lief, A. (1948). *The Commonsense Psychiatry of Adolf Meyer.* New York, NY: McGraw-Hill.

Lipowski, Z.J. (1983). Current trends in consultation-liaison psychiatry. *Canadian Journal of Psychiatry, 28,* 329–338.

Lipowski, Z.J. (1988). Somatization: The concept and its application. *American Journal of Psychiatry, 145,* 1358–1368.

Lipsitt, D.R. (1984). Not by beds alone. Presentation in Symposium: General hospital psychiatry: Change and challenge. 137th Annual Meeting of the American Psychiatric Association, Los Angeles, CA. May 9, 1984.

Lipsitt, D.R. (2001). Psychodynamic perspectives on hypochondriasis. In V. Starcevic & D.R. Lipsitt (Eds.). *Hypochondriasis: Modern Perspectives on an Ancient Malady.* (pp. 265–290). New York, NY: Oxford University Press.

Lipsitt, D.R. (2003). Difficult patient-doctor encounters. In W. Branch (Ed.). *Office Practice of Medicine.* (4th edition, pp. 1215–1222). Philadelphia, PA: Saunders.

Lipsitt, D.R., Joseph, R., Meyer, D., & Notman, M. (2015). Medically unexplained symptoms: Barriers to effective treatment when "nothing is the matter" *Harvard Review of Psychiatry, 23,* 438–448.

Marin, C.G., & Carron, R. (2002). The origin of the concept of somatization [Letter to the editor]. *Psychosomatics, 43,* 249–250.

Medical Tribune. (1964). General hospitals increasing care of mentally ill. December 9, p. 8.

Moore, G.L. (1978). The adult psychiatrist in the medical environment. *American Journal of Psychiatry, 135,* 413–419.

Peabody, F. (1927). The care of the patient. *Journal of the American Medical Association, 88,* 877–882.

Pratt, J.H. (1922). The principles of class treatment and their application to various chronic diseases. *Hospital Social Services, 6,* 401–411.

Prince, M. (1905). *The Dissociation of a Personality: A Biographical Study in Abnormal Psychology.* New York, NY: Longmans, Green & Co.

Rosenzweig, S. (1974). *The Historic Expedition to America (1909): Freud, Jung and Hall the King-Maker.* St. Louis, MO: Rana House.

Schur, M. (1955). Comments on the metapsychology of somatization. *The Psychoanalytic Study of the Child, 10,* 119–164.

Schwab, J.J., Fennell, E.B., & Warheit, G.J. (1974). The epidemiology of psychosomatic disorders. *Psychosomatics, 15,* 88–93.

Shorter, E. (1992). *From Paralysis to Fatigue.* New York, NY: Free Press.

Sifneos, P. (1996). Alexithymia: past and present. *American Journal of Psychiatry, 153*(7 Suppl), 137–142.

Waller, E., Scheidt, C.E., & Hartmann, A. (2004). Attachment representation and illness behavior in somatoform disorders. *Journal of Nervous and Mental Disease, 192,* 200–209.

Worcester, E., McComb, S., & Coriat, I.H. (1908). *Religion and Medicine; the Moral Control of Nervous Disorders.* New York, NY: Moffat, Yard.

6

BEGINNINGS OF CONSULTATION AND LIAISON

But where's the man who counsel can bestow, Still pleas'd to teach, and yet not proud to know?

—*Alexander Pope,* An Essay on Criticism, *1711, line 71*

Our journey continues with the consultation. Each consultant brings with him or her an amalgam of personal experience; attitudes; beliefs; skills; knowledge; and social, cultural, and religious influences. Education has had both conscious and unconscious elements, from family immersion to formal institutional exposure. Our focus here is not to plumb these many facets of personal consultancy but to define, in a limited way, consultation (and liaison) as a process as it has been contributed to by those historical domains that have been described.

The joke about the consultant in any branch of medicine is that she or he is "the specialist from out of town who comes with slides and does the rectal." Parsing this lighthearted jibe for other meaning, we might note that it implies someone with uncommon (out-of-town) knowledge, who is academically oriented (slides), and who does the work that others are unable or don't care to do (the rectal). Consulting psychiatrists are seen ambivalently by those requesting their services, expecting either some "miraculous" intervention or suspecting complete uselessness. The "rectal" of psychiatric consultation is the request that someone take responsibility for the task no one wants, as in calling for "clearance of suicidal ideation" prior to a patient's discharge. Ambivalence toward psychiatrists is noted when the "wise-ass" psychiatrist, invited to assess the patient's mental status, makes the "medical" diagnosis that was missed by the consultee. The latter's embarrassment may diminish future consultation requests from that consultee.

Clearly, the exercise of consultation is not consistent "smooth sailing," but performing psychiatric consultation is nevertheless most often a gratifying experience and received appreciatively by most as a useful contribution to total patient care. Psychiatrists who choose this domain of specialized activity find the challenges stimulating, the efforts mostly salutary, and the engagement personally rewarding (Strain, 1981). Traditionally, most consulting work is carried out in an inpatient setting, although later expansion of consultation-liaison services has extended to emergency rooms, outpatient clinics, and even private physicians' group practices (Friedman & Molay, 1994).

Origin and Definition of Consultation

What is a psychiatric consultation, and what is its history? Chroniclers of the history of psychiatry (Alexander & Selesnick, 1966) state that "psychiatry began when one man attempted to relieve another man's suffering by influencing him" (p. 37). Thus, in its broadest interpretation, consultation occurred eons ago, even before anyone put a name to it. Perhaps apocryphal is the story of Hippocrates having consulted on Democritus (460 BC) during a "mad" episode (Sjostrand, 2001); a wealthy man who thought and laughed a lot and believed the world was made up of invisible atoms could readily be thought "crazy." Legend has it that Hippocrates, after interviewing him, corrected this public image.

Another historical account has Avicenna (AD 980–1037) offering advice to physicians on the care of patients, without assuming responsibility for the patient, perhaps a forerunner of "liaison" as much as "consultation." Freud certainly tendered his "extreme" recommendations to physician colleagues, long before formulating his psychoanalytic theories. Testimony to the act of consultation in medicine by the eighteenth century figures prominently in the many prints, cartoons, and drawings of those times, captioned as such; the caricaturist Daumier was especially adept at lampooning physicians in consultation.

Different cultures may define consultation differently. In the United States, when a patient seeks advice from a physician, that has generally been referred to as a "visit" or an "appointment," or an "examination," maybe even a "second opinion"; only rarely does the patient request a "consultation." In Britain most particularly, the physician's office is referred to commonly as the consulting room, and each visit of the patient to the doctor is regarded as a consultation, the process sometimes referred to as consultancy.

The dictionary defines consultation as the act of asking for advice. Does that mean that when one has not *requested* a consultation—as in the case of a patient visited by a physician—none has occurred? Or is the consultation actually only *for the physician* who has requested it of another doctor? In other words, is advice that no one wants considered a consultation, or does the consultee have to invite it? Probably psychiatrists, even as alienists, were giving advice to general practitioners before anyone knew much about mental illness.

A more specialized definition (Campbell, 1996, p. 155) states that psychiatric consultation is

> expert advice sought by the attending physician or, sometimes, by the patient. . . . The consultant may or may not meet directly with the patient, but ordinarily, he does not take actual charge of a case; instead, he advises or counsels the attending physician. . . . Caplan limits the term consultation to . . . a process of interaction between two professionals, the mental health consultant and the consultee who seeks the consultant's help in regard to a current work problem, . . . a coordinate relationship . . . in which the consultant accepts no direct responsibility for implementing remedial actions for the client.
>
> *(p. 155)*

The idea that consultation is the "interaction between two professionals" overlooks the possibility that a consultation may involve several members of a caretaking staff.

An early example of "psychiatric consultation" may have occurred in Bernard de Mandeville's remarkable 1711 *Treatise of the Hypochondriack and Hysterick Passions*, all written in old English. De Mandeville purports to follow the style of Seneca, as he recounts the "dialogues" of a physician with his patient. The patient, Misomedon, opens with "I have sent for you, doctor, to consult you about a distemper, of which I am very well assured, I shall never be cured" (p. 1). What ensues may well be not only techniques of treating hypochondriacal patients but also an example of what Michael Balint considered an "extended consultation." Misomedon anticipates a problem of contemporary medicine when he asks his physician, Philoperio, "Are you in haste, pray? Can you hear a man talk for half an hour together, and perhaps not always to the purpose, without interrupting him?" (p. 2). Such "consulting" on the clinical aspects of patients' mind-body experience in the 1700s can rightfully be said to have formed the latticework for the evolution of consultation-liaison psychiatry, although more defined recognition probably did not materialize until the 1920s.

A Unique Specialty?

All medical and surgical practitioners are generally available for consultation when requested by colleagues, but I am unaware of a medical specialty other than psychiatry that employs the word "consultation" as an adjective to grace its subspecialty specifically—in this case, as *consultation* psychiatry. Allusion to consultation in other medical specialties is referred to as consultation *in* internal medicine, *in* neurology, or *in* surgery (e.g., Harrington, 1990). Few texts allude to the consultation process itself as a subject of inquiry, especially as it embraces an understanding of the patient-doctor relationship, communication, patients' reactions, and perceptions. Rarely, apart from psychiatry, do texts address these issues. An exception is the small, informative volume by a professor of general practice in Australia (Usherwood, 1999).

A situation that may well warrant and benefit from a consultation is the following:

> If one doctor doctors another doctor
> Does the doctor who doctors the doctor
> Doctor the way the doctor he is doctoring doctors?
> Or does the doctoring doctor doctor the doctor the way
> The doctored doctor wants to be doctored?
> The doctoring doctor doctors the doctor the way
> The doctoring doctor wants to doctor the doctor,
> Not the way the doctored doctor wants to be doctored.

This folkloric tongue-tangler probably grew from recognition of how complex doctor-patient relations can be and how they often require consultative assistance.

The beginnings of formalized consulting services in general hospitals is attributed by Lipowski (2002) to George Henry (1929–1930), describing the beginning of consultation-liaison psychiatry very much as we know it today (Lipowski, 2002, p. 5) Henry described his experience of initiating a psychiatric consulting service through his encounters with 300 general hospital inpatients. Although Henry mentions only "consultation," never "liaison," in his 1929 paper, he concludes that most of the problems he encountered could be adequately handled by a *properly educated* general physician or house officer. The thrust of his remarks is therefore to the pedagogical ("liaison") aspect of psychiatric consultation. Henry's description of the essential skill of the effective psychiatric consultant can be little improved on even 85 years after its appearance (see prologue).

Already as a young instructor in psychiatry at Cornell Medical School, in addition to spelling out the urgent need for psychiatric education of nonpsychiatrists and medical students, Henry astutely cautions the intended psychiatrist consultant bringing his or her wares to the general hospital neighborhood: proceed cautiously, listen attentively, avoid jargon, use simple introductions, avoid strict adherence to theories, and write concise and informative nontechnical notes.

Before psychiatric C-L services were formally declared, "psychiatric" consultation with nonpsychiatrist physicians was a fairly robust endeavor carried out by doctors other than psychiatrists. James Jackson Putnam, for example, a neurologist credited with bringing psychoanalysis to America in the early 1900s, provided consultation to medical and surgical patients at Massachusetts General Hospital. Writing of the origins of C-L psychiatry, Hackett (1978) traces "the origin of organized interest in the mental life of patients at Massachusetts General Hospital to 1873" (p. 3) when Putnam (1910), excited by psychiatry and psychoanalysis in a European trip, returned to offer assistance to physician colleagues and their "patients whose maladies defied diagnosis and treatment, in short, 'the crocks' " (Hackett, 1978, p. 3). Hackett opines that "today's liaison psychiatrist [might] find a familiar *anlage* in J.J. Putnam" (p. 3). At Boston's Peter Bent Brigham Hospital in the late 1920s and 1930s, consultation to medical and surgical patients was provided by a young, unpublished psychiatrist named Donald McPherson, according to historian Sanford Gifford, of the Boston Psychoanalytic Institute (personal communication). It is very likely that psychiatric consultation was being provided by psychiatrists in other institutions without referring to themselves as C-L psychiatrists and without being recorded as such in the professional literature.

War and Consultation

Offering consultative assistance to nonpsychiatrist physicians was in evidence even in the midst of a war. Maurice Levine (1943), chair of psychiatry at Cincinnati General Hospital, a mecca of future C-L psychiatrists and psychosomaticians, published a seminal book on psychotherapy in medical practice "in response to a recurrent need [of] general practitioners, internists, surgeons and others, [who] often ask for information about the handling of the personality problems of their patients" (p. vii). Grounded in practical approaches to common problems of the medical practitioner, Levine, trained in both psychiatry and psychoanalysis, emphasized how he avoided, in his teaching, "burdening the general practitioner with much material about psychodynamics" (p. 174). His example served as a template for future C-L psychiatrists who eventually spread to institutions like Rochester's Strong Memorial Hospital (Romano, Engel), New York's Einstein Medical Center (Rosenbaum, Reiser), and Boston's Beth Israel Hospital (Kahana, Snyder), in a virtual diaspora of C-L psychiatrists.

Wars are not generally known for their good results. However, the involvement of psychiatrists in assessing the "unfit" of military service in both world wars may have hastened and catalyzed the development of consultation psychiatry as a field of special interest and skill. Furthermore, their success at treating, with brief interventions (consultations), the many mental repercussions of combat sufficiently impressed nonpsychiatrist colleagues with new interest in and respect for the field, followed by a desire for increased training in "psychological medicine." This rallied interest was coincident with the years of psychosomatic medicine's development in the 1940s and 1950s, many reports of "psychosomatic" war casualties appearing in the new journal *Psychosomatic Medicine*. The wartime studies and clinical experiences of 1942–1945 were compiled in a volume titled *Wartime Psychiatry* (Lewis & Engle, 1954).

Soon after the war, in February 1945, a group of psychiatrists with teaching skills gathered in a hotel in Hershey, Pennsylvania, to design educational programs for general practitioners whose interest had been peaked during their service years and who would also be treating the many veterans returning from war with the emotional residue of that experience. Supported by the National Committee for Mental Hygiene and the Commonwealth Fund, a group of prominent psychiatrists (Douglas Bond, Henry Brosin, Donald Hastings, M. Ralph Kaufman, John M. Murray) launched a postgraduate course in "psychotherapeutic medicine" for two weeks in April 1946 at the University of Minnesota, in the shared belief that "psychiatry had something that could and must be shared with general medicine . . . and the urgent need of collaboration from general medicine in the care of the psychoneuroses" (Witmer, 1947, p. 3; Lipsitt, 2000).

Federal Contribution

With the value of psychiatric consultation in general medicine having been demonstrated, the postwar momentum in matters of mental health was carried forward with President Truman's signing of the National Mental Health Act in July 1946, authorizing the formation of the National Institute of Mental Health (NIMH). Besides being charged with conducting mental health research, NIMH was also entrusted with the support of the training and education of mental health professionals and the development of community mental health services, of great developmental relevance to the foundations of C-L psychiatry. And in 1948, the Hill-Burton Hospital Construction Act provided funds for establishing psychiatric units in general hospitals, thus providing a home base for future C-L psychiatrists. The general hospital as a fertile resource for enlarging C-L services was readily grasped by writers like Kaufman and Margolin (1948) and Kubie (1944).

C-L Expansion

Articles describing experiences of psychiatric consultation in many institutions were already appearing in abundance in the 1950s by recognized writers.[1] By the 1960s, literature on C-L psychiatry revealed markedly increased interest and activity. It more likely described the discipline and its attributes as well as the requisite skills of the C-L psychiatrist than the experiences of the recipients of consultation. Many of the earliest descriptions alluded simply to "consultation psychiatry," while the amalgamated term "consultation-liaison" assumed greater prominence in later years. However, the first "handbook" of psychiatric consultation by Schwab (1968) reveals his visits to "over 30 Consultation-Liaison Programs [*sic*] in the United States and Canada in 1962–64" (p. ix), indicating that there was already a robust movement to establish such services in general hospitals. Familiar names in psychiatry appeared in Schwab's descriptions: Knight Aldrich, Klaus Berblinger, Henry Brosin, George Engel, Shervert Frazier, Thomas Hackett, W.E. Meyer, and Eric Wittkower.

Mendel and Solomon's (1968) *The Psychiatric Consultation* asserted that "the increasing importance of psychiatry in many aspects of modern life has brought about the emergence of a new psychiatric discipline, consultation psychiatry"

(p. 215). While we know the rudiments of liaison psychiatry had their beginnings much earlier than this, perhaps this notation evidences an increasing formal acceptance of the discipline. Special designation of the "discipline" appears warranted since consultation to inpatient medical and surgical services requires different skills than those of the psychiatrist practicing mostly psychotherapy in a defined outpatient setting.

In concert with the federal measures of the 1940s, the American Psychiatric Association (APA) acknowledged the need for C-L psychiatry by formally establishing the General Practitioner Education Project, directed by Howard M. Kern, Jr. An outgrowth of this activity was the creation in 1956 of a "liaison committee," titled Committee on Psychiatry and Medical Practice, to sponsor with the Academy of Medical Practice training programs for general practitioners.

Most general hospital C-L services do not provide consultation to health care agencies, industry, or schools, although considerable literature highlights the utility of such psychiatric consultation to these areas (Caplan, 1963). The contributory relationship of general hospital psychiatry and psychosomatic medicine to C-L psychiatry is well known and widely celebrated, but the catalyzing impact of community mental health consultation is regarded more like a "country cousin." In 1963, President John Kennedy, strongly committed to the mental health of Americans, signed into law the Mental Retardation Facilities and Community Mental Health Centers Construction Act. This legislation intended to acknowledge transfer of mental health care from state institutions to community centers and general hospitals. It also designated the objective of *consultation and education* (U.S. Department of Health, Education & Welfare, #1478, 1964), perhaps accelerating interest and activity in C-L services, both in medical schools and in general hospitals.

Throughout the 1960s, this consultation/education component spawned a flood of papers on consultation in the literature, although most were not directly related to consultation in general medical settings. Community mental health centers were not considered entirely successful, but the increased focus on psychiatric consultation redounded to the benefit of C-L psychiatry's growth. The notion that psychiatrists alone could not address the massive mental health needs of the country gave rise to heightened awareness of the need to train other caregivers to assist in the task of "teams." This need impelled greater involvement of primary care physicians, whose education and training in mental health matters posed a task well suited to the skills of C-L psychiatrists.

Consultation and the Primary Care Movement

The 1960s and 1970s saw an energized focus on the role of the C-L psychiatrist in the primary care movement. Textbook publishing flourished with a proliferation of volumes to help primary care physicians integrate mental health interventions in their practices. Michael Balint's (1951) book *The Doctor, His Patient and the*

Illness attracted new interest as Balint Groups sprouted to help general practitioners improve their relationships with patients by enhancing interviewing and communication skills.

An APA Task Force Report on Psychiatric Education and the Primary Physician (APA, 1970) summarized the results of seven "Colloquia for Postgraduate Teaching of Psychiatry" held throughout the 1960s (APA, 1967). In the 1970s, recognizing the primacy of the consulting psychiatrist in these endeavors, the sponsoring Committee on Psychiatry and Medical Practice was renamed the Committee on Psychiatry and Primary Care, soon to be changed again to Committee on Consultation-Liaison Psychiatry and Primary Care Education, thus essentially recognizing and solidifying the evolution from "consultation psychiatry" to "consultation–liaison psychiatry."

Consultation Today

The *Handbook of Consultation-Liaison Psychiatry* (Leigh & Streltzer, 2007) states that "consultation-liaison (CL) [*sic*][2] psychiatry refers to the skills and knowledge utilized in evaluating and treating the emotional and behavioral conditions in patients who are referred from medical and surgical settings" (p. 3). While this describes the broader field, it does not specify who requests the consultation. In this instance, the patient appears the passive recipient of the C-L psychiatrist's ministrations, for in fact it is a rare occurrence in hospital practice that the patient requests psychiatric consultation.

The consultative experience differs in many respects from that of the office psychotherapeutic encounter. While the psychotherapist must deal with the transferences and resistances of only one (or more) patient, the consultant needs to learn to deal tactfully with these aspects and behavioral idiosyncrasies of all constituents of the consultation process. Table 6.1 delineates these differences.

Even the well-trained general psychiatrist, lacking the experience of working with the complex medically ill will require specialized experience and training to qualify as a consulting psychiatrist. Guidelines for such training have existed since the 1970s (Russell, Weinstein & Houpt, 1976–77; Orelans, Houpt & Trent, 1979), further enhanced through C-L or psychosomatic fellowships. When our younger son Steven first entered school, already aware that his older brother knew how to read but not how he arrived at that ability, he said to the teacher, "I'm not like Eric; I have to learn how to read." So it is with C-L fellows who have had little training in consultative techniques, having spent most of their residency learning psychotherapy, psychopharmacology, and other special aspects of psychiatric practice, with perhaps a minimum of experience working in medical settings. Consultation skill does not come automatically—it must be learned. And, having long since completed their training, leaving the rigors of medical and surgical wards of a general hospital, their experience has been largely confined to psychiatric settings, spaces, and personnel. Some may have even repressed the unpleasant

TABLE 6.1 Contrasting/Comparing Consultation-Liaison and Office Psychiatry

C-L	Office
Medical setting; system oriented	Outpatient setting; dyad oriented
Eclectic (not theory)	Theory based
No selection criteria	Selection criteria
Other driven	Patient driven
Low motivation	High motivation
Regressed ("sick role")	Relatively well adapted
Catch-as-catch-can	Consultation room
Variable times	Specific times
Poor confidentiality	Good confidentiality
Patient ill-prepared	Patient well-prepared
Rapid alliance	Attenuated alliance
"Nonworking"	"Working"
Brief intervention	Attenuated intervention
Mostly supportive (abreaction, suggestion, "manipulation")	Mostly expressive (interpretive, insight, "reconstructive")
Transference interpretation rare	Transference interpretation often
Enhance patient-doctor relationship	Enhance coping skills
Improve medical outcome	Improve adaptation
Correct misattributions	Explore fantasies
Shore up defenses	Identify defenses
Diagnosis—"personality," dynamic	Diagnosis—psychiatric, dynamic
Share data with others (staff, MD)	Not shared (to a fault?)

Don R. Lipsitt, M.D.

aspects of internship and need to work through certain reservations about "being back on the wards."

Peteet and Reich (1980) have cogently described the problems in learning C-L psychiatry. Residents who spend most of their training time in dyadic or even group experiences may be less aware of basic consultative work that relies not only on assessment of the patient but also on the involved staff, the consultee, and the particular setting in the general medical hospital. Striking omissions in many residency training programs include diagnosis of organic brain syndromes, stress reactions to illness and hospitalization, appreciation of the value of abbreviated patient contact, and benefits to the caretaking staff members.

Consultation Models

In time, several models of consultation have been defined, each with slightly different focus. Since the expanded definition of C-L psychiatry includes a pedagogical component, each model implicitly or explicitly addresses the nature of the doctor-patient relationship and the physician's contribution to the "problem" (Kahana, 1959). Most models have been built on the original taxonomy by Strain and colleagues (Strain, Pincus, Houpt, Gise & Taintor, 1985) describing six definable models: consultation, liaison, bridge, hybrid, autonomous, and postgraduate. Others have described the patient-centered consultation, the colleague- (or consultee-) centered consultation, the situation-oriented consultation, and the agency-centered consultation (Caplan, 1963; Greenberg, 1960; Schwab, 1968; Solomon, 1968).

The "plain" consultation model has been equated with the fire alarm model in which the response is to a crisis of more or less urgency. Little more is expected of the psychiatrist than to assess the patient's circumstances and make ameliorating recommendations.

The liaison model involves a more comprehensive assessment of the patient's surroundings, staff, and interactions related to his or her illness and reason for requesting the consult. This model includes an expectation on the part of the psychiatrist to provide some level of education, instruction, demonstration, and clarifying explanation to the consultee and staff to assist in the understanding and "management" of the patient's predicament, with special emphasis on the patient-doctor relationship.

The bridge model usually is applied to the consultant's ongoing engagement on a peer-level basis with primary care physicians or with teams functioning in specialized services (e.g., intensive care or cardiac care units, cancer care, obstetric wards, hemodialysis programs, and transplant services). In this model, the psychiatrist functions on a day-to-day basis with the team members.

The hybrid model parallels the bridge model but focuses more on collaborative teaching along with representatives from other disciplines, like psychology, social work, and different medical specialties.

In the autonomous model, an independent psychiatrist may be employed by a medical group to provide consultative service exclusively to that group. While this may be part of the general hospital structure, the psychiatrist most often is not officially part of the hospital's psychiatry department.

The postgraduate specialization model is seen in those instances where a graduate primary care physician will commit to extended training in psychiatry, focused largely on C-L types of services. It can also apply to combined residency training—for example, in medicine and psychiatry or pediatrics and psychiatry.

Many of the elements of good consulting should, of course, be part of every physician's armamentarium, if only there would be sufficient time, adequate training, and appropriate attitude. Psychiatrists would then be available to supplement only those aspects of the interview (consultation) that expand, embellish, and fulfill the "history-taking" exercise. Elements such as identifying transference and countertransference issues, unconscious fantasy, distorted illness attribution, cultural variation, and emotional conflict would then "round out" a proper holistic exploration of the patient's and consultee's needs.

Performance of a good interview/consultation can be not only informative for caretakers but also formative for patients, as they experience interest, respect, attentiveness, listening, and clarification unlike any they may have had in a lifetime! Elements of such experience may include such inquiries as to why the patient comes at a particular time for advice or why his or her physician thinks the patient would benefit from a psychiatrist's visit; what was happening at the time of the visit/hospitalization/consultation; and what the patient thinks is the matter ("attribution"). It may also include more searching inquiries into their fears, feelings, and thoughts; what they have done to obtain relief; and to whom they have talked about their discomfort. The physician's exclusive focus, empathy, and support may themselves go far in relieving much discomfort, fear, anxiety, and uncertainty. Many medical educators have warned students that these aspects of care can easily be overshadowed by technological and pharmacological aids and may be too soon forgotten in the care of the patient (Peabody, 1927).

The quality of a consultation may hinge on the interview itself. Interviewing, as taught in medical school, relates largely to "history taking," not so much to the nuances of personality, patterns of coping, family relations, life experience, and narrative ability of the patient, all of which contribute to illness and disease experience. Skilled techniques are learned in psychiatric training, through intensive supervision of therapeutic intervention. Harry Stack Sullivan's (1953) extensive experience of interviewing psychiatric patients is carefully described in a series of lectures contained in the book *The Interpersonal Theory of Psychiatry*. Sullivan emphasizes the nature of communication and the evolving relationship between the parties involved, a process in which "patterns of living are to be clarified and that in the process benefit may accrue to the client" (p. ix). A skilled interviewer notices mannerisms, linguistic nuance, and nonverbal reactions, not "just answers." Michael Balint is famously quoted for his remark that if the physician (interviewer) only asks questions, all he or she will obtain is answers and nothing else.

A technique developed by Felix Deutsch and William Murphy (1955), derived from psychoanalytic percepts and called the "associative anamnesis," has been employed effectively by interviewers with interest and experience in psychosomatic and psychoanalytic dimensions of medicine. Offering maximum latitude to the patient to respond, the interviewer uses few words to keep the narrative flowing, triggering, without the patient's awareness, revelation of important psychological data. Gerald Caplan (1963)—whose experience has been more with schools, industry, and institutional consulting—has nonetheless written widely of consultation essentials. For example, Caplan cautions that developing as a consultant requires opportunities to reflect on one's own professional life (pp. 21–25).

Psychiatrists attend to this personal aspect through supervision in training as well as through group interaction with primary care physicians in Balint Groups (Lipsitt, 1999) or personal experience in psychotherapy or psychoanalysis. Familiarity with the foundations of the field, as addressed here, broadens the C-L psychiatrist's range of interest and skills as well as appreciation of the life experiences of patients.

Over time, the experience of multiple practitioners with the rudiments of consultation has been consolidated into accepted specific guidelines for effective consultation (Cohen-Cole, Haggerty & Raft, 1982; Gitlin et al. (1996). With the approaching century's end, Lipowski (1991) noted that

> C-L psychiatry has achieved the status of a full-fledged subspecialty of psy-
> chiatry . . . whose main contribution [is] . . . to draw attention of clinicians
> and researchers to psychosocial aspects of physical illness, and to the compli-
> cations of such illness and of the medical and surgical therapies.
>
> *(p. 68)*

Liaison: Secret No Longer

When and how did "liaison" enter the picture? What is the origin of this curious amalgamated specialty called consultation-liaison psychiatry?

As soon as psychiatrists began consulting to their psychiatrically naïve colleagues, they recognized the need for an educational component to their services. While the choice of the word "liaison" may not have been the most felicitous, it had a historical use in the literature for a variety of interactional activities (see, for example Barrett, Pratt, Henry). The word adhered, and, while it may suitably characterize some of the experiences of C-L psychiatrists, it has in some respects become arguably the nemesis of C-L psychiatry (Dimsdale, 1991; Neill, 1983; Strain, 1983).

Following World War II, according to Schwab, changes in concepts of illness and increasing scientific influences catalyzed a surge of interest in "psychiatric consultation work." In their description of the organization of a psychiatric consultation service, Hackett and Weisman (1960, p. 280) described four fundamental principles of the "work": (1) rapid evaluation; (2) the psychodynamic formulation of the major conflict; (3) an effective program for therapy; and (4) the active implementation of that program by the psychiatrist. No mention was made of liaison. In time, increasing experience with such "work" revealed that optimal benefit of a consultation involved more than the doctor-patient interaction; "ancillary" staff other than the consultee were critical participants in a patient's care: ward staff including nurses, house officers, attending physicians, even record-keeping secretarial staff. Different models as described above emerged in different situations, some requiring more emphasis on a systems approach, others minimal involvement of additional personnel. To carry out consultant suggestions often required specialized psychological or psychiatric knowledge not typically part of most physicians' skill set. It became evident that every consultation required more-or-less educational effort in addition to suggestions for management of the patient. In its application to the general hospital setting, the emphasis on education came to be referred to as "liaison." By around 1980, what had previously been referred to simply as "consultation psychiatry" was now referred to as "consultation-liaison psychiatry" (Lipowski, 1970; Schwab, 1968) as a recognized special activity of a select group of psychiatrists.

The "consultation and education" component of the community mental health movement described above stated, "All types of consultation [have] two elements in common, 1) solving a problem and 2) helping involved others to 'improve skills and broaden knowledge' " (U.S. Department of Health, Education & Welfare, #1478, 1964, p. 3), the latter presupposing a "liaison" function of the consultant.

As psychiatry began embedding itself more visibly in the general hospital, psychiatrists gladly assumed the age-old doctor's role as teacher. The word "liaison" to describe this pedagogical function of psychiatric activity had lurked around for many years. Albert Barrett (1922) may have been the first to describe the collaborative clinical work of psychiatrists, probably using language acquired during time in the military during WWI (Lipsitt, 2000, p. 199).

With a multiplicity of engaging meanings, the word was incorporated only four years after Barrett's use in an article by George Pratt (1926), prophesying the psychiatrist's role as a "liaison agent," who would "become the integrator that unifies, clarifies and resolves all available medical knowledge concerning that human being who is the patient, into one great force of healing power" (p. 408). The word had cachet and in just three more years was attached by George Henry (1929–1930) to the concept of "liaison psychiatry" (p. 494). And only a decade later, the first designated "psychiatry liaison service" was founded at the University of Colorado (Billings, 1939), followed closely by a similar program at Massachusetts General Hospital. Descriptions, elaborations, and modifications of C-L services have proliferated in the psychiatric literature as their popularity has risen and fallen.

Roget's twenty-first century thesaurus (Kipfer, 1999, p. 137) offers a wide selection of synonyms for the word liaison: encounter, amour, entanglement, fling, illicit romance, interlude, intrigue, communication, connection, contact, fixer, hookup, interchange, interface, intermediary, link.

As such, the word may apply to many of the challenges of the pedagogical aspects of psychiatric consultation in the work of the C-L psychiatrist. There are those who might see it as "sneaky," insurers as illicit, but for those who engage symbiotically, a pleasant tryst. For the consultant who encounters resistance on the medical ward, effective liaison may require similar skill of wartime negotiations. The linkage, cooperation, and communication at the interface is the most salubrious of all. One writer has referred to the relationship of psychiatry to medicine as a "romance" characterized by "on-again-off-again" relationships (Moore, 1978, p. 413).

Less appreciative terms like "gossip," "hanging around," "busybody," or "wasting time" are extended characterizations of recent times by liaison psychiatrists disappointed in the results and reimburseability of more traditional functions of the liaison service (Dimsdale, 1991; Murray, 1979; Neill, 1983). While American psychiatrists tend to devalue the liaison component of their work, the British, perhaps with Churchillian perseverance, continue to extol great utility in it (Creed, 1991; Guthrie, 2006; Mayou, 1987).

To assure a psychiatric liaison as problem-free as possible, several proponents offer sage advice: do not be pushy or proselytizing (Lipowski, 1968, p. 416); avoid assuming a manipulative role (Greenhill, 1977, p. 179); do not use cute (jargon) or fanciful (psychoanalytic) language (Henry, 1929–1930, p. 492; Oken, 1983)—advice worthy of partners in a secret affair.

Our custom throughout this book will be to refer to the linked C-L discipline without further extensive description. Excellent reviews of the liaison component exist for the interested reader (Oken, 1983; Lloyd, 1987; Lipowski, 2002; Greenhill, 1977; Friedman & Molay 1994). A superb detailed step-by-step account of the consultation process is available in Stotland and Garrick's *Manual of Psychiatric Consultation* (1990), a small volume that might profitably be in the library, if not pocket, of every beginning C-L psychiatrist or fellow. Another helpful account of the consultation technique is the chapter by Lackamp in *Psychosomatic Medicine and Consultation-Liaison Psychiatry* (Amos & Robinson, 2010). A more lighthearted but thoroughly competent exegesis of the consultation process can be found in *Sigmoidoscopy: Medical-Psychiatric Consultation-Liaison: The Bases* (Robinson, 1999).

Approaching the turn of the century, with the role of psychiatric consultation well ensconced in the training experience, considerable deliberation and robust controversy over questionable distinctions between liaison, consultation, and psychosomatic medicine had ensued, and the stage was set to entertain ideas of specialty recognition. Subsequent chapters will address the foundations of this meandering path from "consultation" to "psychiatric consultation" to "consultation-liaison" to "psychosomatic medicine."

Notes

1 Cushing, 1950; Bibring, 1956; Butler & Perlin, 1958; Greenhill & Kilgore, 1950; Grotjahn & Treusch, 1957; Kaufman, 1953; Kahana, 1959; Schiff & Pilot, 1959; Schmale, 1958; Schwartz, 1958.
2 This book uses the abbreviation C-L throughout (cf. Lipsitt, 1991) rather than any used by others.

References

Alexander, F.G., & Selesnick, S.T. (1966). *The History of Psychiatry*. New York, NY: The New American Library (Mentor).

American Psychiatric Association. (1967). *Colloquium for Postgraduate Teaching of Psychiatry.* Washington, DC: American Psychiatric Association.

American Psychiatric Association Task Force. (1970). *Report on Psychiatric Education and the Primary Physician.* Washington, DC: American Psychiatric Association.

Balint, M. (1951). *The Doctor, His Patient and the Illness.* New York, NY: International Universities Press.

Barrett, A.M. (1922). The broadened interests of psychiatry. *American Journal of Psychiatry, 79,* 1–13.

Bibring, G.L. (1956). Psychiatry and medical practice in a general hospital. *New England Journal of Medicine, 254,* 366–372.

Billings, E.G. (1939). Liaison psychiatry and intern instruction. *Journal of the Association of American Medical Colleges, 14,* 375–385.

Butler, R.N., & Perlin, S. (1958). Psychiatric consultations in a research setting. *Medical Annals of District of Columbia, 27,* 503–506.

Campbell, R.J. (1996). *Psychiatric Dictionary.* (7th edition). New York, NY: Oxford University Press.

Caplan, G. (1963). *The Theory and Practice of Mental Health Consultation.* New York, NY: Basic Books.

Cohen-Cole, S., Haggerty, J., & Raft, D. (1982). Objectives for residents in consultation psychiatry: Recommendations of a task force. *Psychosomatics, 23,* 699–703.

Creed, F. (1991). Liaison psychiatry for the 21st century: A review. *Journal of the Royal Society of Medicine, 84,* 414–417.

Cushing, J.G. (1950). The role of the psychiatrist as a consultant. *American Journal of Psychiatry, 106,* 861–864.

De Mandeville, B. (1711[1976]). *A Treatise of the Hypochondriack and Hysterick Passions.* London, UK: Dryden Leach (New York, NY: Arno Press).

Deutsch, F., & Murphy, W. (1955). *The Psychiatric Interview.* New York, NY: International Universities Press.

Dimsdale, J.E. (1991). Challenges, problems and opportunities in consultation-liaison psychiatry. *Psychiatric Medicine, 9,* 641–648.

Friedman, R.S., & Molay, F. (1994). A history of psychiatric consultation in America. *Psychiatric Clinics of North America, 17,* 667–681.

Gitlin, D.F, Schindler, B.A., Stern, T.A., Epstein, S.A., Lamdan, R.M., McCarty, T., . . . Stiebel, V.G. (1996). *Psychosomatics, 37,* 3–11.

Greenberg, I.M. (1960). Approaches to psychiatric consultation in a research hospital setting. *Archives of General Psychiatry, 3,* 691–697.

Greenhill, M.H. (1977). The development of liaison programs. In G. Usdin (Ed.). *Psychiatric Medicine.* (pp. 115–191). New York, NY: Brunner/Mazel.

Greenhill, M.H., & Kilgore, S.R. (1950). Principles of methodology in teaching the psychiatric approach to medical house officers. *Psychosomatic Medicine, 12,* 38–48.

Grotjahn, M., & Treusch, J.V. (1957). A new technique of psychosomatic consultations: Some illustrations of teamwork between an internist and a psychiatrist: A practical approach to psychosomatic medicine. *Psychoanalytic Review, 44,* 176–192.

Guthrie, E. (2006). Psychological treatments in liaison psychiatry: The evidence base. *Clinical Medicine, 6,* 544–547.

Hackett, T.P. (1978). Beginnings: Liaison psychiatry in a general hospital. In T.P. Hackett & N.H. Cassem (Eds.). *Massachusetts General Hospital Handbook of General Hospital Psychiatry.* (pp. 1–13). St. Louis, MO: C.V. Mosby Co.

Hackett, T.P., & Cassem, N.H. (Eds.). (1978). *Massachusetts General Hospital Handbook of General Hospital Psychiatry.* St. Louis, MO: The C.V. Mosby Co.

Hackett, T.P., & Weisman, A.D. (1960). Psychiatric management of operative syndromes. I. The therapeutic consultation and the effect of noninterpretive intervention. *Psychosomatic Medicine, 21,* 267–282.

Harrington, J.T. (1990). *Consultation in Internal Medicine.* Toronto: B.C. Decker, Inc.

Henry, G.W. (1929–1930). Some modern aspects of psychiatry in a general hospital practice. *American Journal of Psychiatry, 9,* 481–499.

Kahana, R.J. (1959). Teaching medical psychology through psychiatric consultation. *Journal of Medical Education, 34,* 1003–1009.

Kaufman, M.R. (1953). The role of the psychiatrist in a general hospital. *Psychiatric Quarterly, 27,* 367–381.

Kaufman, M.R., & Margolin, S.G. (1948). Theory and practice of psychosomatic medicine in a general hospital. *Medical Clinics of North America, 32,* 611–616.

Kipfer, B.A. (Ed). (1999). *Roget's Thesaurus.* (2nd edition). New York, NY: Barnes & Noble.

Kubie, L.S. (1944). The organization of a psychiatric service for a general hospital. *Psychosomatic Medicine, 6,* 252–272.

Lackamp, J.M. (2010). The consultation process. In J.J. Amos & R.G. Robinson (Eds.). *Psychosomatic Medicine: An Introduction to Consultation-Liaison Psychiatry.* (pp. 1–14). Cambridge, UK: Cambridge University Press.

Leigh, H., & Streltzer, J. (2007). *Handbook of Consultation-Liaison Psychiatry.* New York, NY: Springer.

Levine, M. (1943). *Psychotherapy in Medical Practice.* New York, NY: The Macmillan Company.

Lewis, N.D.C., & Engle, B. (1954). *Wartime Psychiatry: A Compendium of the International Literature.* New York, NY: Oxford University Press.

Lipowski, Z.J. (1968). Review of consultation psychiatry and psychosomatic medicine. III. Theoretical issues. *Psychosomatic Medicine, 30,* 395–422.

Lipowski, Z.J. (1970). New perspectives in psychosomatic medicine. *Canadian Psychiatric Association Journal, 15,* 515–525.

Lipowski, Z.J. (1991). Consultation-liaison psychiatry 1990. *Psychotherapy and Psychosomatics, 55,* 62–68.

Lipowski, Z.J. (2002). History of consultation-liaison psychiatry. In M.W. Wise & J.R. Rundell (Eds.). *The American Psychiatric Publishing Textbook of Consultation-Liaison Psychiatry: Psychiatry in the Medically Ill.* (pp. 3–11). Washington, DC: American Psychiatric Publishing.

Lipsitt, D.R. (1991). Coming of age: Hyphen or slash? Editorial. *General Hospital Psychiatry, 13,* 149.

Lipsitt, D.R. (1999). Michael Balint's group approach: The Boston Balint group. *Group, 23,* 187–201.

Lipsitt, D.R. (2000). Psyche and soma: Struggles to close the gap. In R.W. Menninger & J.C. Nemiah (Eds.). *American Psychiatry after World War II. 1944–1994.* (pp. 152–186). Washington, DC: American Psychiatric Press.

Lloyd, G. (1987). Developments in liaison psychiatry in the United Kingdom. *Psychotherapy and Psychosomatics, 48,* 90–95.

Mayou, R. (1987). A British view of liaison psychiatry. *General Hospital Psychiatry, 9,* 18–24.

Mendel, W.M., & Solomon, P. (1968). *The Psychiatric Consultation.* New York, NY: Grune & Stratton.

Moore, G.L. (1978). The adult psychiatrist in the medical environment. *American Journal of Psychiatry, 135,* 413–419.

Murray, G.B. (1979). Ethical problems in liaison psychiatry. *Psychiatric Annals, 9,* 75–79.

Neill, J.R. (1983). Once more into the breach: Doubts about liaison psychiatry. *General Hospital Psychiatry, 5,* 205–208.

Oken, D. (1983). Liaison psychiatry (liaison medicine). *Advances in Psychosomatic Medicine, 11,* 23–51.

Orelans, C.S., Houpt, J.L., & Trent, P.J. (1979). Models for evaluating teaching in consultation-liaison psychiatry: III. Conclusion-oriented research. *General Hospital Psychiatry, 1,* 322–329.

Peabody, F. (1927). The care of the patient. *Journal of the American Medical Association, 88,* 877–882.

Peteet, J., & Reich, P. (1980). Problems in learning consultation/liaison psychiatry. *McLean Hospital Journal, 5,* 33–36.

Pope, A. (1711). *An Essay on Criticism.* Retrieved June 21, 2015 via Wikipedia.org.

Pratt, G.K. (1926). Psychiatric departments in general hospitals. *American Journal of Psychiatry, 82,* 403–410.

Putnam, J.J. (1910). Personal experiences with Freud's psychoanalytic method. *Journal of Nervous and Mental Disease, 37,* 630–639.

Robinson, D.J. (1999). *Sigmoidoscopy: Medical-Psychiatric Consultation-Liaison: The Bases.* Port Huron, MI: Rapid Psychler Press.

Russell, M.L, Weinstein, H.M., & Houpt, J.L. (1976–1977). The application of competency-based education to consultation-liaison psychiatry: III. Implications. *International Journal of Psychiatry in Medicine, 7,* 321–328.

Schiff, S.K., & Pilot, M.L. (1959). An approach to psychiatric consultation in the general hospital. *Archives of General Psychiatry, 1,* 349–357.

Schmale, A.H., Jr. (1958). Relationship of separation and depression to disease. I. A report on a hospitalized medical population. *Psychosomatic Medicine, 20,* 259–277.

Schwab, J.J. (1968). *Handbook of Psychiatric Consultation.* New York, NY: Appleton-Century-Crofts.

Schwartz, L.A. (1958). Application of psychosomatic concepts by a liaison psychiatrist on a medical service. *Journal of the Michigan Medical Society, 57,* 1547–1552.

Sjostrand, L. (2001). Hippocrates's evaluation in the madness of Democritus. *Svensk Medicinhistoriska Tidskrift, 5,* 117–130.

Solomon, P. (1968). The psychiatric consultation in private practice. *Medical Annals of the District of Columbia, 37,* 322–323.

Stotland, N.L., & Garrick, T.R. (1990). *Manual of Psychiatric Consultation.* Washington, DC: American Psychiatric Press.

Strain, J.J. (1981). Benefits of liaison psychiatry. *American Journal of Psychiatry, 138,* 1636–1637.

Strain, J.J. (1983). Liaison psychiatry and its dilemmas. *General Hospital Psychiatry, 5,* 209–212.

Strain, J.J., Pincus, H.A., Houpt, J.L, Gise, L.H., & Taintor, Z. (1985). Models of mental health training for primary care physicians. *Psychosomatic Medicine, 47,* 95–110.

Sullivan, H.S. (1953). *The Interpersonal Theory of Psychiatry.* New York, NY: W.W. Norton & Co.

U.S. Department of Health, Education & Welfare. (1964). Consultation and education. *Public Health Service Publication #1478.* Washington, DC: US Department of Health, Education and Welfare.

Usherwood, T. (1999). *Understanding the Consultation: Evidence, Theory and Practice.* Buckingham, UK: Open University Press.

Witmer, H.L. (1947). *Teaching Psychotherapeutic Medicine.* New York, NY: Commonwealth Fund.

SECTION II
Crises and Benefactors

Preamble: *However contributory to the foundations of C-L psychiatry have been philosophy, physiology, psychoanalysis, psychosomatic medicine, and epidemiology—each in its own way—the ultimate growth and sustenance of the field relies heavily on fiscal realities. C-L psychiatrists came late to an appreciation of the importance of money in sustaining their enterprise. They were originally accustomed to plying their skills in eleemosynary institutions where "money was not the issue," and, had it not been for the funding support of occasional benefactors, the whole endeavor may not have survived. This section reviews the ins and outs and ups and downs of economic windfalls and perils that have continually plagued the field. Foundation support has indeed been "foundational."*

Nevertheless, money alone is not sufficient. Without the interest, innovation, curiosity, and creativity of dedicated individuals, the early seeds of C-L psychiatry may not have taken root. This section also pays tribute to those early benefactors who have established the pedestal upon which others have built. It concludes with a review of the fiscal trials and tribulations with which C-L psychiatry has contended throughout its history.

7

"FOUNDATIONAL SUPPORT"

When They Say It Isn't the Money

Introduction

Medical education before the mid-twentieth century did not prepare graduates well for the economics of their profession, with both good and bad consequences. Rarely did we inquire how care was paid for or indeed how we ourselves might be compensated. We were privileged to be able to enter the profession and to focus on caring for patients, especially in hospitals where faceless "administrators" necessarily looked after the essentials of running an institution. On the plus side, our naiveté freed us to learn, to take time with patients, to attend to paperwork that essentially recorded data related only to patient care, rarely to requirements of billing departments or external regulators and insurers. The downside was the peril of trying to maintain a system where finances influence survival.

Certainly, the growth and development of C-L psychiatry has relied on suitable financial support. The vicissitudes of funding decidedly represent a profound foundational aspect of the history of the specialty. As an administrator of a psychiatry department, with all of its many demands, the matter of institutional and economic support required a disproportionate allocation of my time. Negotiating with administrators, insufficiently compensated staff, other department heads, billing departments, insurers, and managed care companies was a taxing and vexing activity. A lack of suitable supportive "talking points" from valid research made the task all the more difficult!

For the most part, C-L psychiatry depended on "the kindness of strangers" to keep it afloat. Rarely did practitioners themselves delve into these murky waters. Atypically, in 1937, Billings's clinical group in Colorado made early forays into calculating the cost and value of consulting a medical patient in the general hospital. At the time, this was a kind of curiosity, something to prove its practicality and to be noted in the breach, not in its quotidian application. With patients whose average hospital cost was $52, Billings wrote that psychiatric consultation shaved an impressive $4.68 off that total cost! (Billings, McNary & Rees, 1937).

C-L psychiatry was fortunate to be the early beneficiary of several major sources of financial support: the Rockefeller Foundation via the young Dr. Alan Gregg, Kate Macy Ladd and the Josiah Macy Jr. Foundation, and perhaps, to a lesser extent, foundations like the Commonwealth Fund. Subsequently, the Education Branch of the National Institute of Mental Health, under Dr. James Eaton's directorship, provided a major financial thrust. It was perhaps only when the latter funding was exhausted that C-L psychiatrists were jolted into awareness that their very livelihood and that of the profession could not survive without research that could demonstrate the specialty's value. I will address each of these seminal events.

I. Alan Gregg and Rockefeller Largesse

> *To give away money is an easy matter and in any man's power. But to decide to whom to give it and how large and when, and for what purpose and how, is neither in every man's power nor an easy matter.*
>
> —*Aristotle (nptrust.org)*

The First World War had left the economy reeling and short of funds, so that in the years between 1920 and 1940 services were especially dependent on non-governmental support. Not only philanthropic largesse but also developments in medicine, political turmoil, and war conflated to bring change to the fields of medical research and practice. In addition to the United States, Europe and the Far East became as much an interest to philanthropists as did the more domestic issues. The Rockefeller Foundation (RF) was not the only philanthropy interested in world events; others included the Josiah Macy Jr. Foundation, the Milbank Memorial Fund, the Commonwealth Fund, and the Rosenwald Fund.

But Rockefeller stood out, especially in its support of psychiatry. Philanthropies were focused on projects that would have worldwide influence. Rockefeller wealth extended to many studies, fellowships, and projects in Europe, Latin America, and China in pursuit of John D. Rockefeller Senior's admirable but arguably grandiose notion of introducing "scientific medicine" to the entire world. Some critics had referred to the laudable instincts of a "robber baron," while others attributed this behavior to charitable commitments instilled in him since childhood.

While Rockefeller interests ranged far and wide, our focus here will be largely on ways in which they affected psychiatry. With psychiatry in a high degree of disarray in the 1930s, the infusion of funds by Doctor Alan Gregg of the Rockefeller Foundation offered a saving grace. The profound influence of the Rockefeller family, both directly and indirectly, upon the establishment of C-L psychiatry cannot be underestimated. Although it was Dr. Alan Gregg, a socially minded Harvard Medical School graduate, through whom the Rockefeller largesse flowed, the vicissitudes that nurtured and directed this flow comprise in itself a fascinating story.

Tracing the "genealogy" of psychiatry's benefaction in the behemoth philanthropic Rockefeller Foundation is no easy task. Chernow (1998) had written that "to delve into the voluminous Rockefeller papers is to excavate a lost continent" (p. xv). During the early years of psychiatry's development, Rockefeller philanthropies were likely the largest in the world, surpassing even the Carnegie Foundation, from which it took its inspiration. The father of the senior John D. Rockefeller, William "Doc" Rockefeller, had been publicly exposed as a snake-oil salesman, "styling himself a 'botanic physician' or 'herbal doctor' " (p. 11), a con man with a history of imposturing, fake "credentials," bigamy, even an unlitigated rape charge (pp. 28–29). Until the press sleuthed him out as "Dr. Levingstone," living and "working" in North Dakota, he had remained a "family secret" of which John Senior had been much ashamed and embarrassed. Assiduously dodging any open discussion of his father, he nonetheless harbored a vigorous conflictual ambivalence toward him, feeling curiously indebted to "Doc Bill" for his self-reliance and penchant for earning money on the one hand but decrying his miscreant amoral behavior on the other (p. 32).

During his long life, John experienced many minor ailments and turned largely to patent medicines and herbals, and—after meeting a homeopathic physician whom he befriended for life—he became a robust advocate of homeopathic medicine, a form of medicine that had gained some popularity in the latter part of the nineteenth century. His homeopathic physician friend was branded by others a likely charlatan or at least an inept physician. Shades of old Doc Bill! Nonetheless, John not only defended his friend but, in the philanthropic phase of his life, supported the establishment of the Homeopathic Medical College, becoming a trustee and vice president of that institution.

John shunned regular physicians in preference for "alternative" treatments until, during a prolonged absence of his homeopathic physician, he allowed himself to be treated by a Harvard Medical School physician who cured a recurrent hydrocele that his homeopath told him was entirely incurable. He subsequently nurtured greater respect for physicians of a more orthodox stripe, but he never relinquished his interest in "traditional" practitioners, in spite of advice from people in his family and his employ that homeopathy was "quackery" and that he should abolish his reliance on such medical deception.

Even in his reverence for this preferred homeopathic "treatment," it was testament to his respect for his advisors that he nonetheless was able to defer to and heartily support those responsible for allocating his philanthropic funds to what he regarded as "the best minds" and researchers that could be found in medical science. Rockefeller money was funneled first through the General Education Board (GEB), founded in 1902, and, later, the RF, founded in 1913, seeding not only the University of Chicago but also the Rockefeller Institute for Medical Research (RIMR).

Simon Flexner was recruited to direct the RIMR, later named head of Rockefeller University; Flexner recommended Richard Pearce to direct the Division of Medical Education; Pearce had actually been hired at University of Pennsylvania by Simon Flexner when the latter was head of the Department of Pathology before moving to head RIMR. Pearce recruited Raymond Fosdick, Abraham Flexner, Simon's brother, and Alan Gregg to the GEB. Pearce hired Gregg as his assistant; Gregg would ultimately become director of the Division of Medical Sciences. Fosdick later became a president of the foundation. It all sounds rather "incestuous," but the foundation had many irons in the fire and wished to take advantage of these brilliant, multitalented people in a variety of roles. The multiple interests of these few inner-directed pioneers at times became a problem for Gregg; his private letters often referred to the crossed boundaries, headstrong positions, or distracting pursuits of his colleagues. And when he and his wife purchased a home in Scarsdale, he wrote to a friend how good it felt to be able to hammer a nail in the wall or pull a flower from the garden without having to go through other controlling hoops. Although Abraham Flexner had been "squeezed out" of his place in the GEB in 1928 to found the Institute of Advanced Studies at Princeton, he nonetheless continued to offer sometimes unwanted "advice" to Gregg from that perch.

When John Senior was edging into retirement during World War I, John Junior began to assume responsibility not only for the business aspects of the Rockefeller fortune but more especially for the philanthropic objectives of John Senior's life. Young John (Junior) had been plagued with uncertainties and anxieties about his responsibilities, searching for his own identity in his adoring yet strained relationship with his father.

Junior cultivated an interest in mental illness. He himself had suffered a variety of ills, on at least one occasion experiencing deep depression and exhaustion, described as a "breakdown," for which he sought help from "nerve specialists" in Europe. He had weathered his own father's "breakdown" years earlier. And a sister, Edith, plagued with many phobias, had been treated in Europe—not entirely successfully—by Karl Jung. The senior Rockefeller, having met Jung on one occasion, openly regarded the practice of psychoanalysis with some suspicion and as so much "mumbo jumbo." He nonetheless "tolerated" this treatment of his daughter in response to her husband Harold's reports that such intervention had rendered her a "new woman" and had been helpful to him as well. They had both sought help at the Burgholzli in Zurich after the devastating loss of their four-year old son from scarlet fever. Affected by the loss of a favorite grandchild, John Senior dealt with his sorrow by helping to set up a memorial fund to study the causes of scarlet fever. Edith became a strong disciple of Jung and subsequently, with Jung's encouragement, a psychoanalyst herself, establishing a rather unorthodox practice in Switzerland and later in Chicago. Senior was always fascinated with medicine, although one may speculate how much was related to compensatory feelings about his father's dubious activities and how much to the death of Edith and Harold's child, his favored grandson.

Dr. Alan Gregg's "Preparation"

Louis Pasteur said, "[C]hance favors only the prepared mind." In that regard Alan Gregg was certainly prepared to believe that psychiatry and psychosomatic medicine were potentially fruitful beneficiaries of Rockefeller philanthropy.

It is challenging to speculate how Junior's experience influenced him to endorse Dr. Alan Gregg to oversee the dispensing of funds in support of research into psychosomatic medicine. In the 1930s, after the stock market crash and the ensuing depression, psychiatry began to locate in general hospitals as an outgrowth of criticism of the asylum system of care, increasingly viewed by organized psychiatry as at least inadequate and probably unethical and inhumane. Although general hospitals had predated mental asylums, they curiously experienced a period of most rapid growth through the depression years. Rising public disgruntlement with the squalid conditions of asylums and a surge of moral concern began a long examination of state hospitals and a desire for alternative treatment.

Mental patients began to be diverted from asylums to settings capable of providing more humanitarian and comprehensive care closer to their communities. In 1873, a government survey counted fewer than 200 hospitals. But by 1910 over four thousand had been established, their numbers swelling to more than 6,000 by 1920, believed to be due in part to the difficulty of family members to care for the sick at home (Starr, 1982, p. 75). Interest in hospitals and health care was also fueled by social and political debate over the desire for universal health insurance (a debate that never ceases!).

The depression years saw 2,500 banks fail and five million people unemployed. A popular song was "Brother, Can You Spare a Dime?" In the news was Amelia Earhart's transatlantic solo flight, the kidnapping of Charles Lindbergh's baby, the election of Franklin Delano Roosevelt, and the repeal of prohibition. While Hitler's menacing policies began to envelop Europe, people in the United States were being entertained by the *Wizard of Oz* and *Fantasia*. The Three Stooges became a popular comedy act, and hit tunes of 1934 included "Cocktails for Two" and "On the Good Ship Lollipop." Roosevelt signed the Social Security Act in 1935 and was reelected in a landslide in 1936. In this setting, FDR's proposals for Social Security and welfare programs met with enthusiastic endorsement. With a mix of fear and uncertainty, people looked to their government for aid and comfort. The times were good and bad.

For psychiatry in the 1930s, Dr. Alan Gregg emerged as a virtual "white knight." He was a major decision maker in the allocation of Rockefeller funds, but it was not as though his interests were parochially fixated on the needs of psychiatry. He made large philanthropic concessions to the humanities, to agriculture, to education, to public health, and to other worthy causes. His interest in and support of psychiatry at a time when its reputation was not all that glowing was a bold and courageous gesture, but he must have known that it would gain the approval of John Junior if not John's father. And indeed it did, in spite of Senior's insistence on the importance of homeopathy.

What series of events prepared Gregg's mind to be so open to the problems and prospects of psychiatry? As a Harvard College undergraduate, he had attended Freud's epochal lectures at Worcester's Clark University in 1909, even attending the postlecture gathering at James Jackson Putnam's farm in New Hampshire, where the psychiatric eminent congregated. Gregg graduated Harvard Medical School in 1916 and completed one year of postgraduate training in internal medicine at Massachusetts General Hospital. There he once again encountered Professor James Jackson Putnam, the neurologist who had arranged the Freud visit and lectures and was responsible for the early development and acceptance of psychoanalysis in America. Putnam was also described as a kind of psychiatric consultant at "the General" (Hackett, 1978, pp. 2–3).

In his general medical experience, Gregg had exposure to Dr. Francis Weld Peabody (1927), the highly revered professor of medicine whose humanitarian sensitivities found expression in the much-quoted paper "The care of the patient." Young Gregg was also intrigued with the neurophysiological work of Walter Cannon at Harvard and with Charles Scott Sherrington when he received an honorary Harvard degree in 1906 for his work on neuronal synapses.

Judging himself a relatively poor student in the basic science years, Gregg blossomed in the clinical years at Harvard. When he was particularly critical of his own performance, his morale was bolstered by encouraging comments from his older psychiatrist brother Donald. Alan developed a habit of writing his observations in notebooks and was especially sensitive to the qualities that made "good" and "bad" doctors. On one occasion, he noted how he was "thunderstruck" at the "colossal rudeness and stupidity . . . of a certain professor of medicine in a well-known American medical school" (Penfield, 1967, p. 68). In another entry, he observed in himself "a very definite ignorance of the complexities and the elusiveness of psychosomatic conditions although I had already acquired a very definite interest in psychiatry" (p. 69). Pursuing that interest, he chose a fourth-year elective at the Boston Psychopathic Hospital (the "Psycho"), where he wrote of the "intelligent way" things were done there and where he had been tutored by Dr. Elmer Southard, the hospital's chief and Harvard's professor of neuropathology, with whom he was able to discuss cases. He wrote in his notebook, "I just reveled in this complete freedom, and with it I was able to develop a major interest in psychiatry, a new field at that time where practically nobody was at work" (p. 69).

Gregg particularly enjoyed discovering the "hidden struggles of mind and body" in his patients. He wrote, "[W]hat you learn applies to the minds of the sick as well as to their bodies" (Penfield, 1967, p. 74). It comes as little surprise that the woman he courted and subsequently married was training at Smith College and later Johns Hopkins to become a psychiatric social worker; she would treat emotionally disturbed soldiers returning from war (p. 101). In another entry, he wrote, "They were being instructed [at Hopkins] by Freudian analysts, but also by the best of the conservative psychiatrists, such as Professors McFie Campbell [later moving to Boston's "Psycho"—au.] and the great Adolf Meyer" (p. 101).

Gregg practiced medicine for only a year, and part of that was with the Harvard Medical Unit attached to the British Army in World War I between 1917 and 1919. Returning from the war, he somewhat reluctantly approached the head of Rockefeller's International Health Commission (IHC), whose director offered him a choice of several public health projects around the world. He enthusiastically chose Brazil, throwing himself energetically into studying and treating hookworm. There he met Dr. Richard Pearce, who as a member of the Foundation's IHC had been dispatched several times to Brazil on the hookworm project.

Gregg and Pearce found common interests as both were Harvard medical graduates, Pearce having interned at Boston City Hospital. He was a pathologist and had done graduate study in Leipzig in infectious disease, at which institution there was great interest in psychiatry. Pearce became director at the foundation of a newly established division to study medical education and, very impressed with Gregg, arranged for him to come to the RF in 1922 to serve as his assistant. Gregg felt inadequate for the job but wanted to be back in the United States and closer to his family, where his father was ailing, so he eagerly accepted. With Pearce away much of the time, Gregg dealt with most of the business and felt at times that he was simply "minding the store" rather than developing new plans. His father died a short time later, and, at the age of 32, just a few months later, Alan married.

With hardly time either to grieve or to enjoy his new marriage, his first assignment as Pearce's assistant was as a traveling fellow, surveying medical education in Ireland, Italy, Norway, Iceland, Russia, Sweden, Finland, and Greece in the years 1925 to 1930. He remained Pearce's associate director of the Division of Medical Education (DME) from 1922 to 1930. Pearce died in 1930, the Board of Trustees renamed the DME the Division of Medical Science, and Gregg was appointed director of that division.

Rocky Times at the Institute

All institutions, the Rockefeller organization being no exception, experience internal squabbles, politics, rivalries, ambitions, and competitions in ideas, objectives, and finances. Another newly established division, the Division of Natural Science, was angling to absorb not only biological but also social sciences, and Gregg was concerned that, in his new position, he might lose some of his base. He had been given a mandated mission to focus support for medical research over and above the customary institutional grants. Both he and Pearce, through their travels to Europe and other countries reviewing medical education systems, were probably the best informed of such activities of any in the world.

When Gregg first arrived on the Rockefeller scene, he encountered the Flexner brothers, who became a source of some consternation for him. Simon was head of the RIMR and a member of the Board of Trustees, and younger brother Abraham had joined the General Education Board about the time Gregg came on board. Much excitement was stirring over the reaction to Abraham Flexner's

1910 Report on Medical Education in the United States and Canada, later simply referred to as the "Flexner Report." The excitement drained attention away from other foundation projects, and, as Chernow summarized, at this important moment of transition at the RF, "medicine and education had merged as the top priorities of the Rockefeller philanthropies when the two trends fruitfully dovetailed" (Chernow, 1998, p. 491). The lessons learned from the Flexner Report, funded initially by the Carnegie Foundation, were now being implemented by the RF. Abraham was encouraged to begin a process of upgrading selected medical schools around the country, with improvement in many schools and the closing of others. Stringent requirements and guidelines were established, following the Johns Hopkins model. "Medical schools that wanted Rockefeller grants had to upgrade entrance standards, institute four year programs, and adopt the full-time teaching approach" (p. 491). Johns Hopkins Medical School, where Simon Flexner had first begun teaching as professor of pathological anatomy, would become an important contributor to American psychiatry as well as to C-L psychiatry.

Flexner's ambition tended to overshadow other projects. He wanted to continue to fund medical schools, but it was part of Pearce's legacy that he thought there should be support of individual investigators, not just institutions and programs, a notion that Gregg strongly embraced. It was a difficult setting in which a newcomer was challenged to hold on to strong ideas, although what seemed good for medical schools seemed good for psychiatry. By some serendipitous coincidence, Raymond Fosdick had become president of the foundation at the time that Gregg became director of the Division of Medical Science, and Fosdick supported him in his interests and objectives. Fosdick and Max Mason, successive presidents of the foundation, had both had psychiatric problems in their families, which may have furthered the move to keep psychiatry as a central focus. Both wives had committed suicide, and Fosdick's wife had tragically killed their children (Schneider, 2002, p. 38).

"This movement to universalize the Johns Hopkins model proceeded even though it had one highly disgruntled critic: John D. Rockefeller, Sr., who still waged a lonely battle for an alternate form of medicine. 'I am a homeopathist,' he complained" (Chernow, 1998, p. 492), probably in obeisance to old "Doc Bill." He wanted to be assured that all medical schools to which he contributed would show fair and liberal treatment toward homeopaths. But he did not contradict those whom he employed to make important decisions about medical education. In his deference to them, he said that he was "too soft-hearted" to judge such matters.

Flexner intended to eliminate all schools of homeopathy, in spite of Senior's interest in them. The ensuing tumult in the foundation nearly overshadowed the work of Pearce and Gregg in the Medical Science Division, but Gregg's instinct for making estimable decisions between 1930 and 1951 must have pleased both the Junior and Senior Rockefellers, for he was made vice president of the foundation in 1951.

By the time Abraham Flexner left the Rockefeller Foundation in 1928, he had been able to attract $78 million to promote the scientific development of medical education. "The sum total of these developments resulted in nothing less than a revolution in medical education. Doc Rockefeller's son had banished laggards from the profession and introduced a new era of enlightenment in American medicine" (Chernow, 1998, p. 493), dispensing over $130 million since the Flexner Report. The report, according to Chernow, dealt a "lethal blow" to homeopathic schools (p. 492).

In this heady and competitive climate, many of the programs of the Division of Medical Education had been stripped away by other divisions, and psychiatry was one of the few remaining. At one point, Gregg, in despair and weary of the strains in the New York office, had expressed thoughts of resigning and returning to public health. Schools of public health had been founded at Harvard and Johns Hopkins at the same time the Rockefeller Foundation was chartered. Gregg's experience in public health had been strong, and he was considered for an assistant deanship at Johns Hopkins School of Public Health. In such moments of discouragement he was again supported by his psychiatrist brother Donald. In spite of his dedicated purpose, it seemed at times almost by default that Gregg was able to focus on psychiatry as his predominant funding interest. The transition from hookworm to psychiatry may seem a strange evolution, but his autobiographical descriptions note that his two special interests were psychiatry and public health.

The Picture Brightens

When the Board of Trustees began to see that after the war many of the institutions they had been funding were beginning to be able to support themselves, they approved the idea of supporting individuals who showed exceptional promise and who might influence the direction of medical education through a younger group of medical scientists. Gregg was pleased with the reorganization that eliminated much fragmentation. Abraham Flexner had left for Princeton University; the Division of Medical Education had been completely folded into the Division of Medical Sciences; a new president of the foundation was in place; and Gregg had full support of John Junior to proceed with his own ideas. Junior had begun to have more involvement, and his friend Raymond Fosdick, brother of Riverside Church's Reverend Harry Emerson Fosdick, was a strong advocate for strengthening the dedication to the development of psychiatry. A member of the board, Dean David Edsall of Harvard Medical School, chaired a committee to develop a plan of action for the work in the medical sciences, approving a shift in direction toward individuals, groups, and departments "to advance research and medical knowledge" (Schneider, 2002, p. 33). Edsall expressed interest in Gregg's ideas about psychiatry at board meetings, identifying it as one of four subjects requiring general help in developing research. In this new vibrant climate, Gregg's hopes were revived!

Actually, the board had already been introduced to Gregg's interest in psychiatry in the mid-1920s and had begun to show "some evidence of a new general interest in the 'science of the mind' " (Schneider, 2002, p. 40). While Gregg was doing his surveys in Europe for Pearce, he had visited Emil Kraepelin's clinic and other research institutes. On return, with Simon Flexner's strong support, he and Pearce persuaded the foundation to fund both Kraepelin's Institute for Psychiatric Research in Munich and an institute of brain research in Berlin. Flexner's support was based on his belief that helping a few clinics in Europe could serve as training models for Americans to promote psychiatry in their own country (p. 40). Pearce, having shifted his interest away from funding large institutions, had not been enthusiastic about this allocation of resources but was nonetheless agreeable to Gregg's conviction that the division should support "the concentrated investigation of a single subject in medicine" (p. 40). In 1925, Gregg recorded in his personal notes, "The beginnings of a study of the field of psychiatry, which my visit to Kraepelin's clinic provided, is something I have in mind developing, in relation to other branches of medicine" (Schneider, 2002, p. 39). This small triumph gave Gregg renewed impetus to engage the foundation's officers and trustees to debate and consider new priorities, including psychiatry and mental health. The shift from attention to reforming medical schools a la Flexner toward the support of individual researchers themselves had begun (p. 33).

The transition to a new orientation had actually begun before Pearce's death, when he had given Gregg a large swath in which to pursue new ideas. As one observer remarked, it was striking that even in spite of the foundation's "large size, conservatism, and fear of the future . . . trustees [who are] more likely to do nothing than to adopt a bold new course of action should place psychiatry high in their priority list" (Schneider, 2002, p. 35). Gregg wrote to his wife at this time, "I find myself responsible for diminishing the hours, days, and years of suffering and incapacity of I wonder how many people who may through the aid of Rockefeller Foundation money initially, be eventually affected by discoveries and improvements of the real people in the practice of medicine and the prevention of disease" (Schneider, 2002, p. 37).

With organizational and personnel changes in 1928 and increased focus on the United States and Canada, Gregg was more determined to move psychiatry ahead, to gradually help it to "become integrated into American medicine" (Schneider, 2002, p. 40). The foundation was trending away from largely institutional support, and its president opined that the United States "badly needs psychiatric clinics." The fact that board members' brothers, sisters, spouses, and wives had personal encounters with the field probably exerted subtle, perhaps silent, influence on new directions (p. 38). On one occasion, Gregg had written to his brother for advice about books on insanity, which a trustee had requested of him. Alluding to the trustee (but not by name, although it was Fosdick), Gregg said that Fosdick had had some tragedy in his family and that the trustees as a group "showed some considerable interest in an effort to make some headway in the general field of

World War II, Rockefeller, and Psychiatry

Although war had put a crimp in Rockefeller philanthropy, the foundation's largesse continued to exert influence. A number of psychiatrists (and psychoanalysts) who had benefitted from Rockefeller philanthropy joined the war effort, where they made a marked impression on nonpsychiatrist physicians. Many of the latter had never encountered a psychiatrist or were accustomed to negative characterizations of them from psychiatry's "bad old days" before the 1930s. A positive collaborative experience treating soldiers at or near the battlefield won new respect for what psychiatry, properly applied, could accomplish. Starr (1982), a chronicler of changes in medicine, writes that "the recognition of psychiatry during the war was, quite likely, its greatest achievement" (p. 344). Such experience, publicized by Public Health Service psychiatrists and mental health lobbyists, had much to do with the passage of legislation for the National Mental Health Act in 1946, to fully emerge as the National Institute of Mental Health (NIMH) in 1949. The postwar publication of Albert Deutsch's (1948) book *The Shame of the States*, on the abysmal conditions of state asylums, added impetus to the movement to address the nation's mental health; Deutsch wrote, "It is because modern psychiatry is a stranger to so many mental hospital wards that many more patients don't return to their communities as cured" (Starr, 1982, p. 354). And the arrival of European refugee psychiatrists also contributed to the "growth of a more influential psychiatric profession" (Starr, 1982, p. 345).

Picking up, in a sense, where Rockefeller left off, federal support and funding was now available not only for research and training but also for mental health clinics. From 1948 to 1962, NIMH funding for research increased from $374,000 to $42.6 million, with training grants escalating from $1.1 to $38.6 million, in an effort to attract more trainees to psychiatry. Atypically, training stipends to residents in psychiatry were higher than those in other specialties (Starr, 1982, p. 346). Special enticements were made to general physicians returning from war to encourage them to switch to psychiatry.

Thus, Rockefeller money had indirectly exerted a powerful influence on psychiatry's recognition as a valid and respectable specialty. Following the war, the soil had been cultivated in general hospitals for psychiatrists to address the needs of returning soldiers and others to be assisted in their journey of recovery.

The Final Years

The postwar changes in the foundation affected its philanthropic targets and, once again, left Gregg unhappy and inclined to leave the foundation. On more than one occasion he had to be dissuaded from submitting his intention to resign. His work had been held in extremely high regard, and, to retain him as a member of the foundation, he was made a vice president and member of the Board of Trustees in 1951. In this new role, he wrote and lectured worldwide on medical education and research until his retirement in 1956. For his impact on psychiatry and other achievements, he was given the Lasker Award in 1956, with the accompanying caption that he was "a physician who hasn't treated a patient in thirty-five years, a medical educator who has never taught a class, a research man who has done no research. Yet . . . he accomplished more for medical research, medical education and the practice of medicine than if he had been personally outstanding in all three" (Engel, 1956, *New York Times*, Nov. 4, pp. 6,11; Schneider, 2002, p. 5). *Time* magazine wrote, "No man alive has had a wider or deeper influence on both the practice and teaching of medicine than Dr. Gregg" (*Time*, Nov. 26, 1956). He died less than a year later on June 19, 1957.

He was much praised for his support of psychiatry during his years at the foundation, and expressions of appreciation were amplified following his death. Assessing the totality of his work, Schneider wrote of Gregg, "He certainly was responsible for making an impact on the practice of psychiatry and related neurological fields, especially in the U.S. But the main importance of these grants was the introduction of psychiatric departments in medical schools and hospitals" (2002, p. 52). It was something of a disappointment to Gregg that his efforts to promote psychiatric research on a more scientific basis did not yield more results. Most "breakthroughs" in psychiatric research seemed to come from the pharmaceutical industry beginning in the mid-1950s.

Nevertheless, according to Schneider, in a review of Rockefeller philanthropy and its influence on medicine, Richard Pearce and Alan Gregg were "among the most influential men in the world of medical research and education, and in the process they set the model for the current relationship between medical centers and external funding sources" (2002, p. 7). Although Gregg did not achieve all he had hoped for, his earliest beneficiary and later biographer, Wilder Penfield, wrote, "In any case his strategy, modified though it was, was crowned with a remarkable degree of success" (Lipsitt, 2006, p. 11). Psychiatry, he said, under Gregg's influence, had moved from asylums to general hospitals and had achieved greater scientific "respectability among the other academic departments of medicine." Some psychiatrists had been assisted to perform their own basic research, while teachers of psychiatry adopted a more modern approach "to teach this old specialty" in a manner that would interest medical students. In addition, and of great significance going forward, "the close association between psychiatry and internal medicine proved to be of great benefit and has brought to American psychiatrists, and to physicians in general, the maturity and balance of judgment necessary today" (Penfield, 1967, p. 283).

Gregg's colleague and successor as director of the Division of Medical Sciences, and a later biographer, Robert Morison, wrote of Gregg that he was "the physician's physician, the psychiatrist's psychiatrist, the administrator's administrator. . . . A good deal of the acceptance gained for psychiatry from other branches of

s Come to America

perhaps of more than passing interest that early studies in psychosomatic
found a home with the Macy Foundation, with its legacy of Quaker-
ing religious freedom, many sought refuge in America in its early days.
that group were many avowed Quakers, considered blasphemous for
osition to the teachings of the Church of England. One Thomas Macy
d in 1635 from England to New York and subsequently moved to New
Four years later, he and nine other men purchased land from New York,
with the Indian name Nantucket, off the coast of Cape Cod, Massa-
where they established a large Quaker community. There, many of the
ts engaged first in farming and then the whaling industry, accumulating
ble wealth. As Quakers, they were very committed to assisting others
and their respect for the female members of the sect was well known
were accepted as "priests" of the sect). The elder Macy raised a very large
f which sea captain Josiah Macy, 200 years later, was a sixth-generation
escendant.

58, Josiah Macy, Jr. was born and grew on the island, moved to New York
e married the daughter of a wealthy leather merchant from Brooklyn,
ded New York's first oil refinery in 1860, subsequently sold to John D.
ler, Sr. (another Macy started the well-known department store in New
y). Of interest is that the Macys and the Rockefellers became business
s and then friends.

unior Josiah had a much beloved daughter, Catherine Evirit "Kate"
1863. Kate was 13 when her father died of typhoid and left her a trust
isisting largely of Standard Oil securities. At the age of 20, she married
raeme Ladd, a yachtsman who called himself a "merchant." Ladd also
m a very wealthy family and seems mostly to have dabbled in a variety
pations" until his wife became ill; he devoted the rest of his life to taking
er. There is no record of any children of Kate's marriage. Together they
ying up land in Raritan, New Jersey, eventually to amass one of the larg-
s in the state, named Natirar (Raritan backward—for some reason they
nchant for spelling things backward, naming his boat Etak after his wife)
eapack-Gladstone area, where they lived in a specially built 40-room
, occupying separate bedrooms. There, on the property, beginning in
te established a convalescent facility, Maple Cottage, where "deserving
men who are compelled to depend upon their own exertions for sup-
l be entertained, without charge, for periods of time while convalescing
ess, recuperating from impaired health, or otherwise in need of rest"
2012, p. 13), a concept of health care perhaps modeled after her own
ce of illness.

r Ladd died in 1933, and on the 50th anniversary of his death, according
us covenants of his will, the Ladds' Natirar was sold to King Hassan II of

academic medicine came from Alan Gregg's suc
like a reasonable bet" (Penfield, 1967, p. 284). G:
could be unsparingly critical but unconditionally
supportive (p. 284).

Strange Coincidence

In my own training in the late 1950s, I was unk
major contributions by Alan Gregg and the Roc
Milton Rosenbaum at Einstein Medical Center,
of the early Rockefeller fellowships. In my late1
Bibring, introduced to Boston psychiatry by Star
beneficiary who had made such valued contrib
tion to general medicine. Psychiatry was a vibra
the field were highly coveted. And over my desk
sculptress, hung a bas relief of Simon Flexner, di
tute, where it all began, keeping an eye on a bene
specialty of psychiatry.

II. The Josiah Macy Jr. Foundation: Whe
Psychosomatic Medicine

There was little systematic research into the inte
functions, and not much thought for the need to
lems from the psychosocial point of view.

Although psychiatry had long distanced itself from
cal roots, echoes of religion remain very much a p:
the field. William James comes to mind with his
experience. James was a philosopher, psychologist,
be president twice of the American Psychological
ered father of American psychology. His father wa
Adolf Meyer's father was also a minister. The fa
his wife were ecclesiasts. And the Emmanuel mov
started by Rev. Elwood Worcester, pastor of the
supported by psychoanalyst Dr. Isadore Coriat as
The Mind Cure Movement, as described in *The Va*
greatly influenced the beginnings of medical psy
epidemiology and beginnings of medical psychoth
pursued religious studies even as she strengthened
analysis, and psychosomatic medicine.

Quake

Thus, it
medicin
ism. See
Among:
their op
emigrat
England
an islan
chusetts
inhabita
conside:
in need
(womer
family,
Quaker
In 18
where I
and fou
Rockefe
York C
associat

The
Macy, ii
fund co
Walter
came fr
of "occ
care of
began t
est esta
had a p
in the
mansio
1908, I
gentlev
port sh
from il
(Tudic
experie

Wal
to curi

Morocco, then passed on his death in 1999 to his son Mohammed VI, then repurchased by the Somerset County of New Jersey, and finally leased to Sir Richard Branson, owner of the Virgin Group, who developed it into a spa resort. The significance of this history is that it left Josiah's daughter Kate with copious amounts of money with which she endowed the Josiah Macy Jr. Foundation, founded in 1930 before Ladd's death, in honor of her deceased father.

Kate's Doctor, the Patient, and Her Illness

Kate had been very attached to an older sister who died in 1893 and devoted herself to her sister's care throughout her illness with cancer. Historical accounts suggest that Kate "collapsed" after this loss and became a virtual invalid, with symptoms that could not be diagnosed by the usual medical techniques (perhaps now referred to as medically unexplained symptoms [MUS]). She spent much of her time in bed or wheelchair, eventually suffering atrophy of her leg muscles, making walking impossible. She nonetheless oversaw the operations of the foundation, appointing as the first president her own physician, Ludwig Kast, a Viennese-born-and-trained doctor who tended her from 1917 when she was 54 until his appointment as president and overseer of the foundation in 1930. By the time of her death at 82 (b. 1863) in 1945, four years after Dr. Kast, still an invalid, she had already resourced the Macy Foundation fund with $19 million, with additional funds bequeathed on her death.

Kast remained president of the foundation until his death in 1941. Little information is available about Kast's medical orientation. The few papers written by him indicate a strong interest in lipid metabolism and atherosclerosis and do not reveal evidence of his psychological interests. As a member of the New York Medical Society, he was instrumental in establishing integrative colloquia and lectures, with a permanent lectureship established in his name by appreciative colleagues. He carried on a lively correspondence with Dr. Henry Sigerist, preeminent medical historian and humanist, about topics of medical history and other matters of mutual interest. With Kast's broad exposure to ideas in medicine, it is virtually inconceivable that he was not familiar with the discoveries and papers of Freud, especially having trained at the University of Vienna. As an observant physician, it would seem unlikely that he would not perceive Kate's symptoms as of an emotional nature, although probably unable to offer much in the way of rehabilitation. One might wonder whether he held a negative opinion of Freud's controversial hypotheses or whether he was cautiously politick, holding too active an interest in "psychiatric" illness in abeyance, lest he antagonize his patient. Miss Ladd's "puzzling" ailments would seem to have been a prime subject for a trial of new psychoanalytic approaches.

Whatever the explanation, it is noteworthy that the early philanthropic focus of the Macy Foundation, under Kast's directional presidency, was on psychosomatic medicine, with large commitments of funds to psychosomatic medicine pioneers like Franz Alexander and Flanders Dunbar. Describing the early years of the foundation, Clarence Michalis (1955), chairman of the Board of Directors, wrote:

> Dr. Kast's vision and wisdom gave clarity to her purpose. . . . He devoted his great resources of professional knowledge, his sound judgment, philosophic outlook, and understanding of organization procedure to the guidance of the enterprise. Through it, his ideals of service to medical science were translated into action.
>
> *(pp. 2–3)*

Dr. Willard Rappleye succeeded Kast on his death as president of the foundation, about whom Michalis wrote:

> [H]is understanding of the responsibilities and opportunities of the physician as a servant of mankind, his enthusiastic acceptance of Mrs. Ladd's views of the use to be made of her benefactions have insured continuation of the work so well begun by his predecessor.
>
> *(p. 3)*

If, indeed, actions speak louder than words, then dedication to support of psychosomatic medicine was a very important field of exploration by these functionaries and the foundation. Rappleye (1955), continuing the dedication of the foundation to psychosomatic medicine, wrote:

> The development of dynamic psychiatry, with the recognition of the role of unconscious motivation in behavior, has brought new understanding and possibility of prediction to the study of man's social nature. It is now demonstrated that the insights that illuminate psychosomatic problems in the individual also throw light on the genesis of social tension.
>
> *(p. 10)*

Describing her vision for the foundation, Kate Ladd, with her strong heritage of Quaker humanitarian roots, wrote:

> It is my desire that the Foundation in the use of this gift should concentrate on a few problems rather than support many undertakings, and that it should primarily devote its interest to fundamental aspects of health, of sickness, and of methods for the relief of suffering. To these ends the Foundation might give preference in the use of this fund to integrating functions in medical sciences and medical education for which there seems to be particular need in our age of specialization and technical complexities. The

Foundation will take more interest in the architecture of ideas than in the architecture of buildings and laboratories.

(Josiah Macy Jr. Foundation Report, 1955, pp. 5–6)

During Kast's tenure, the foundation did indeed focus a great deal of its attention on psychosomatic medicine.

Kate Ladd Meets Flanders Dunbar

Kate Ladd said that "far more aid was being given to biochemical and physiological research than to psychobiological and sociological [research]" (Rappleye, 1955, p. 5); it must have been a serendipitous meeting of Kate Ladd and Flanders Dunbar. Exactly how Dunbar and Kate Ladd had knowledge of each other is not exactly known, but it is not surprising she became a beneficiary of Macy largesse. Josiah Macy, Jr. was connected to John Rockefeller as an associate in Standard Oil. Kate was an admirer and friend of Harry Emerson Fosdick, a founding member of the Board of Directors of the Rockefeller Foundation. Fosdick was the Presbyterian pastor of Riverside Church, built by Rockefeller, which may account for Kate's switch from Quakerism to Presbyterianism, even though she was not a churchgoer. Fosdick's brother Raymond was in charge of philanthropy for the Rockefeller Foundation under John D. Junior in 1913, so that it was only "six degrees of separation" for Kate Ladd to become aware of Flanders Dunbar, with her dual interests in religion and psychosomatic medicine. Harry Emerson Fosdick was a major proponent and practitioner of pastoral counseling and of the church's cooperation with psychiatry and the popular Alcoholics Anonymous (Encyclopedia Britannica, 1910–1911).

Although Kate did not emphasize religion in her philanthropic plans, she did say the fund was to be "an integrating force in medical research, promoting a concept of healing which saw the patient as a complete individual, healthy only when he possessed a wholesome unity of mind and body" (Rappleye, 1955, p. 6), concepts that were of both secular and religious relevance. "In an enlightened democracy," she wrote, "philanthropy could best serve by investigating new ideas and methods" (p. 6).

Further reflections of Mrs. Ladd's philanthropic inclinations are stated in the history of the foundation (Michalis, 1955):

Although depressing statistics furnished by state and federal agencies for years have shown mental illness to be the nation's biggest public health problem, less money is devoted to research into causes and treatment of mental disability than to research in any other major field of human illness. Mrs. Ladd's injunction to her trustees to assist especially projects that call for the integration of biological, medical, and social sciences has been the central theme of the Foundation's activities throughout its two and a half decades, unifying all its interests so that with slightly shifting emphasis through the years that theme is still dominant.

(pp. 98–99)

Although Mrs. Ladd had not specifically made reference to religion in her philanthropic plans, *historians* of the foundation refer to her funding interests in

how psychosomatic interrelationships, improvement of social work education, use of adult education in personality adjustment, exploration of emotional factors in the learning process, personality development in children, *consideration of the role of religion in illness and health*, impinge upon the great area of human relations.

(p. 99; emphasis by au.)

Over the years, the Macy Foundation contributed to Franz Alexander's studies on fatigue; Walter Cannon's physiological studies on "fight or flight" (as part of an interest in the war effort to learn more about war neuroses and shell shock); psychologist John Bowlby's work on attachment and separation; animal studies of maternal-child relations and the effects of early trauma on later emotional problems in children; Dr. Howard Liddell's studies at Cornell University on the biological basis of psychological trauma in animals as it relates to the vulnerability of newborns to environmental stress; and Gregory Bateson's anthropological studies of communication in the doctor-patient relationship.

Fulfilling Kate's charge for integrated approaches, in 1936 the foundation sponsored a four-day conference to bring together "representatives of medicine and the social sciences, *with psychiatry as a unifying discipline*, to the consideration of biological and social studies of man's relations with his fellows" (Michalis, 1955, p. 85; emphasis by au.)

As with the Rockefeller Foundation, World War II somewhat curtailed the philanthropic activities of the foundation. Nonetheless, a 1941 conference in partnership with the National Institute of Health's Unit on Gerontology stressed that "older persons with emotional and psychosomatic difficulties respond well to psychotherapeutic measures" and that "understanding of psychosomatic mechanisms is as important for the practice of geriatrics as for all other branches of medicine" (Michalis, 1955, p. 85). This focus on aging is likely one of the last endeavors spearheaded by Dr. Kast as Kate entered her 80s and shortly before his own demise.

Continuing this interest in promoting integration, interpersonal and interdisciplinary communication, and postwar activities under a new president, Dr. Rappleye included a series of conferences convening "a select group" of representatives from established medical departments, under the chairmanship of Boston's Dr. John Murray, a psychoanalyst and professor of psychiatry at Boston University Medical

School, recently returned from his consultancy in neuropsychiatry to the Army Air Forces (Michalis, 1955, p. 100), and an advisor to Alan Gregg on issues related to psychoanalysis.

There is little question that philanthropic support by Kate Ladd's disbursement of funds through the Macy Foundation was germinal in establishing psychosomatic medicine in the United States. While the verities of life (and death) always emerge in time, what Gregg refers to as "Great Medicine" would not be where it is today without the vision and charity of the Rockefellers, Macys, Greggs, and Ladds. Alan Gregg and Kate Macy Ladd both understood that philanthropic support is insufficient to maintain social achievements. According to Gregg, "We must also face the fact that we seem to understand neither the accomplishments nor the potentialities of medicine and are unwilling, therefore, to pay for it" (Gregg, 1956, p. 16). And Kate Ladd wrote that "the ideas for sustained undertakings which may emerge [from philanthropic support] in turn should be taken over and maintained by the public" (Rappleye, 1955, p. 6). To the extent that a public is not willing or able to do this, it is fortunate that other resources appear episodically.

III. Commonwealth Fund

Although not as vigorously supportive of psychiatry per se as the Rockefeller and Macy Foundations, the Commonwealth Fund early contributed substantially to projects and individuals (with fellowships) whose objective was to promote comprehensive health care, partly through application of psychiatry and other disciplines to improvement in the delivery of primary care. Many psychiatry residents from 1912 to 1934 at Boston Psychopathic Hospital received Commonwealth support as did more senior psychiatric educators (Gifford, 1978, p. 372). Dr. M. Ralph Kaufman received a fellowship grant (1928–1931) for analytic training and analysis by Wilhelm Reich at the University of Vienna. On return, he was briefly director of McLean Hospital before establishing a training program at Boston's Beth Israel Hospital (1933 to 1942) with Lydia Dawes in child psychiatry and Felix Deutsch in psychosomatic research, a model of general hospital psychiatry, with teaching and training for medical and surgical house officers, replicating a program begun by Stanley Cobb in 1934 at Massachusetts General Hospital. Kaufman left the Beth Israel in 1942 for military service and on return established a very strong C-L program at New York's Mount Sinai Hospital.

In the early 1950s, the Commonwealth Fund provided major support for an "experiment in comprehensive care and teaching" at New York Hospital–Cornell Medical Center with the aim of "providing physicians who are better prepared to cope with the complex demands of modern medicine" (Reader & Goss, 1967, p. 8). Although not specifically focusing on psychiatry or psychosomatic medicine, one of its clinics designed for "broader medical care" included staff of Drs. Harold Wolff, Stewart Wolf, Thomas Rennie, and Herbert Ripley, who "trained a host of young internists in research techniques as well as the practice of psychosomatic medicine" (pp. 16–17).

In granting support to this project, the Commonwealth Fund followed the philosophy outlined in the organization's annual report of 1949, expressing the need to counteract the trend toward (super)specialization causing medicine to fail to "deal with people whole instead of in parts" (Reader & Goss, 1967, p. 18). Scientific progress in medicine, they stated, was welcome, but that the discoveries of such pioneers as Pasteur, Claude Bernard, and Virchow were leaving "too many people undeniably not helped by laboratory study and accomplished surgery" and that were "allowed to develop ailments that medicine, either alone or in partnership with various kinds of social manipulation, could prevent" (p. 18). This forerunner of what might later become an integrated approach to biopsychosocial medicine unfortunately floundered when the fund, in 1960, "stipulated that no further funds would be provided for patient care or teaching, but only for research activities" (p. 19). Once again, as foretold by Gregg and Ladd, failure of public support would seriously deter progress.

IV. James Eaton and the Psychiatry Education Branch

In the Mount Rushmore of C-L psychiatry, James S. Eaton, Jr. can be placed in the same class with Alan Gregg and Kate Macy Ladd for his cultivation of the field in which other seeds could grow. In fact, as chief of the National Institute of Mental Health's (NIMH) Psychiatry Education Branch (PEB), he probably was responsible for the most extensive evaluation of C-L psychiatry programs ever launched.

Eaton's story of how he came to the special discipline of C-L psychiatry sheds light on how one selects that pathway. His childhood illnesses of pneumonia, asthma, and allergy instilled an early interest in illness, while his psychological struggles around a speech impediment and sexuality prompted a capacity for introspection. The outgrowths of psychological-mindedness and humanism led quite naturally, if haltingly, to psychiatry as a career choice. Following the prescribed training in both specialties of psychiatry and internal medicine at Tulane, he found himself "in the right place at the right time" (personal communication). Having completed residency training, he remained on as faculty at Tulane and Charity Hospital, teaching students, house officers, and attendings an integrated approach to patient care.

As we have seen, serendipity accounts for many of the twists and turns in the trajectory of C-L psychiatry. Jim's ascendency to the position as chief of the PEB was such an event. On an occasion when his chairman at Tulane, Dr. Robert Heath, was unable to attend a regional meeting of Southern Professors of Psychiatry in Charleston, South Carolina, Jim, only recently out of residency, was sent in his stead. He was apparently adventurously voluble in his comments about medical student education and was subsequently invited by Bernard Bandler, attending the meeting and at the time chief of the branch, to interview for a position at NIMH. He was hired on, and, when Bandler left NIMH to return to Boston University, Jim was first appointed acting chief and, after a national search, chief of the service. In that position from 1974 to 1983, he became a man with a mission!

If ever there was a fine meshing of objectives with need, it came in the 1970s with this opportunity to fuel his lofty intent to narrow the mind-body dualism extant in medicine; what he did in his personal career he hoped to do for the broader profession. This "impossible" task was precisely what touched Jim's heart, and for at least the next decade he would tackle this endeavor with relish, optimism, and innovation.

Full of determination to "reacquaint medicine with psychiatry and psychiatry with medicine," he embarked on a personal quest to learn what could be done to achieve his goal. He familiarized himself with C-L programs that included Massachusetts General Hospital with Avery Weisman and Tom Hackett; Strong Memorial Hospital with George Engel and John Romano; Montefiore/Einstein Medical Center with Mort Reiser, Ed Sachar, and Herb Weiner; University of Southern California with Bill Kiely and Don Naftulin; University of Florida with John Schwab; Mount Sinai Hospital with M. Ralph Kaufman and James Strain; University of Pennsylvania with Mickey Stunkard and Joe DiGiacomo; Columbia Physicians and Surgeons Hospital with Don Kornfeld; Harvard's Mount Auburn and Cambridge Hospitals with Don Lipsitt; and others to garner as great an awareness as possible of C-L activities and psychosomatic medicine as existed at the time. He joined the American Psychosomatic Society to understand more about C-L research.

Opportunities for innovation did not have to wait long. One of his first responsibilities was to review 530 grant awards to 205 institutions due to expire on June 30, 1975 (Eaton, Haas, Abraham, Reus & Goldberg, 1976). Clearly, there was little time for one or two staff to review all of these programs applying for support beyond 1975, before governmental threat to discontinue funding. To supplement the 2.5 full-time equivalent personnel of the branch, Jim estimated he would need approximately 100 consultants to assist with the task. A thorough set of standards was established, and thus was begun the Kafkaesque enterprise to satisfy government mandates that precluded funding without adequate review, at the same time not allowing government endorsed "guidelines." Reviewers were entirely voluntary and were reimbursed travel expenses only. They included department chairs, deans, academic teachers and researchers, and directors of C-L services (of both child and adult psychiatry and primary care education).

Timing was problematic. Jim's entrance into government service came at the nexus of the Nixon and Ford administrations. Strict enforcement of accountability and "cost-effectiveness" had been amplified to a near-paranoid degree. Regulatory opposition to any federal guidelines hampered the establishment of a review process and required deftness in the extreme to traverse the tight interstices of administrative control. With considerable assistance of a sympathetic division director, Dr. Neal Waldrop, and very carefully worded documents, Jim moved the project forward.

A document, *Points of Concern for Site Visitors*, was produced to establish some degree of standardization; the large number of volunteer reviewers were vetted and recruited; orientation sessions were scheduled; and the intense process was launched. Goals, as set forth in the document, sought the best integration of psychological, behavioral, and social issues in a wide spectrum of medical curricula, spanning the first year of medical school to specialty residencies, fellowships, and continuing graduate educational programs (e.g., general practitioner training in psychiatry). To increase objectification, site visit teams of two or three visitors were established with assignments to review each grant in institutions throughout the country (including Puerto Rico). This process was able to thoroughly evaluate and report on most programs in medical student education in psychiatry and behavioral sciences, as well as those for postgraduate training of psychiatrists and general practitioners and for consultation-liaison programs.

Not only were site visitors able to "Johnny Appleseed"[1] ideas about education and training, but they were reciprocally able to improve their own knowledge of such programs to take back to their institutions. The élan and genuine excitement shared by reviewers brought great enthusiasm to the project.

Access to a dean's office is never more readily accomplished than when the anticipation and prospect of funding of an institution hangs in the balance. All programs in each institution were intensely reviewed over periods of several days and involved the program directors, medical students, house officers, attending physicians, full-time faculty, administrators, and in some cases patients. Reports included institution demographics, local politics, curricular content, as well as assessment of program effectiveness in each individual institutional program.

With flexibility, the "points of concern" document was not a mere checklist to be slavishly followed but rather an expectation that "visitors would inevitably employ their own individually unique operational styles of data gathering, and would exercise appropriate latitude of judgment in choosing which areas of a program to focus most heavily on, which ones to skim over lightly." Consultants and program directors were both assured that "a good site visit would be conducted . . . in much the same way that an experienced clinician selectively concentrates his attention on certain signs and symptoms, making full use of his judgment, reasoning abilities, and past experiences" (Eaton et al., 1976, p. 442). In all likelihood, no equivalent evaluative survey of psychiatric education programs had been achieved ever before or since (Eaton, Daniels & Pardes, 1977). But, indeed, it was done in less than a year, in spite of structural, organizational, and political barriers and "advice" from many that it could not be done.

As expected, not all programs would live up to established criteria. Findings resulted in many programs being defunded because of deficiencies, but the thorough reviews catalyzed development of criteria for programs whether or not they were supported by grant money. The entire field of C-L psychiatry as well as other educational programs was immensely improved and expectations established for future grantees.

With sharpened criteria to judge C-L programs, Reifler and Eaton (1976) reviewed 50 applications (of 150) to NIMH's PEB for financial support in fiscal year 1977. They personally visited 13 programs. Training tools used by the programs included didactic seminars (39/50) and/or case conferences (29), evaluation forms (24), videotaped interviews (15), knowledge exam (12), chart audit (10), career follow-up (5), and attitude ratings (5). Conclusions drawn from the survey included the impression that program directors poorly understood educational objectives, evaluation procedures, or use of their findings to modify their own programs (Reifler & Eaton, 1976).

Astute politically as well as clinically, Eaton recognized the hurdles to be mounted if advances in training and mental health services were to be assured. In a climate where public accountability was being demanded and "sociopolitical, economic, and philosophical pressures . . . threaten[ed] [psychiatry's] existence as a valued medical specialty" (Eaton & Goldstein, 1977, p. 642), it became clear to Eaton and his associate Leonard Goldstein (1977) that both professional and public alert were imperative, as detailed in their 1977 article "Psychiatry in crisis" in the *American Journal of Psychiatry*. Drawing on PEB's overview of national training programs, they acknowledged the work of the PEB in helping to stimulate "a great renewal of interest in upgrading and revitalizing psychiatric educational programs throughout the United States" (p. 644). As realists, with an appreciation of the evanescence of federal funding, it was as though they were writing a last will and testament for the field. Offering the opinion that "the uniquely important role of the psychiatric physician is frequently overlooked" (p. 644), and noting that the federal support for psychiatric training had decreased from more than $41 million in fiscal year 1969 to only $25 million in 1976, they anticipated the destructive impact on mental health care of further cuts to funding for psychiatric education.

With growing demand stimulated by federal laws that established community mental health centers, increased primary care training in psychiatry, and escalating demand for mental health care, "well-trained psychiatrists will be able to demonstrate their value in the mental health and health fields" (Eaton & Goldstein, 1977, p. 645). Recognizing the need to educate the public as well as trainees about psychiatry's value, they offered suggestions: Psychiatrists must take the lead in counteracting "dataless assumptions and antiprofessional bias" (p. 644). There was need to gather "honest, objective data" about decreasing graduates entering psychiatry, about attitudes of medical students toward the specialty, about the role of foreign medical graduates, as well as about the "anticipated effect of decreased training monies," and need to analyze "the impact of the present and future policies of state and federal health and mental health agencies on psychiatric education" (p. 644).

"We must," they concluded, "be prepared to demonstrate this difference, worth, and uniqueness in a variety of service delivery, research, and educational settings;

where 'the squeaky wheel gets the grease' is where quality training programs make the difference" (Eaton & Goldstein, 1977, p. 645). To achieve this purpose, Eaton counseled academic psychiatry to become involved in the "political marketplace." The general public would need to be persuaded about psychiatry's relevance to research and education (Eaton, 1978), and toward that objective Eaton initiated an administrative fellowship in which he mentored several future leaders in academic psychiatry. One of Eaton's administrative fellows, in a published reminiscence, has reflected on Eaton's impact: "He had a major impact not only on my career but on the careers of many others as well, including those of Jay Scully, Burton Reifler, and Victor Reus. As Chief of the Psychiatry Education Branch at NIMH . . . [he was] one of the most influential people in academic psychiatry in the country" (Faulkner, 2007). Scully, having taken a student elective in consultation psychiatry with Eaton at Tulane, switched interest from surgery to psychiatry, later to become medical director of the American Psychiatric Association. Other fellows included Mort Silverman, Susan Blumenthal, Richard Goldberg, Art Nielson, Harry Wright, and Barry Fenton, all outstanding contributors to psychiatric research and education. The fellowship had been initiated over the "official" prohibitions of the program.

Jim Eaton, in his thoughtful approach to training and education, has served as a veritable "super-ego" of C-L psychiatry, with his urging of accountability, clarity of definitional boundaries in the field, proper teaching, and relevant research. He and his associates have field-tested an evaluative paradigm for the practice, research, and teaching of C-L psychiatry, which unfortunately, because of cessation of funds, could not be sustained (Eaton, 1980). For his impressive contribution to the field of C-L psychiatry, Eaton was awarded the Academy of Psychosomatic Medicine's Thomas P. Hackett Award in 1987.

While the "osmotic" process of information sharing exceeded the actual availability of funds, Eaton's entire enterprise was both "cost-effective" and frugally catalytic of excitement and interest, especially in C-L and medical student education programs, the core interests of PEB. Unfortunately, as long as programs are reliant on the vagaries of politics and economics and the imagination and creative energies of a single individual, sustainability is always at risk. Nevertheless, much forward movement of C-L's relevance has been achieved by Eaton, as it had been by Alan Gregg and Kate Ladd at different times and different places. The discipline is indebted to all for its survival. Whether recognition of C-L as a specialty can lessen the leap-frogging from crisis to crisis and future existence remains to be seen.

Unless our field generates an Alan Gregg, a Kate Macy Ladd, or a James Eaton every few years, the fate of C-L psychiatry always rests uneasily in the balance. As Eaton began to read the federal writing on the wall in the 1980s, with impending cessation of federal funding, he expounded on the "unfinished business of C-L psychiatry" (Eaton, 1986). Gradually, it appeared necessary to leaders in the field to seek recognition in a more sustainable way; that realization contributed to the eventual quest for specialty designation.

Note

1 Jim's instruction to his fellows and reviewers to "Johnny Appleseed" their ideas was an apt metaphor for the pedagogical passion he instilled.

References

Billings, E.G., McNary, W.S., & Rees, M.H. (1937). Financial importance of general hospital psychiatry to hospital administrators. *Hospitals, 11,* 400–444.

Chernow, R. (1998). *Titan: The Life of John D. Rockefeller, Sr.* New York, NY: Random House.

Cobb, S. (1936). *Foundations of Neuropsychiatry.* Baltimore, MD: Williams & Wilkins.

Deutsch, A. (1948). *The Shame of the States.* New York, NY: Harcourt, Brace.

Eaton, J.S., Jr. (1978). Academic psychiatry in the political marketplace. *Archives of General Psychiatry, 35,* 1145–1149.

Eaton, J.S., Jr. (1980). The psychiatrist and psychiatric education. In H.I. Kaplan, A.M. Freedman, & B.J. Sadock (Eds.). *Comprehensive Textbook of Psychiatry III.* (pp. 2926–2946). Baltimore, MD: Williams & Wilkins.

Eaton, J.S., Jr. (1986). Consultation-liaison psychiatry: Unfinished business. *Psychosomatics, 27,* 323–324.

Eaton, J.S., Jr., Daniels, R.S., & Pardes, H. (1977). Psychiatric education: State of the art, 1976. *American Journal of Psychiatry, 134* (Suppl), 2–6.

Eaton, J.S., Jr., & Goldstein, L.S. (1977). Psychiatry in crisis. *American Journal of Psychiatry, 134,* 642–645.

Eaton, J.S., Jr., Haas, M.R., Abraham, A.S., Reus, V.I., & Goldberg, R. (1976). The development of criteria for evaluating psychiatric education programs. *Archives of General Psychiatry, 33,* 439–442.

Encyclopedia Britannica. (1910–1911). *Harry Emerson Fosdick.* Chicago, IL: Encyclopedia Britannica. Retrieved from Britannica.com

Engel, L. (1956). Rx for medicine. *New York Times.* November 4, 6, p. 11.

Faulkner, L.R. (2007). Personal reflections of a career of transitions. *Journal of the American Academy of Psychiatry and Law, 35,* 253–259.

Flexner, A. (1910). *Medical Education in the United States and Canada: A Report to the Carnegie Foundation for the Advancement of Teaching.* Bulletin No. 4, New York, NY: The Carnegie Foundation for the Advancement of Teaching.

Gifford, S. (1978). Medical psychotherapy and the Emmanuel movement in Boston, 1904–1912. In G.E. Gifford, Jr. (Ed.). *Psychoanalysis, Psychotherapy, and the New England Medical Scene, 1894–1944.* (pp. 106–118). New York, NY: Science History Publications.

Gregg, A. (1956). *Challenges to Contemporary Medicine.* New York, NY: Columbia University Press.

Hackett, T.P. (1978). Beginnings: Liaison psychiatry in a general hospital. In T.P. Hackett & N.H. Cassem (Eds.). *Massachusetts General Hospital Handbook of General Hospital Psychiatry.* (pp. 1–13). St. Louis, MO: C.V. Mosby Co.

James, W. (1902). *The Varieties of Religious Experience: A Study in Human Nature.* New York, NY: Longmans, Green & Co.

Lipsitt, D.R. (2006). Psychosomatic medicine: History of a "new" specialty. In M. Blumenfield & J.J. Strain (Eds.). *Psychosomatic Medicine.* (pp. 3–20). Philadelphia, PA: Lippincott Williams & Wilkins.

Michalis, C.G. (1955). *Josiah Macy Jr. Foundation 1930–1955: A Review of Activities.* New York, NY: Josiah Macy Jr. Foundation.

Peabody, F.W. (1927). The care of the patient. *Journal of the American Medical Association, 88,* 877–882.

Penfield, W. (1967). *The Difficult Art of Giving: The Epic of Alan Gregg.* Boston, MA: Little Brown.

Rappleye, W.C. (1955). At the quarter century mark. In *The Josiah Macy Jr. Foundation 1930–1955: A review of activities.* New York, NY: Josiah Macy Jr. Foundation.

Reader, G.G., & Goss, M.E.W. (Eds.). (1967). *Comprehensive Medical Care and Teaching.* Ithaca, NY: Cornell University Press.

Reifler, B., & Eaton, J.S., Jr. (1976). The evaluation of teaching and learning by psychiatric consultation and liaison training programs. *Psychosomatic Medicine, 40,* 99–106.

Schneider, W.H. (Ed.). (2002). *Rockefeller Philanthropy and Modern Biomedicine: International Initiatives from World War I to the Cold War.* Bloomington, IN: Indiana University Press.

Starr, P. (1982). *The Social Transformation of American Medicine: The Rise of a Sovereign Profession and the Making of a Vast Industry.* New York, NY: Basic Books.

Tudico, C. (2012). *The History of the Josiah Macy Jr. Foundation.* New York, NY: Josiah Macy Jr. Foundation. Retrieved from www.macyfoundation.org

Major Sources

Chernow, R. (1998). *Titan: The Life of John D. Rockefeller, Sr.* New York, NY: Random House.

Gifford, S. (1978). Medical psychotherapy and the Emmanuel movement in Boston, 1904–1912. In G.E. Gifford, Jr. (Ed.). *Psychoanalysis, Psychotherapy, and the New England Medical Scene, 1894–1944.* (pp. 106–118). New York, NY: Science History Publications.

Michalis, C.G. (1955). *Josiah Macy Jr. Foundation 1930–1955: A Review of Activities.* New York, NY: Josiah Macy Jr. Foundation.

Penfield, W. (1967). *The Difficult Art of Giving: The Epic of Alan Gregg.* Boston, MA: Little Brown.

Schneider, W.H. (Ed.). (2002). *Rockefeller Philanthropy and Modern Biomedicine: International Initiatives from World War I to the Cold War.* Bloomington, IN: Indiana University Press.

Starr, P. (1982). *The Social Transformation of American Medicine: The Rise of a Sovereign Profession and the Making of a Vast Industry.* New York, NY: Basic Books.

8

A "LACK OF MEANS"

At a time when funding for health care is under serious scrutiny, consultation-liaison services throughout the United States have experienced increasing pressure to justify their existence.

—*Hall, Rundell & Popkin, 2002, p. 25*

Introduction

The noted sociologists Anne and Herman Somers of the Brookings Institution could not have been more prescient when they wrote in their 1961 report, "It is hard to believe that effective coverage [of mental illness] will ever prove practical unless accompanied by rather extensive changes in the *organization of psychiatric services and its maximum integration with general medical care*" (Somers & Somers, 1961, p. 391; emphasis by au.).

The Brookings Report accurately predicted that "the many difficult issues surrounding this complex field [medical care] will remain at the center of public affairs for a long time" (Somers & Somers, 1961, p. ix). The authors speculated that the problems of financing medical care were thrust front and center because "medicine has penetrated mysteries of the human body and mind and mastered techniques of diagnosis, surgery, chemotherapy and psychiatry that were scarcely dreamed of a century ago" (p. xi). Nothing fails like success!

With this "progress," things had become so complicated that "the individual legislator, doctor, or insurance executive, who seeks a broad overview as guidance for dealing with problems not wholly within his own specialized competence, may give up in despair" (p. xii). The "retrenchment" of payment for psychiatric services was due largely, the report stated, to "*no medically acceptable definition of mental illness or mental health"* (p. 390; emphasis by au.). Furthermore, with emotional disturbances "the distinction between health and illness becomes blurred, and the concept of medical need increasingly difficult to pinpoint in space or time" (pp. 148–149). It would appear that insurers have seized upon this blurriness to deny care for those in need.

Even before the Brookings Report, a special article in the *New England Journal of Medicine* (NEJM) called attention to the fact that health insurance programs "excluded from these benefits [health insurance] . . . the one group of [psychiatric] disorders that disables the largest number of people" (McKerracher, 1959, p. 474). And today the beat goes on . . . logarithmically! More than 50 years later, C-L psychiatry and mental illness coverage continues to face this challenge of fiscal sustainability!

Were it not for our naiveté, we should not be surprised about where we are. Another *New England Journal of Medicine* special article appeared in 1967 titled "Medicine, money and manpower: The challenge to professional education" (Darley & Somers, 1967). The introduction to this paper states that "the health professions are beginning to meet the formidable challenges inherent in the affluent, demanding, new health-care economy" (p. 1471). The authors date the onset of this trend to the era of specialization that grew out of the Flexner Report of 1910. Consultation-liaison psychiatry does not appear in this movement!

Who Will Pay?

George Henry (1929–1930) wrote:

> [T]he staff of every general hospital should have a psychiatrist who would continue the instruction and organize the psychiatric work of interns and who would attend staff conferences so that there might be a mutual exchange of medical experience and a frank discussion of the most complicated cases.
>
> *(p. 494)*

When he wrote this, he most likely never pondered the expense of such an enterprise or who might pay for it.

Certainly, insurers would be loath to reimburse consultations to medical and surgical patients who typically did not regard themselves as "psychiatrically sick" and who did not request psychiatric attention. And liaison especially, involving education of medical staff, was not a service offered and billed by other medical specialties. More fortunate institutions like Mount Sinai Hospital in New York and Beth Israel Hospital in Boston enjoyed the services of attending staff who volunteered their teaching, time, energy, and interest to the programs. Why would insurers pay for liaison that was provided "free" as an adjunct to consultation? In

Boston, émigré psychoanalysts were happy to find a new home where they gratefully could reengage in clinical service (Levin & Michaels, 1961). Such service now is as rare as hen's teeth.

Research Evidence

Why has research evidence not been accepted? Evidence of cost savings with psychiatric intervention has existed at least since Billings's simplistic demonstration in 1937 (Billings, McNary & Rees, 1937). Edward Billings had established the first American C-L service in Colorado, coined the term "liaison psychiatry," and published a paper on the financial advantages of such services to general hospitals (Billings et al., 1937). He speculated that liaison services could save the hospital $8,400 a day based on a per diem rate of $3.49 at the time (in 1930s dollars; this is closer to $100,000 today) (Billings, 1941). Because it was the heyday of philanthropic support of psychiatry by the Rockefeller and Macy Foundations, perhaps there was little curiosity to ponder the relevance of Billings's paper (Thompson & Suddath, 1987). Psychiatrists of my own generation were not taught to think of the cost of medical care before health care insurance became a major industry; hospitals had been founded as eleemosynary institutions.

Subsequent economic benefits of psychiatric consultation were also reported in the literature (Follette & Cummings, 1967; Jones & Vischi, 1979; Mumford, Schlesinger & Glass, 1982; Mumford, Schlesinger, Glass, Patrick & Cuerdon, 1984; Pincus, 1984; Schlesinger, Mumford, Glass, Patrick & Sharfstein, 1983). For example, the review by Mumford and associates of 34 controlled studies (Mumford et al., 1982) showed that psychological interventions helped surgical and cardiovascular patients do better than controls on ratings of anxiety, pain, distress, speed of recovery, use of analgesics, physical complications, and length of hospital stay. And another study by Schlesinger and associates (Schlesinger et al., 1983) demonstrated that 7 to 20 outpatient psychotherapy visits could reduce subsequent rates of hospitalization for patients with such physical disease as chronic obstructive pulmonary disease, diabetes, heart disease, and hypertension. In light of such evidence, it is curious that insurance companies are not persuaded to support psychiatric consultation and liaison. Nonetheless, much of this literature remained in the shadows as some C-L programs suffered diminished funding or total closure. Administrators, legislators, and insurance companies were "deaf" to arguments that reimbursement and support of C-L programs is a cost-saving investment in comprehensive health care. Although all medical specialties experienced "cutbacks" of funding in the 1980s, psychiatry as a whole, not only C-L, was considered "hardest hit" (Levitan, 1983).

Hackett (1981) editorialized, "How do we loosen the economic noose that threatens our training, our research, and our clinical practice?" (Levitan, 1983, p. 26). The solution to the problem, according to Hackett, was to once again to demonstrate the values of our therapies. If we are worth our salt we must prove it, not just to our patients, but also to our fellow physicians, hospital administrators, [and] third party payers as well as to our state and national legislators.

(p. 26)

The odyssey persists in this search for "proof." Just how to "prove it" has been elusive for decades as C-L psychiatrists strive to show they are "worth their salt."

In a series of lectures at Columbia University shortly before his death, Alan Gregg (1956), the great benefactor through Rockefeller support of C-L psychiatry in the 1930s and 1940s, recognized that philanthropy (charity) was finite and advocated for prepayment for health care. This, he trumpeted, should be as essential as the costs one incurs for food, shelter, and clothing (Gregg, 1956). Insurance companies, he speculated, prefer *life* insurance with its certainty of death rather than *health* insurance where "health" and "living" are too vague and "forever" to attract their interest. "Biological" rather than "biopsychosocial" psychiatry appeared to be the preferred model of care with insurers. The advent of psychopharmacology brought support for "drug studies" but not so much for the psychosocial repercussions of illness.

More compelling arguments would be required! Previous philanthropic support may have induced complacency, but prospects of funding from other sources were disappointing. It gradually became clear that support would have to be devised through the ingenuity of the "stakeholders" themselves. Depending on the "kindness of strangers" can be temporarily gratifying, but nothing compares to the constancy of a permanent relationship. Thus, the economics of C-L psychiatry is every bit as "foundational" as, say, philosophy, psychoanalysis, or physiology. The clarion call linking research to funding had gone out over the decades but was seldom heard by those capable of action. When the message is not heard, the impulse is usually to shout louder.

A Lack of Means

Over 100 years ago, S. Weir Mitchell, in his famous 1894 address, noisily castigated psychiatrists for their "torpor," characterizing his audience as "trammeled by custom, *lack of means*, and above all, in some cases (and this is saddest and most shameful of all [original—au.]), directly or indirectly by politics"(Mitchell, 1994, p. 30; emphasis by au.).

The "lack of means" to satisfy the need has been ever thus; lack of means has always been a top concern for C-L psychiatry, and psychiatrists have not been known for their economic prescience. Mental health has never garnered either the financial or the political support it warrants, considering its impact on personal, community, and global events. Whenever budgets need to be "trimmed," the paring knife seems to go first to "human services," including mental health. As chair of a department of psychiatry, I felt that much of my administrative time was spent deterring cannibalization of departmental turf and budget. The administrative rationale was that "we need the resources for revenue-producing services," which psychiatry decidedly was not.

In 1951, the neurologist Merrill Moore, at Boston City Hospital, wrote of that hospital's resistance to psychiatric service, because " 'crazy' patients are not wanted here." This was in spite of the fact that an estimated "50 to 80 per cent of all admissions consisted of patients with psychoneuroses or psychosomatic disorders" (Moore, 1951, p. 135). "Emotional disorders," he wrote, "may be the main reasons for the admission of many patients, or they may constitute a burdensome complication in addition to whatever medical diseases affect them" (p. 135). Psychiatric patients were already being admitted but inadequately recognized and treated, Moore claimed. He acknowledged that gaining approval for adequate psychiatric care would revolve around "the problem of finding trained personnel, *money*, space, time and assistants with energy, interest and proper training to carry on such a project once it was started" (p. 136; emphasis by au.). Research was not mentioned!

Others, in distant lands, believe that the United States never has a lack of means. I recall how, in 1975, before drastic cuts in funding, following my presentation of a description of liaison services to an international audience, a European colleague remarked on the "enviable funding and staffing" of American C-L programs in contrast to those of his own country. By the 1980s, in a talk to a similar audience, conditions had changed, if not totally reversed. Those services that had previously been shored up by private foundations and federal agencies had taken a downward course in the United States while European C-L services were enjoying governmental encouragement and support (Huyse, 1996), illustrative of the oscillating nature of funding characterizing the field.

More recently, assessment of funding for C-L services took place not only in the United States but in other countries as well. German universities and general hospitals in 2000 were now experiencing economic pressure to justify their services, calling for the "need to carefully address and evaluate the financial base of the services they provide," during a decade of cost-control that threatened to impact the rationing of care. In a worldwide review of cost analysis for C-L services, the authors note the paucity of relevant studies in German-speaking countries and suggest that research addressing management of somatizers, considering their high utilization of health resources, would demonstrate both clinical and socioeconomic benefits (Gundel, Siess & Ehlert, 2000).

An Irish study compared coding by psychiatrists with that of nonmedical billing personnel and noted the disparity, with professional billers missing billable codes for complex med-psychiatric diagnoses. The authors concluded, "Given the marked increase in case complexity associated with psychiatric comorbidities, future funding streams are at risk of inadequate payment for services rendered" (Udoh, Afif & MacHale, 2012). And a Swedish study in 2003 surveyed all psychiatry departments in the country to assess reimbursement schemes for C-L services, revealing a vast array of (dis)organizational systems mostly relying on "gentlemen's agreements" regarding funding (Wahlstrom, 2003). A Japanese survey by Noguchi and associates (2014) of general hospital psychiatry states, "Most institutions have not obtained merit from the current payment systems because of an excessively high requirement for the qualification of reimbursement" (p. 182).

Although Mitchell may have felt physicians were too preoccupied with a "lack of means," nothing drives the machine like adequate finances. More than 20 years after Moore's NEJM editorial, Lipowski (1974), the chronicler of progress of C-L, reassessed its status. Noting the economic stringencies of the time, he wrote that "under the prevailing conditions, no psychiatrist can earn an average income by confining himself to consultation-liaison work" (p. 626). Such conditions, he added, deterred the establishment of dedicated C-L services and "teams" that could meet the clinical and educational needs of the institution. Essential to this achievement, Lipowski advocated, would be funds from the psychiatry department, other nonpsychiatry departments being serviced, and insurance companies that recognized the value of time spent as part of the "atypical" medical service offered by C-L services. A formidable ideal, to be sure!

Crisis, Crisis, Crisis!

A "lack of means" has continuously dogged C-L services; financial support and reimbursement disparities have been a virtual nemesis of C-L psychiatry since its origins. By the 1970s, the situation with funding was already being addressed as a crisis. Once Rockefeller and Macy funds ceased, some C-L programs were "downsized" or totally eliminated. NIMH funding temporarily filled the void during the 1970s to early 1980s, largely through the commitment of James Eaton, but a subsequent blow with cessation of this funding by the 1980s sent C-L psychiatrists scurrying to find new means of support (Lazarus & Sharfstein, 1998). The extent to which C-L psychiatry depended on external financial support had become glaringly apparent (Levitan, 1983). "Hung out to dry," practitioners of the field began a search for remedial action if their interests were to continue to be served. Even department chairs in psychiatry were reluctant to drain their slim resources to sustain programs that were not revenue producing.

Insurance companies refused to reimburse a poorly defined clinical activity provided to patients who did not request it by physicians with ill-defined identity. Research data supporting the efficacy and utility of consultative services were apparently inadequate. Furthermore, the poor public image of psychiatry had carried over from the nineteenth century, when it was essentially custodial, taking place in distant asylums administered by "alienists" or "mad doctors," many of whom had no psychiatric training; private practice of psychiatry was virtually nonexistent. Even with minimal, if any, support of asylums by state, federal, and philanthropic resources, the neglect in these facilities was well known. As far as the attitude of the rest of medicine toward the mentally ill was concerned, "out of sight" was "out of mind," an attitude prevailing for decades in medicine. If general hospitals supported psychiatrists at all in certain roles, the practice of C-L psychiatry was essentially unknown. Unsurprisingly, the public had little comprehension of what a C-L psychiatrist was or did!

There was little incentive by politicians and administrators to look for newer, more viable ways to provide the public with mental health services. Thus, when psychiatric services more robustly transitioned from rural locations to community health centers and general hospitals in the 1970s, reimbursement problems escalated and continued to bedevil C-L psychiatry, presenting a serious impediment to its development. Recognition of this situation as a crisis (Kovan, 1974) may have been the bellwether of multiple funding crises to come, for indeed, eight years later in 1982, Viederman (1982), a C-L psychiatrist at Cornell, editorialized that the situation was still a crisis.

In the 1980s, prominent C-L psychiatrists nervously declared the subspecialty "at a crossroads," with an uncertain future unless fiscal, political, and identity challenges could be met (Pasnau, 1982). Concurrent with fiscal crises, psychiatry was in the throes of a shifting theoretical focus, from one that was "brainless" (psychodynamic) to one that was "mindless" (psychopharmacologic) (Eisenberg, 1986; Lipowski, 1989). Psychiatry as a discipline was itself assessing the differential benefits of an organic versus a psychosocial approach to mental illness, possibly further catalyzed by the pharmaceutical industry. Perhaps the identity confusion of psychiatry with its vacillating orientations from "mind oriented" (brainless) to "brain oriented" (mindless) presented a "moving target" for funding and reimbursement agencies, with resulting hesitancy to support either one.

With better education of psychiatrists about correct coding of comorbidities, charting, and identification of DRGs (diagnostic related groups), and establishment of specialized psychiatric billing services, reimbursement had improved somewhat (Strain, Fulop & Hammer, 1992). But each change in insurance policies and regulations thrust the situation back again into crisis mode (Kassirer, 1996). Without adequate funding, not only were patients denied proper treatment, but facilities to treat them were constantly in jeopardy. In 1986, the 2nd Annual Rosalynn Carter Symposium on Mental Health Policy invited economists and mental health professionals to consider "financing mental health services and research," culminating in an anemic summary that "we face the paradox that as the prospects for achieving solutions have heightened, coordinated support for the care and treatment of the mentally ill has worsened" (p. 98), not dissimilar from the Brookings Report summary. Recurrent crises spawned The Hospital Cost and Utilization Project of 1988 (HCUP-US.ahrq.gov), initiated as a federal-state-industry partnership to establish a database that could address issues of medical insurance and others, with painfully slow results.

It may be risking an accusation of paranoia to suggest that hesitation to pay for psychiatric services is based on a large "conspiracy" related to more than stigma (Greenblatt, 1975). C-L services have been held to a "higher standard" of demonstrated efficacy, cost-benefit and cost-offset, and matters of good patient care than, say, social service, nursing, or even chaplaincy. Strain and others (Strain, Easton & Fulop, 1995; Strain, Lyons, Hammer, Fahs, Lebovits, Paddison & Nuber et al., 1991), forceful advocates of improved funding, saliently identified barriers to funding and suggested "marketing" efforts to overcome them (Strain, 1987; Wise, 1987). Arguing that "the reduction of psychiatric comorbidity in and of itself should be sufficient to warrant funding support for C-L training and staffing" (Strain, Easton & Fulop, 1995, p. 187; Strain, Fulop & Hammer, 1994), they correctly state that "it seems an unfair burden that a C-L intervention should also need to demonstrate, in addition, cost offset capability"; other interventions, even including cardiac surgery or Medicare-supported social work services, have not had to "pass the test" before receiving financial support from third-party payers. A virtual frenzy of cost-offset, cost-benefit, or cost-effectiveness studies have been largely unable to change this perspective on C-L services (Strain, Hammer & Fulop, 1994).

There are few nowadays who would deny the prevalence of mental health problems in society reflected in comorbidities in general hospital populations. Yet, to justify adequate reimbursement or staff support for liaison services, the more definitive demonstration or "organization" of such specific services continues to be demanded by those who hold the purse strings. Hospital administrators resist incorporating charges for C-L services in already elevated per diem rates (as is done for social service and other patient care disciplines). Politicians and policy makers refuse funding for fear of "increasing national deficits" (and losing elections); department heads budget "more demanding" and remunerative aspects of departmental structure; and insurers ignore cost-savings benefits, readily and repeatedly demonstrated, because such savings will accrue not to them but "downstream" to other agencies and facilities.

(Un)Managed Care

If C-L psychiatrists were not already feeling put upon by the health care system, managed care was the "frosting on the cake," proposing that behavioral health care be "split off" by "carve-outs," for separate management and pricing. Managed care, introduced in the early 1980s, was broadcast as a "cost-saving measure" but was considered by the opposition as nothing more than a cost-saving measure for the "managers" (Iglehart, 1996; Shore & Beigel, 1996). A story in *The Wall Street Journal* (Goldberg, 1997) quoted a managed care executive saying, "[W]e see people as numbers . . . we're a mass-production medical assembly line and there is no room for the human equation in our bottom line" (Goodman, 2005).

Managed care treated psychiatry differently from medicine through these "carve-outs," removing "complicating" aspects of mental health from what were considered "medically necessary" services. It was designed to pay only for "medically necessary" psychiatric treatment, and some said it helped to "remedi-calize" psychiatry, while others saw it widening the chasm between medicine and psychiatry. On the assumption that psychosocial rehabilitation can readily take place apart from medical care, any intent to reintegrate mental patients in soci-ety was severely compromised by carving out their behavioral needs. Managed care left comprehensive care *un*managed, and even after two decades cost savings were questionable. Some observers are of the opinion that psychiatrists accepted "carve-outs" too passively.

Surviving the regulatory phases in health care reform of managed care, DRGs, and E&M (evaluation and management) coding, C-L psychiatrists persisted in their quest for ways to assure reimbursable services. Medicine in general was first introduced to the "resource-based relative value scale" proposed in 1988 by Dr. William Hsiao of Harvard as another plan to reign in the costs of health care. It was unclear just how this would affect reimbursement for C-L services. Physicians had to learn to navigate around new concepts of Health Maintenance Organizations (HMOs), Preferred Provider Organizations (PPOs), and other alphabetized programs as well as a "capitation environment" (Massachusetts Med-ical Society, 1996).

In the 1990s, insurers and government health agencies were criticized for look-ing more to benefit overhead entities like administration than benefit patient care (Friedman & Molay, 1994). Managed care pushed for briefer treatment interven-tions, more pharmacologic treatment, fewer follow-up visits, and earlier discharge from hospital. The need to obtain "authorization" for treatment and approval of recommendations antagonized physicians and gave short shrift to patients. Physi-cians wearied of endless phone calls and resented the entrance of "third-party" intrusion into clinical decision making, often by personnel without medical cre-dentials. Certain managed care plans had freedom to almost willy-nilly decide who could and could not be a provider, with certain services assigned to "lower-cost" professionals like social workers and psychologists. Consultations by any service were often limited to one a day, inducing a "race" by competing services to be the first to consult (Shore & Beigel, 1996). And follow-up consultations were not allowed.

C-L psychiatry's core objective of comprehensive care was shattered!

The Academy of Psychosomatic Medicine (APM)—with support from the Center for Mental Health Services, the Substance Abuse and Mental Health Services Administration, and the Center for Mental Health Policy and Services Research of the University of Pennsylvania—was prompted in 2000 to assess the impact of managed care on mental health care (Alter, 2000). Noting the lack of necessary funding for mental health care, they report that "none of the docu-ments reviewed address the significant economic barriers to providing care, and none call for the review of contractual arrangements, which clearly define how reimbursement will occur" (p. 7). Recommendations included holding managed care and managed behavioral health organizations (MC/MBHO) "accountable for the integration of medical and psychiatric care, *regardless of financial risk*" (p. 40; emphasis by au.), a rather strong and optimistic imperative!

All medical entities scrambled for solutions to massive system reforms. In a defensive move to counter health reform changes, hospitals in the 1990s moved toward mergers and acquisitions (NEJM, Editorial, March 14, 1996). Private industry, especially insurance companies, became the driving force in medicine. Consultation-liaison psychiatry, unfamiliar . . . and probably unwanted . . . became the loser in this mélange (Gonzales & Randel, 1996).

What to Do?

As untold aphorisms declare, crises also present opportunities. William James (1906), in a letter to a friend (May 6, 1906), wrote that "great emergencies and crises show us how much greater our vital resources are than we had supposed." With the necessity of funding assuming greater import, the need for C-L psychiatry to establish its bona fides loomed large. Although Lipowski (1974) had predicted in the 1970s that liaison psychiatry would present a viable model for all of psychiatry, this prediction, like so many before it, seemed overblown and on a distant horizon, especially if ways could not be found to finance it. With Hackett's admonition in mind, C-L psychiatrists were still implored to prove their worth.

With frustratingly little improvement in funding through extant research findings, philanthropic funding, or changed attitudes in administrators, insurers, or politicians, what pathways were available to C-L psychiatrists to remedy dire circumstances? Advisors in the field recommended (A) more robust research; (B) more creative ways to "waltz" administrators, politicians, and payers, and (C) greater understanding of the economics of medicine.

(A) Salvation by Research? Searching for Alice

With an equivalence of the political slogan "It's the economy, stupid," frustrated C-L psychiatrists began "shouting," "It's the research, stupid." Following the tsunami of funding problems in the 1980s, improved C-L research was perceived as a remedy, resulting in a proliferation of papers promoting research strategies, methodology, and statistical techniques (Saravay & Strain, 1994). Implied was that more rigorous studies would demonstrate cost-effectiveness and patient benefits from psychiatric consultation and assure increased reimbursement and improved policy making, with a promise of enhancing C-L psychiatry's sustainability and insurability (Levenson, 1990). Acknowledging that a "marketplace model" was not viable, Fenton and Guggenheim, assessed funding problems and dreamily asked, "Why can't Alice find Wonderland?" (Fenton & Guggenheim, 1981; Guggenheim, 1978). Guggenheim was indefatigable in his search for "Alice" and obtained approval from APA's president John Talbot to create the Task Force on

C-L Funding. Members included Jim Strain, Arthur Barsky, Stephanie Cavana-ugh, G. Richard Smith, Cheryl McCartney, and Emily Mumford.

The intense focus on the economics of C-L shifted research attention to "outcome studies" to show how benefits of C-L service could justify funding (Borus, Barsky, Carbone, Fife, Fricchione & Minden, 2000). Although "cost-benefit" studies had already appeared in the literature of past decades, none seemed to have impressed insurers, administrators, or policy makers, who, in a curious mix of metaphors, apparently "wore blinders" and were "tone deaf" about mental health services.

I well recall the aggravation of trying to persuade insurance company reviewers that by treating chronically ill patients with comorbid psychiatric illness in one-half hour sessions once a month, it was possible to decrease their utilization of emergency rooms, office visits, medication, and hospitalization (all willingly paid for under medical insurance), but "utilization review" held that such infrequent visits probably meant that patients "did not need psychiatric input at all" (Lipsitt, 1964). Questions of stigma, civil rights, improved health, or other factors did not enter the equation! Short-sightedness prevailed! Profit motive was king, and insurers could not acknowledge the savings to be garnered by a least expensive psychiatric approach to care.

One of the first studies to heed the renewed call for better research was that of Levitan and Kornfeld (1981). A thoughtfully designed, controlled study showed that liaison involvement in the care of patients with fractured femurs could save patients, hospitals, and insurers days of hospitalization and therefore considerable sums of money. The authors concluded that such intervention offered a clear cost-containment mechanism for medical care in general. The finding was clung to by advocates of C-L psychiatry like a drowning man to a life preserver. Hailed as heroes in the field, these researchers were credited with a "breakthrough" for other C-L psychiatrists to emulate.

To persuade "stakeholders" of the need and to encourage more C-L research, the National Institute of Mental Health, their own federal funding for C-L services diminishing or nonexistent, in 1982 published a large compendium of evaluative tools for the novice (C-L) researcher. An exploratory foreword stated that the "purpose of this anthology is to assist public policy makers, hospital administrators, clinical and academic department chairmen, and individual physicians to learn what progress is being made in C-L psychiatry programs that eventually results in that most important goal—improved patient care" (Trent, Houpt & Eaton, p. iii).

Perhaps less global and more to the point, Pardes, then-director of NIMH and a "recovering C-L psychiatrist," stated in his prefatory note, "[T]his book presents ways in which various programs have tried to answer [these questions about C-L services] and provides a thorough discussion of problems inherent in any measurement of health and mental health care education" (p. iv). In addition to assessing the responsiveness of C-L services to the needs of nonpsychiatric health care, the volume presents examples of research methodologies of specific services around the country to adequately train psychiatrists in the special skills of the C-L practitioner.[1]

Recognizing that improved research depended greatly not only on observation and numbers but also on measurement and data gathering, efforts were made to design instruments that could accomplish this purpose. A major innovative project was created by James Strain and colleagues (Hammer et al., 1993) called Micro-Cares, developed as a software computerized system and delivered to over 100 medical school psychiatry departments in the United States and around the world. The program recorded systematized data on not only numbers of consultation requests but also diagnoses, types of patients, costs, supervision hours, and the like, greatly facilitating a variety of research projects as well as uses for training and supervision.

Each new change in insurance policies called forth new demands on C-L services to comply and to focus research on ever-changing conditions as, for example, during the DRG era (Strain et al., 1992). Intended to more precisely refine diagnosis, use of DRGs required that reimbursement be determined on the basis of diagnosis rather than time spent with a patient (Mitchell & Thompson, 1985).

In spite of emerging research with well-designed studies that began showing improved patient function, more appropriate hospital utilization, more successful physician effort, cost savings, and the like, they were nonetheless generally dismissed by insurers. Smith opined that a narrow definition of "serious mental disorder" had marginalized clinical entities like somatization and comorbidities (Smith, 1998). Introducing "liaison screening" was recommended at or early in admission of patients to general hospitals, where 30–60% of patients have comorbid mental health problems, assuming that improved case finding and consultation would prove valuable; but reimbursement has not followed and has only now begun to be valued, mostly in countries other than the United States (Huyse, Saravay & Smith, 2008).

Continuing Malaise

Increased research in the field seemed unable to reverse the tide. By 1985, the continuing disappointing "progress" and general "malaise" around funding issues was noted by Guggenheim (1985) in a paper discussing cost, cost cutting, and cost efficacy issues and describing potential remedies. Clearly, once again, it was asserted, more and better research was in order.

To reinforce the Levitan/Kornfeld findings for doubters, Strain and associates replicated findings a decade later with a multisite study utilizing modified methodology (Strain, Fulop, Hammer & Lyons, 1991). Besides the savings from decreased length of hospital stay, other hospital costs of care for hip fracture patients were considerably reduced with inclusion of a liaison component to consultation, cost of which was met with cumulative revenues generated. Of course, when hospital days could be decreased by a variety of other institutional and administrative changes, savings from psychiatric consultation for this achievement lost its valence, and administrators no longer found this ("expensive") service essential to cut lengths of stay. Other more convincing benefits would have to be demonstrated!

McKegney and Beckhardt (1982) summed up the challenge facing C-L psychiatry. While the "'psychosomatic' or 'biopsychosocial' model makes eminent sense, . . . its acceptance by the health care system, and physicians in particular, will depend upon scientific demonstration that psychological and social factors influence biologically defined medical illness" (p. 198). In reviewing C-L research for the decade from 1970, they traced the shift from largely descriptive studies to more outcome-oriented research, especially as patients, the recipients of C-L interventions, were affected (McKegney & Beckhardt, 1982). This excellent review of extant research literature at the time acknowledges the failure of most studies to account for "time spent" in carrying out service, a feature that is decidedly associated with cost. Future studies, they advise, will need to consider whether "cost-benefit" or "cost-effectiveness" considerations are essential (p. 213). Cost-effectiveness, they predict, may be more "valuable" since it assesses more complex outcomes than strictly fiscal benefits of the service. And, in fact, by 2000 (echoing McKegney and Beckhardt [1982]), Borus and associates (2000) questioned whether studies that pursued the "holy grail" of cost-offset or cost-benefit were actually on the wrong track to sustainability and urged that research should look more to patient care and well-being as valued outcomes in their own right.

Papers continued to be published extolling the cost-effectiveness and cost-benefits of C-L services. Pincus summed up a series of studies confirming the cost-effectiveness of C-L services (Pincus, 1984). Reiterating Pincus's assertions a year later, Lyons and colleagues (Lyons, Hammer, Wise & Strain, 1985) emphasized that the potential clinical and economic benefits of consultation-liaison psychiatry accentuate the need for increased research using valid statistical methods by the purveyors of C-L services themselves. The authors review eight strategies of cost-effectiveness research and discuss their relative strengths and liabilities.

C-L psychiatry benefitted under the NIMH directorship of Herb Pardes in the early 1980s. With his own background in psychiatric research, psychosomatic medicine, C-L psychiatry, and psychoanalysis, he promulgated the value of the NIH-NIMH Intramural Research Center as a valued spur to enhanced studies at the interface of medicine and psychiatry (Pardes, 1983). Considerable interest was fostered through NIMH-sponsored research symposia, workshops, and conferences (e.g., Larson et al., 1987; Sharfstein, 1982). Psychiatrists' dilatory attitudes about fiscal matters began to take on new relevance in the viability of C-L services through research. Nevertheless, in spite of this promising upsurge of research interest by 1991, Dimsdale (1991) alluded to the relative underdevelopment of creditable C-L research, with case reports and small series studies still predominating. A research focus, he speculated, was lagging as a result of "distractions" in the field, such as the "continuing debate between advocates of consultation vs. liaison, competition with behavioral medicine practitioners, and the quest for sub-specialization status." His dire prediction was that "unless the development of a firm research base is equally emphasized, one wonders about the long term intellectual development of this important area" (p. 641). And, of course, sullying the promise of improvement, funding sources were being cut!

A reassessment of the status of C-L psychiatry (Cavanaugh & Milne, 1995) made a number of observations: A survey of 119 university programs revealed decreased funding over five years in more than 30% of programs, with no changes in 54% and some increase in 14%. Even with some hopeful signs, 57% described major problems in financial support; increased needs of the acutely ill, geriatric patients, transplant units, and HIV-infected, drug abuse, and delirium patients had escalated service burden even as they were being cut or diminished. Understaffing was reported by 51% of the programs, and liaison activities had ceased or were reduced in 70% of the programs (Cavanaugh & Milne, 1995).

Lest the focus on funding obscure the accomplishments of C-L psychiatric services, attention is drawn to the 1996 publication of Donald Kornfeld's Hackett Award Lecture in 1994, wherein he revisits the many successful contributions of C-L research to the practice of medicine and surgery: cardiac medicine, cancer treatment, ICU experience, treatment of pain and other "medical syndromes," the surgical experience, and in particular cataract surgery. Reports of such studies have been published in esteemed medical-surgical (as contrasted to psychiatric) periodicals like *New England Journal of Medicine, Lancet, Archives of Internal Medicine*, and *Journal of the American Medical Association* (JAMA), where they have had an impact on how physicians view emotional aspects of their work (Kornfeld, 1996). However, most of these studies were funded by research *grants*, not reimbursable services. A distinction must be made between reimbursement and funding. The latter may derive from a variety of resources, whereas reimbursement refers solely to revenue received for services rendered in consultative practice. In the survey by Cavanaugh and Milne (1995), only 13% of financial support for C-L service derived from patient fees, and funding from all sources included only 6% from other departments served.

Most funding for fellowships and general operations of C-L services in the years 1990–1995 was provided by psychiatry departments and the general hospital (about 74%). Editorializing concerns, Saravay (1995) opines, "In the face of educational, clinical, and administrative concerns . . . the erosion of liaison activities is a worrisome development" (p. 92).

Wise and Strain (1996) noted the lack of C-L reviews in Cochrane Reports, due to an absence in the literature of randomized clinical trials. The studies alluded to by Kornfeld had been mostly descriptive reports of clinical observation, about which the editorialists stated, "[D]espite the recognition that psychological factors enhance the morbidity and mortality in various medical disorders, further data is needed to convince policy makers and physicians who are developing clinical guidelines in other specialties that psychiatric intervention should be included" (p. 499). And so it goes again, with the ever-present need "to convince policy makers."

Indeed, by the turn of the century, notwithstanding certain advances in the field including recognition of psychosomatic medicine as the seventh specialty of psychiatry, the fiscal bugaboo persists. As noted in muted tones by Ali, Ernst, Pacheco, and Fricchione (2006), "the main rate-limiting step in this clinical expansion of C-L psychiatric services is the relative lack of behavioral health reimbursement." Again, they anticipate that the future holds promise as "the recent initiative by the Academy of Psychosomatic Medicine [builds] a consortium [that will] allow the gathering of large enough samples of subjects to power studies dealing with questions of comorbidity and may help to attract the funding necessary to carry out such large-scale studies" (p. 220).

(B) Waltzing Holders of the Purse

The process of educating or "convincing" a hospital's administrative structure is an arduous, but not impossible, one. When I was recruited in 1969 to found a department of psychiatry at Mount Auburn Hospital, the Board of Trustees wanted me to generate my salary through fee-for-service consultations, a most unattractive offer that would require essentially no commitment of the institution. I was able over several meetings to persuade them of the inefficiency of such an arrangement, one that would be of less utility to the hospital and to me as an educator. By accepting my proposal, they demonstrated rare flexibility and a capacity to tolerate a degree of uncertainty and risk while gaining experience with a totally new project. Being on salary, meager as it was, allowed me the freedom to do "whatever is necessary" to provide service and engage in teaching and exploration of new boundaries. Hours became endlessly expanded, but not having to think about hourly recompense permitted greater latitude to service institutional and personal objectives without worrying about "bookkeeping" issues. Such work conditions, with long service hours, did compromise my ability to have dinner with my family every night, but their forgiving appreciation of the work I did made life tolerable.

Lessons learned included the importance for C-L of establishing a "presence," making friends with house staff and attendings, and seizing opportunities to be helpful in any way possible, invaluable features of the work rarely achievable in "hit-and-run" consultations. Demonstrating the utility of a hospital-based consultation service and increased requests for consultation allowed for the eventual recruitment of a "fellow" assistant and decreased utilization of outside "one-shot" consultants whose primary allegiance was not to hospitalized patients but to office practice. Such service met with appreciation by consultees (and some disdain by "outside consultants") of rapidly accessible expert psychiatric assessment of their "difficult" patients, an essential ingredient of acceptance and expansion of C-L services. Collaborative support of a chief of medicine was an essential ingredient (Lipsitt, 2013). Still, general hospital administrators are reluctant to pay for full-time staff to provide "free range" services without generating revenue. I was put in mind of Dr. Stanley Cobb's comment of how he had to win over one department at a time in establishing his psychiatric service at Massachusetts General Hospital in 1934.

An occasional program director has been successful in convincing hospital and departmental administrators to include C-L services in the hospital's per diem rate. Wise and Berlin (1983), successful in this negotiation, sent a letter to colleagues, urging them to persuade administrators to fund C-L services as part of the general hospital budget. This innovation provided funding support for two fellows and supervision in one of their institutions.

Alan Gregg, in his determination to persuade board members of the Rockefeller Foundation to support psychiatric services in general hospitals, reveals how his appeal to members of the board with family members who had psychiatric problems was a very effective "negotiation."

Other methods designed to enlighten "nonprofessionals" included the broadcast through white papers on C-L psychiatry, produced and distributed by the American Psychiatric Association (APA) Committee on C-L Psychiatry and Primary Care Education as well as by the Academy of Psychosomatic Medicine. This exercise may have been the equivalent of airdropping leaflets in a warzone, hoping the "right people" would get them.

A bold step was taken by the C-L Association of Philadelphia (CLAP) when it was discovered there was no provision for the coverage of psychiatric services for patients with concomitant medical illness in a public sector managed care plan. A brief position paper described the need for such services, types of services typically delivered, the impact of psychiatric input in the medical setting on costs and other outcomes, and a specific set of recommendations. Through a series of actions aimed at ensuring inclusion of such services as part of mental health care, efforts were successful with acceptance of consultation-liaison services as part of the new state-mandated behavioral health carve-out program for Medicaid-eligible persons (Alter, Schindler, Hails, Lamdan, Shakin Kunkel & Zager, 1997).

An untimely economizing move of the APA had threatened to "sunset" the Committee on Consultation-Liaison Psychiatry and Primary Care Education, seeming to mimic the insurance industry in seeing it as not "cost effective." However, serious lobbying by the committee and other advocates emphasized the poor timing precisely when primary care programs needed greater input from psychiatry, demonstrating necessary vigilance even within one's own professional organizations..

The APA annually invites legislators to an educational conference to convey updated knowledge about mental health definitions, treatments, and costs, but any specific focus on C-L issues has been doubtful. Similar activities occur periodically in district branches of the APA, again with scanty, if any, emphasis on C-L issues. Advocacy activities of the APA generally have much "bigger" issues to pursue than the "lesser" issues of C-L funding. Nevertheless, energies devoted to funding for training and education can potentially benefit C-L programs.

(C) Economics 101

C-L psychiatrists, largely unaccustomed to dealing with the fiscal realities of their work, were increasingly importuned by Guggenheim's task force to go, like Willie Horton the bank robber, "where the money is." It was becoming ever clearer that the least likely aspect of C-L practice to be compensated was liaison. Psychiatry as a discipline was itself assessing the differential benefits of a consultative vs. a liaison approach, and an organic vs. a biopsychosocial (holistic) approach, to mental illness. A consensus was building that perhaps a focus for reimbursement purposes should concentrate most specifically on "consultation," with relative abandonment of "liaison."

Liaison: Boon or Bane?

In 1985, Hales summed up the crisis of the moment, optimistically describing the benefits of a C-L service but suggesting liaison activity itself may be a deterrent to proper reimbursement of services (Hales, 1985). He reports a clinical case requiring more than 10 hours' C-L time for proper management and treatment, noting that only a fraction of the justifiable cost was received by the service, the *liaison* component having been excluded. Reflected in this example is the widespread controversy and dispute over the "value" (in terms of financial support) of liaison activity as a part of consultative services (Hackett, 1982; Strain, 1983). "Liaison," being so difficult to objectify and quantify, tends to cast doubt on the entire consultative enterprise, with this component of C-L psychiatry largely responsible for jeopardizing reimburseability. Strain's efforts to more clearly define differences between consultation and liaison for better understanding was probably more instructive for trainees than for potential payers for service (Strain, 1999). But little changed in rates of reimbursement.

What had begun as the unique embellishment of a "proper" psychiatric consultation (i.e., liaison) seemed to become a liability. Liaison was not part of any other medical discipline. Negative criticism seemed to attract so much attention that it jeopardized the whole enterprise of consultation-liaison psychiatry. A number of C-L services began reverting to the original designation of consultation *only*, the act of diagnosing patients with comorbidity and recommending intervention. Psychiatric consultation had been reimbursed at only 30% of its claimed costs, a rate incompatible with sustaining the service (Guggenheim, 1984).

Evanescent characteristics like quality of life, self-esteem, well-being, family adjustment, personal behavior, and financial security do not lend themselves to easy quantification that can justify cost accountability; unfortunately, psychiatric services do not have the quantitative simplicity of a bilirubin level or a bacterially infected urine. Nevertheless, emotional illness has broad implications for a patient's adaptation and function, so that liaison psychiatry must devise ways to assess its ability to diminish life disruption, anguish, noncompliance, and utilization of health services. Pincus (1984) calls attention to the difficulty in performing cost-offset or cost-benefit studies, although C-L services do offer opportunities to show cost-savings effects of psychiatric intervention in medical illness. He states that "the close relationship of C-L psychiatry to illness that is understood and accepted by lay people (e.g. coronary artery disease, renal disease, etc.) provides a compelling basis for demonstrating its potential benefits" (p. 173). Cohen-Cole (1976–1977) adds that it is the more clinically oriented patient-outcome studies that will have the greatest utility in obtaining the firm financial support needed by C-L services.

The problems of reimbursement were not uniquely American. In 1955, British psychiatric colleagues responded to a joint British proposal by the Royal Colleges of both Psychiatry and Medicine for increased liaison services in general hospitals (Royal College of Physicians & Royal College of Psychiatrists, 1995), suggesting that "purchasers" of such services "include the cost of the liaison psychiatry service . . . within the costs of each medical directorate service" (p. 5). The publication elicited an editorial and a barrage of letters responding to it. The editorial by an emeritus professor of psychiatry, Neil Kessel, asked, "Should we buy liaison psychiatry?" Kessel raised questions about the meaning of "generic liaison psychiatric services" and questioned the validity of cost-saving studies (1996, pp. 725–726). Letters promptly followed from British C-L psychiatrists Sharpe, Storer, Lynch and Hill, Kraemer and Jaswon, and Hardie, challenging Kessel's assumptions and "failure to understand the proposal," only adding to the debate over the value of liaison services in the United States.

"Creative Billing"

By the 1990s, a number of authors had begun to propose methods of "creative billing" as a way to acknowledge, within legitimate bounds, the added value of C-L services; techniques included the "upcoding" of comorbidities, previously omitted, for increased insurance coverage (Hall & Frankel,1996). With better education of psychiatrists about correct coding of comorbidities, charting, and identification of DRGs and establishment of specialized psychiatric billing services, reimbursement had improved somewhat. But each change in insurance policies and regulations thrust the situation back again into crisis mode.

Even before the era of managed care, the economics of reimbursement for psychiatric services was a dizzying patchwork quilt of dubious advances and abundant setbacks. With profit making the ascending motive in health care, insurance companies used every device available to reduce reimbursement and to maximize profits, from utilizing nonmedical "quality assurance" reviewers to lobbying policy makers to oppose fair payments for "behavioral medicine" interventions. The "carve-out" was a device to separate out behavioral health from comprehensive health care, the better to "manage" it.

As one effort to better billing practices and reimburseability, the Academy of Psychosomatic Medicine (APM) in 1996 issued a position paper with recommendations for improving recognition and support by managed care "carve-outs." Observing that Medicaid contracts with managed care agencies had not included psychiatric consultation as an available service, the APM Task Force on Medicaid Managed Care contacted all Medicaid plans with their concern. Guidelines defining "medical necessity" included documentation of consultation requests like acute agitation, suicidal ideation, cognitive impairment, and severe noncompliance or treatment refusal, and evidence that the consultation had been requested by an attending physician (rather than house officer or other). Reminders to consultants to code for all psychiatric comorbidities legitimately improved claims for payment (Hall & Frankel, 1996).

Other Options: What to Do?

By this time, the need had been well established. It was time to make changes! Although insurers were not inclined to reimburse psychiatric consultations, physicians of other services had been favorably impressed with psychiatry's vital contribution to beneficial treatment outcomes; while insurers and other payers have considered C-L services not worth the cost, consultees themselves, even when they make little use of the service, feel such service should be reimbursed on a par with other medical/surgical interventions (Cavanaugh & Flood, 1976–1977). Thus, some directors of C-L services have been able to "sell" their services to specialized programs like transplantation (Surman, Cosimi & DiMartini, 2009), hemodialysis units (Strain, Vollhardt & Langer, 1981), and other programs such as cardiac units, HIV/AIDS services, and cosmetic surgery (Phillips & Dufresne, 2000). Partial or complete payment for the salary of C-L fellows assigned to these programs has been a moderately successful approach to funding. Furthermore, of developmental significance, psychiatric affiliation with these programs spawned a number of specialized C-L disciplines, such as psychooncology (Holland, 2004), psychonephrology (Levy, 2008), and psychosomatic ob-gyn (Stotland, 1985), each with its source of funding from its basic discipline.

The primary care movement of the 1970s, with its federally mandated inclusion of "behavioral science" in medical school curricula, seemed to offer a golden opportunity for participation of C-L psychiatrists, but, as Strain (1999, p. 8) demonstrated, most programs employed a variety of "mental health professionals" other than psychiatrists. The coffers of psychiatry departments have also benefitted when complex medical-psychiatric patients are transferred to med-psych, acute, or geriatric inpatient units in the general hospital, where services are better defined and reimbursed (Table 8.1).

TABLE 8.1 Proposed Funding Methods

- Make C-L part of bed rate
- Support from other services
- Fee-for-service
- Grants
- Specialized services like dialysis, transplant, ICU, ER
- Administrative support
- Federal and State funding

Another suggestion for funding includes outpatient C-L services. With a growing emphasis on shorter hospital stays, patients in need of psychiatric consultation are often discharged before effective consultation can be provided; these patients are more easily seen in outpatient liaison clinics. Although not common, examples of outpatient models have existed since at least 1931 (e.g., Phipps Clinic, New York's Mount Sinai Hospital, Boston's Beth Israel Hospital). The benefits of such clinics for clinical care as well as research and training have been described for the Mount Sinai Medical Center Liaison Clinic by Rowan, Strain and Gise (1984). This clinic was able to generate three quarters of a liaison fellow's salary through reimbursable patient visits. Kaplan (1981) notes, "[T]he liaison clinic offers an additional source of income to consultation-liaison service" (p. 512).

Other potential sources of funding are emergency services in general hospitals, where admission of large numbers of patients with psychiatric complications may add to the glut of cases and the slowing down of triage; a program at Yale has begun to demonstrate fiscal benefits of proactive screening in the emergency setting (Sledge et al., 2015). An Australian commentary notes that the "increase of 'psychosomatic' conditions would become a key role for psychiatrists and any reduction in funding of liaison psychiatry would be short-sighted" (Hundertmark, 2002, p. 424).

Assessment in the New Century

Efforts to demonstrate the value of C-L services with a Sisyphean thrust through research encountered disappointing news by the turn of the century. A systematic review of cost-effectiveness studies revealed that, in two decades of consultation-liaison interventions in general hospitals, only two studies met strict criteria to warrant valid outcomes (Andreoli, Citero & Mari, 2003). Disappointingly, the authors conclude that

> it is not yet possible to establish clinical guidelines for cost-effectiveness of mental health consultation-liaison interventions. . . . [F]urther improvement

of experimental studies, including the development of new criteria and measures, is required so that more information on the clinical and economic effects of consultation-liaison interventions can be obtained and models of overall mental health policy in general hospitals can be assessed.

(p. 503)

As we entered a new century with little improvement in funding or reimbursement of C-L services (especially the liaison component), some authors expressed concern that C-L was "barking up the wrong tree" or searching for the wrong "holy-grail" of cost-offset, both metaphors implying that efforts to secure funding were missing the point of effective C-L services (Borus et al., 2000).

Taking note of health care reform in "the brave new world of health care," Mitchell and Lieberman (2014) in *Psychiatric News* optimistically anticipate that

> With the enormous pressure to contain costs, health systems and payers are more receptive to trying new models of care including a new emphasis on early detection and treatment of psychotic disorders. . . . Some psychiatrists are becoming entrepreneurs: developing IT (information technology) solutions or consulting to practices and systems to facilitate these new care models.
>
> *(p. 3).*

Whether this "trend" will carry over to C-L activity remains to be seen.

In this new "health reform," payers will continue to angle for ways to reduce overall cost. Repeatedly, reimbursement rates are challenged. Medicare physician fees are constantly being threatened with reduction. Individual practitioners and their medical societies spend time that they do not have figuring out ways to eliminate or at least postpone such reductions. In 2014, a physician fee reduction of 24.4% was proposed by Medicare (Wilensky, 2014). Previously, physicians were reimbursed based on a resource-based relative value scale, determined by the workload for a particular intervention, expenses of the practice, and an adjustment for geographic site, features difficult to apply to C-L services. With each such adjustment, physicians have looked for ways to maximize reimbursements, by expending energy and time to understand the rules and to find ways to avoid them, sometimes risking bordering on the illegal. Having barely adapted to managed care by the mid-1990s, physicians continue to be challenged by a whole new set of rules, regulations, and definitions like "sustainable growth rate," "bundled services," "aggregate physician spending," and "E/M codes."

Some institutions have experimented with new models of C-L service—the program at UC Davis (Bourgeois, Hilty, Klein, Koike, Servis & Hales, 2003), for example, where "the need for a clinically and educationally robust inpatient CLS [C-L Service] persists despite funding pressures" (p. 262). This program, through various routes of expansion, has sought "diversified sources of funding support." It has cobbled together salary support for a robust C-L service from medical school administration, state agencies, outpatient facilities, specialized services like AIDS, oncology, hemodialysis, and an endowed chair for a professorship, not necessarily all options for other institutions (Bourgeois et al., 2003). Experimental psychiatric prescreening at Yale University Hospital has begun to show savings through earlier discharge and decreased readmission rates (Sledge, Gueorguieva, Desan, Bozzo, Dorset & Lee, 2015).

While C-L psychiatry since its inception has achieved much, financial support has remained a perennial problem throughout its so-called phase of rapid development. Many opportunities exist for future participation of C-L psychiatrists in such areas as public health, telemedicine/telepsychiatry, medical homes, collaborative care, and accountable care organizations. However, reimburseability remains a constricting deterrent and barrier (Ali, Ernst, Pacheco & Fricchione, 2006). Realization of this burdensome impediment has most certainly contributed to the quest for specialty recognition. Most worldwide literature on C-L research, clinical care, and training alludes to the benefits of C-L psychiatry for the rapidly increasing numbers of patients with complex medical disorders; they emphasize the pressing need for funding but offer little advice for making that a reality (Creed, 2003).

President Obama's Affordable Care Act (ACA) has begun to show evidence of lowering national health expenditures, but it is too early to hazard a prediction on future health care spending and how it might impact C-L programs. The new interest in affordable care organizations and "medical homes" proposes better integrated care especially for patients with chronic ailments. These innovations may offer impetus for new pricing systems that would recognize the essential contribution to care by psychiatry in those settings.

Blumenthal, Stremikis, and Cutler (2013) have emphasized the wasteful nature of some "cost-saving" efforts—for example, additional administrative costs and excessive use of acute care in the face of inadequate prevention (p. 2553)—and believe that the situation will improve with better "engineering" of the health care system. Gradual insistence on preventive care, coordination of health services, and recognition of the financial drain by excessively high utilizers of health care by, for example, "somatizers," whose prevalence runs as high as 50% or more (Ansseau et al., 2004) may bring about desired change.

Of all medical specialties, psychiatry continues to be the most discriminated against by insurers, with C-L services, lacking clear definition, even more so. And with a federal budget in 2015 proposing to reduce distribution of funds to NIH to the lowest point in 15 years, prospects for C-L appear bleak!

The struggle endures! While C-L psychiatrists hold patient care at their core, at times they might well enjoin George Bernard Shaw (1905) in his hyperbolic remark: "Money is indeed the most important thing in the world; and all sound and successful personal and national morality should have this fact as its basis" (p. xiv). Many C-L psychiatrists have high expectations that specialty accreditation will yield longed-for remedy.

Note

1 The first chapter, "Objectives for residents in consultation psychiatry," offers a 1976 draft of a review of competency-based skills for the C-L psychiatrist, from the Association for Academic Psychiatry's Task Force on C-L Psychiatry, drawing substantially on the 1976–1977 publication "The application of competency-based education to C-L psychiatry" (Cohen-Cole).

References

Ali, S., Ernst, C., Pacheco, M., & Fricchione, G. (2006). Consultation-liaison psychiatry: How far have we come? *Currents in Psychiatry Report, 8,* 215–222.

Alter, C.L. (Ed.). (2000). *The Behavioral Health Managed Care Initiative: Standards, Guidelines and Competencies: Mental Health Care for Patients with Chronic Medical Illnesses.* Center for Mental Health Policy and Services Research. Philadelphia, PA: University of Pennsylvania.

Alter, C.L., Schindler, B.A., Hails, K., Lamdan, R., Shakin Kunkel, E.J., & Zager, R. (1997). Funding for consultation-liaison services in public sector-managed care plans. The experience of the consultation-liaison association of Philadelphia. *Psychosomatics, 38,* 93–97.

Andreoli, P.B., Citero, Vde. A., & Mari, Jde.J. (2003). A systematic review of studies of the cost-effectiveness of mental health consultation-liaison interventions in general hospitals. *Psychosomatics, 44,* 499–507.

Ansseau, M., Dierick, M., Buntinkx, F., Cnockaert, P., De Smedt, J., Van Den Haute, M., . . . Vander Mijnsbrugge, D. (2004). High prevalence of mental disorders in primary care. *Journal of Affective Disorders, 78,* 49–55.

Billings, E.G. (1941). Value of psychiatry to the general hospital. *Hospitals, 15,* 305–310.

Billings, E.G., McNary, W.S., & Rees, M.H. (1937). Financial importance of general hospital psychiatry to hospital administrators. *Hospitals, 11,* 40–44.

Blumenthal, D., Stremikis, K., & Cutler, D. (2013). Health care spending—A giant slain or sleeping? *New England Journal of Medicine, 369,* 2551–2557.

Borus, J.F., Barsky, A.J., Carbone, L.A., Fife, A., Fricchione, G.L., & Minden, S.L. (2000). Consultation-liaison cost offset: Searching for the wrong grail. *Psychosomatics, 41,* 285–288.

Bourgeois, J.A., Hilty, D.M., Klein, S.C., Koike, A.K., Servis, M.E., & Hales, R.E. (2003). Expansion of the consultation-liaison psychiatry paradigm at a university medical center: Integration of diversified clinical and funding models. *General Hospital Psychiatry, 25,* 262–268.

Cavanaugh, J.L., Jr., & Flood, J. (1976–1977). Psychiatric consultation services in the large general hospital: A review and a new report. *International Journal of Psychiatry in Medicine, 7,* 193–207.

Cavanaugh, S., & Milne, J. (1995). Recent changes in consultation-liaison psychiatry. A blueprint for the future. *Psychosomatics, 36,* 95–102.

Cohen-Cole, S.A. (1976–1977). The application of competency-based education to consultation-liaison psychiatry. *International Journal of Psychiatry in Medicine, 7,* 295–328.

Creed, F. (2003). Consultation-liaison psychiatry worldwide. *World Psychiatry, 2,* 93–94.

Darley, W., & Somers, A.R. (1967). Medicine, money and manpower: The challenge to professional education. *New England Journal of Medicine, 276,* 1471–1478.

Dimsdale, J.E. (1991). Challenges, problems and opportunities in consultation-liaison psychiatry research. *Psychiatric Medicine, 9,* 641–648.

Eisenberg, L. (1986). Mindlessness and brainlessness in psychiatry. *British Journal of Psychiatry, 148,* 497–508.

Fenton, B. J., & Guggenheim, F.G. (1981). Consultation-liaison psychiatry and funding. Why can't Alice find wonderland? *General Hospital Psychiatry, 3,* 255–260.

Follette, W., Cummings, N.A. (1967). Psychiatric services and medical utilization in a pre-paid health plan setting. *Medical Care, 5,* 25–35.

Friedman, R.S., & Molay, F. (1994). A history of psychiatric consultation in America. *Psychiatric Clinics of North America, 17,* 667–681.

Goldberg, R.M. (1997). What's happened to the healing process. *West Virginia Medical Journal 1997, 93,* 172–173.

Gonzales, J. J., & Randel, L. (1996). Consultation-liaison psychiatry in the managed care arena. *Psychiatric Clinics of North America, 19,* 449–466.

Goodman, H. (2005). Salaries of HMO managers and doctors. In H. Goodman (Ed.). *Money and Health: A Study of American Social Values.* (Vol. 1). (*The Wall Street Journal,* June 18, 1997). (p. 171). Indianapolis, IN: Dog Ear Publishing.

Gregg, A. (1956). *Challenges to Contemporary Medicine.* New York, NY: Columbia University Press.

Greenblatt, M. (1975). Psychiatry: the battered child of medicine. *New England Journal of Medicine, 292,* 246–250.

Guggenheim, F.G. (1978). A marketplace model of consultation psychiatry in the general hospital. *American Journal of Psychiatry, 195,* 1380–1383.

Guggenheim, F.G. (1984). Cost effectiveness and consultation psychiatry: Reflecting on, and in, economic terms. *General Hospital Psychiatry, 6,* 171–172.

Guggenheim, F.G. (1985). The national malaise concerning health-care costs in the DRG era. *General Hospital Psychiatry, 7,* 337–340.

Gundel, H., Siess, M., & Ehlert, U. (2000). Consultation and liaison activity from the socio-economic perspective. A plea for cost-benefit analysis in psychosomatics. [Article in German]. *Psychotherapy, Psychosomatic Medicine and Psychology, 50,* 247–254.

Hackett, T.P. (1981). Thunder on the right. (Editorial). *Psychosomatics, 22,* 733–734.

Hackett, T.P. (1982). Consultation psychiatry held valid, liaison invalid. *Clinical Psychiatry News.* January, p. 36 (also Annual Meeting of Academy of Psychosomatic Medicine, Dallas, TX: December 1981).

Hales, R.E. (1985). The benefits of a psychiatric consultation-liaison service in a general hospital. *General Hospital Psychiatry, 7,* 214–218.

Hall, R.C.W., & Frankel, B.L. (1996). The value of consultation-liaison interventions to the general hospital. *Psychiatric Services, 47,* 418–420.

Hall, R., Rundell, J.R., & Hirsch, T.W. (1996). Economic issues in consultation-liaison psychiatry. In J.R. Rundell & M.G. Wise. (Eds.). *American Psychiatric Publishing Textbook of Consultation-Liaison Psychiatry.* (pp. 25–37). Washington, DC: American Psychiatric Press.

Hall, R., Rundell, J., & Popkin, M.K. (2002). Economic issues in consultation-liaison psychiatry. In J.R. Rundell & M.G. Wise. (Eds.). American Psychiatric Press Textbook of Consultation-Liaison Psychiatry. Washington, DC: American Psychiatric Press.

Hammer, J.S., Strain, J.J., Lewin, C., Easton, M., Mayou, R., Smith, G.C., . . . Himelein, C. (1993). The continuing evolution and update of a literature database for C-L psychiatry: MICRO-CARES literature search system. *General Hospital Psychiary, 15,* (6 Suppl), 1S–73S.

Henry, G.W. (1929–1930). Some modern aspects of psychiatry in general hospital practice. *American Journal of Psychiatry, 9,* 481–499.

Holland, J. (2004). IPOS Sutherland memorial lecture: An international perspective on the development of psychosocial oncology: Overcoming culture and attitudinal barriers to improve psychosocial care. *Psychooncology, 13,* 445–449.

HCUP-3. (1998). Healthcare (Prev. Hospital) Cost and Utilization Project 1988-1994. Washington, DC: Agency for Health Care Policy and Research, U.S. Department of Health and Human Services. Available at http://www.ahcpr.gov/ data/hcup-pkt,htm. Accessed February 13, 2015.

Hundertmark, J. (2002). The impact of mainstreaming on patient care in Australian emergency departments and liaison services. (Correspondence) *Australia and New Zealand Journal of Psychiatry, 38,* 424.

Huyse, F. (1996). The European consultation-liaison workgroup (ECLW) collaborative study. I. General outline. *General Hospital Psychiatry, 18,* 44–55.

Huyse, F., Saravay, S.M., & Smith, G. (2008). Internationalization and integration of the "C-L" psychiatry field. *Journal of Psychosomatic Research, 64,* 557–558.

Iglehart, J.K. (1996). Managed care and mental health, *New England Journal of Medicine, 334,* 131–136.

James, William. (1906). Letter to W. Lutoslawski. May 6, 1906. Retrieved from Notablequotes.com

Jones, K.R., & Vischi, T.R. (1979). Impact of alcohol, drug abuse and mental health treatment on medical care utilization: A review of research literature. *Medical Care, 17(Suppl. 2),* ii–82.

Kaplan, K. (1981). Development and function of a psychiatric liaison clinic. *Psychosomatics, 22,* 502–512.

Kassirer, J.P. (1996). Mergers and acquisitions—Who benefits? Who loses? (Editorial). *New England Journal of Medicine, 334,* 722–723.

Kessel, N. (1996). Should we buy liaison psychiatry? (Editorial). *British Journal of Psychiatry, 89,* 481.

Kornfeld, D. (1996). Consultation-liaison psychiatry and the practice of medicine. The Thomas P. Hackett Award Lecture given at the 42nd annual meeting of The Academy of Psychosomatic Medicine, 1995. *Psychosomatics, 37,* 236–248.

Kovan, R.A. (1974). Crisis in consultation: The need to develop accountability. *Hospital and Community Psychiatry, 25,* 536–537.

Larson, D.B., Kessler, L.C., Burns, B.J., Pincus, H.A., Houpt, J.L., Fiester, S., . . . & Chaitkin, L. (1987). A research development workshop to stimulate outcome research. *Hospital and Community Psychiatry (Psychiatric Services), 38,* 1106–1109.

Lazarus, J.A., & Sharfstein, S.S. (1998). *New Roles for Psychiatrists in Organized Systems of Care.* Washington, DC: American Psychiatric Press.

Levenson, J.L. (1990). Methodology in consultation-liaison research. *Psychosomatics, 31,* 367–376.

Levin, S., & Michaels, J.J. (1961). The participation of psycho-analysts in the medical institutions of Boston. *International Journal of Psychoanalysis, 42,* 271–283.

Levitan, S.J. (1983). Evaluation of consultation-liaison psychiatry: Better health at lower cost? In J.B. Finkel (Ed.). *Consultation-Liaison Psychiatry: Current Trends and New Perspectives.* (pp. 25–49). New York, NY: Grune & Stratton.

Levitan, S., & Kornfeld, D. (1981). Clinical and cost-benefits of liaison psychiatry. *American Journal of Psychiatry, 138,* 790–793.

Levy, N.B. (2008). What is psychonephrology? *Journal of Nephrology, 21*(Suppl. 13), S51–S53.

Lipowski, Z. J. (1974). Consultation-liaison psychiatry: An overview. *American Journal of Psychiatry, 131,* 623–630.

Lipowski, Z. J. (1989). Psychiatry: Mindless or brainless, both or neither? *Canadian Journal of Psychiatry, 34,* 249–254.

Lipsitt, D. R. (1964). Integration clinic: An approach to the teaching and practice of medical psychology in an outpatient setting. In N. E. Zinberg (Ed.). *Psychiatry and Medical Practice in a General Hospital.* (pp. 231–249). New York, NY: International Universities Press.

Lipsitt, D. R. (2013). Partners at the interface. *American Journal of Psychiatry, 170,* 1401–1402.

Lyons, J. S., Hammer, J. S., Wise, T. N., & Strain, J. J. (1985). Consultation-liaison psychiatry and cost-effectiveness research. A review of methods. *General Hospital Psychiatry, 7,* 302–308, 349–352.

Massachusetts Medical Society. (1996). *Vital Signs,* September.

McKegney, F.P., & Beckhardt, R.M. (1982). Evaluative research in consultation-liaison psychiatry. Review of the literature: 1970–1981. *General Hospital Psychiatry, 4,* 197–218.

McKerracher, D.G. (1959). On modern psychiatry and the health plans. *New England Journal of Medicine, 260,* 474–478.

Mitchell, G., & Lieberman, J. (2014). The role of psychiatrists in the brave new world of health care. *Psychiatric News.* April 4. Retrieved from www.psychnews.org

Mitchell, W. (1994). Address before fiftieth annual meeting of the American medico-psychological association held in Philadelphia, PA. May 16, 1894. *American Journal of Psychiatry, 151,* 28–36.

Mitchell, W.D., & Thompson, T.L., 2nd. (1985). Research problems for consultation-liaison psychiatry in the DRG era. *General Hospital Psychiatry, 7,* 349–352.

Moore, M. (1951). The need for psychiatry in a municipal general hospital. *New England Journal of Medicine, 244,* 135–136.

Mumford, E., Schlesinger, H. J., & Glass, G. V. (1982). The effects of psychological intervention on recovery from surgery and heart attacks: An analysis of the literature. *American Journal of Public Health, 72,* 141–151.

Mumford, E., Schlesinger, H. J., Glass, G. V., Patrick, C., & Cuerdon, T. (1984). A new look at evidence about reduced cost of medical utilization following mental health treatment. *American Journal of Psychiatry, 10,* 1145–1158.

Noguchi, M., Kobayashi, T., & Satake, N. (2014). A report on the current situation of general hospital psychiatry: The results of the Japanese general hospital survey 2012, *Japanese Journal of General Hospital Psychiatry, 26,* 121–232.

Pardes, H. (1983). Introduction: Research at the interface of medicine and psychiatry. *General Hospital Psychiatry, 5,* 79–81.

Pasnau, R.O. (1982). Consultation-liaison psychiatry at the crossroads: In search of a definition for the 1980s. *Psychiatric Services (Hospital and Community Psychiatry), 33,* 989–995.

Phillips, K., & Dufresne, R.G. (2000). Body dysmorphic disorder: A guide for dermatologists and cosmetic surgeons. *American Journal of Clinical Dermatology, 1,* 235–243.

Pincus, H.A. (1984). Making the case for consultation-liaison psychiatry: Issues in cost-effectiveness analysis. *General Hospital Psychiatry, 6,* 173–179.

Rowan, G.E., Strain, J.J., & Gise, L.H. (1984). The liaison clinic: A model for liaison psychiatry funding, training, and research. *General Hospital Psychiatry, 6,* 109–115.

Royal College of Physicians & Royal College of Psychiatrists. (1995). *The Psychological Care of Medical Patients: Recognition of Need and Service Provision.* London, UK: Royal College of Physicians & Royal College of Psychiatrists.

Saravay, S.M. (1995). Academic consultation-liaison services: The problems and the promise (Editorial). *Psychosomatics, 36,* 91–94.

Saravay, S.M., & Strain, J.J. (1994). Academy of Psychosomatic Medicine Task Force on funding implications of consultation-liaison outcome studies. Special series introduction: A review of outcome studies. *Psychosomatics, 35,* 227–232.

Schlesinger, H.J., Mumford, E., Glass, G.V., Patrick, C., & Sharfstein, S.S. (1983). Mental health treatment and medical care utilization in a fee-for-service system: Outpatient mental health treatment following the onset of a chronic disease. *American Journal of Public Health, 73,* 422–429.

The Second Annual Rosalynn Carter Symposium on Mental Health Policy. (1986). Financing mental health services and research: Current perspectives. November 20 at *Emory University School of Medicine, Department of Psychiatry.* Washington, DC. National Academy of Sciences.

Sharfstein, S.S. (Chair) (1982). Symposium on consultation-liaison research. Annual Meeting of the American Psychiatric Association, May, 1982. Toronto, Canada.

Shaw, G.B. (1905). *The Irrational Knot.* New York, NY: Brentano.

Shore, M., & Beigel, A. (1996). The challenge posed by managed behavioral health care. (Editorial). *New England Journal of Medicine, 334,* 116–118.

Sledge, W.H., Gueorguieva, R., Desan, P., Bozzo, J.E., Dorset, J., & Lee, H.B. (2015). Multidisciplinary proactive psychiatric consultation service: Impact on length of stay for medical inpatients. *Psychotherapy and Psychosomatics, 84,* 208–216.

Smith, G.C. (1998). From consultation-liaison psychiatry to psychosocial advocacy: Maintaining psychiatry's scope. *Australia and New Zealand Journal of Psychiatry, 32,* 753–761; Discussion 762–766. The impact of mainstreaming on patient care in Australian emergency departments and liaison services. (2002). June, 38(3), 424.

Somers, A.R., & Somers, H.M. (1961). *Doctors, Patients and Health Insurance.* Washington, DC: Brookings Institution.

Stotland, N.E. (1985). Contemporary issues in obstetrics and gynecology for the consultation-liaison psychiatrist. *Hospital and Community Psychiatry, 36,* 1102–1108.

Strain, J.J. (1983). Liaison psychiatry and its dilemmas. *General Hospital Psychiatry, 5,* 209–212.

Strain, J.J. (1987). Appraisal of marketing approaches for consultation-liaison psychiatry. *General Hospital Psychiatry, 9,* 368–371.

Strain, J.J. (1999). Liaison psychiatry. In J.R. Rundell & M.G. Wise (Eds.). *Essentials of Consultation-Liaison Psychiatry.* (pp. 3–11). Washington, DC: American Psychiatric Press.

Strain, J.J., Easton, M., & Fulop, G. (1995). Composition and funding. Consultation-liaison psychiatry services. *Psychosomatics, 36,* 113–121.

Strain, J.J., Fulop, G., & Hammer, J.S. (1992). A new tool for consultation-liaison funding: Modified DRGs to reflect psychiatric comorbidity. *General Hospital Psychiatry, 14,* 119–123.

Strain, J.J., Fulop, G., & Hammer, J.S. (1994). Consultation-liaison funding: Issues for service and training. In H. Leigh (Ed.). *Consultation-Liaison Psychiatry: 1990 and Beyond.* (pp. 181–195). New York, NY: Plenum.

Strain, J.J., Fulop, G., Hammer, J.S., & Lyons, J.S. (1991). Research applications of a consultation-liaison psychiatry data base. *Psychiatry in Medicine, 9,* 559–576.

Strain, J.J., Hammer, J.S., & Fulop, G. (1994). Academy of psychosomatic medicine task force on psychosocial interventions in the general hospital inpatient setting. A review of cost-offset studies. *Psychosomatics, 35,* 263–262.

Strain, J.J., Lyons, J.S., Hammer, J.S., Fahs, M., Lebovits, A., Paddison, P.L., . . . Nuber, G. (1991). Cost offset from a psychiatric consultation-liaison intervention with elderly hip fracture patients. *American Journal of Psychiatry, 148,* 1044–1049.

Strain, J.J., Vollhardt, B.R., & Langer, S.J. (1981). A liaison fellowship on a hemodialysis unit. A self-funded position. *General Hospital Psychiatry, 3,* 10–15.

Surman, O., Cosimi, A.B., & DiMartini, A. (2009). Psychiatric care of patients undergoing organ transplantation. *Transplantation, 87,* 1753–1761.

Thompson, T.L., 2nd & Suddath, R.L. (1987) Edward G. Billings: pioneer of consultation-liaison psychiatry. Psychosomatics, 28,153–156.

Trent, P.J., Houpt, J.L., & Eaton, J.S., Jr. (Eds.)

Udoh, G., Afif, M., & MacHale, S. (2012). The additional impact of liaison psychiatry on the future funding of general hospital services. *Irish Medical Journal, 105,* 331–332 [Ireland].

Viederman, M. (1982). The crisis in private consultation. (Editorial). *Hospital and Community Psychiatry, 33,* 969.

Wahlstrom, L. (2003). Psychiatric consultation-liaison in Sweden surveyed. *Larsartidningen, 100,* 120–124 [Sweden].

Wilensky, G.R. (2014). Improving value in Medicare with an SGR fix. *New England Journal of Medicine, 370,* 1–3.

Wise, T.N. (1987). Segmenting and accessing the market in consultation-liaison psychiatry. *General Hospital Psychiatry, 9,* 354–359.

Wise, T.N., & Berlin, R.M. (1983). Psychiatrists' role in consultation-liaison. *American Journal of Psychiatry, 140,* 269.

Wise, T.N., & Strain, J.J. (1996). The need for randomized controlled trials: The Cochran(*sic*) initiative. (Editorial). *Psychosomatics, 37,* 499–501.

SECTION III

The Process of Specialty Recognition

Preamble: *According to Paul Starr, in an exquisite description of the origins and transformation of American medicine, the evolving of a profession depends on many variables, including power, authority, politics, commonalities, and the like. In his definitive book* The Social Transformation of American Medicine (1982), *he states: "Professional claims, of course, should not be taken simply at face value. The rewards of professional status encourage would-be and even established professions to invent or elaborate credentials, sciences and codes of ethics in bids for recognition. Rather than as indicators of professional status, such features should be seen as the means of legitimizing professional authority, achieving solidarity among practitioners, and gaining a grant of monopoly from the state. Occupations may or may not succeed, depending on their means of collective organization and the receptivity of the public and the government" (p. 16).*

These next chapters address the struggles of C-L psychiatry to achieve recognition, visibility, and acceptability as a "sovereign" discipline within organized medicine and psychiatry. The process of legitimizing psychosomatic medicine as its "professional authority" is examined in its complex trajectory.

9
PRELUDE TO SPECIALIZATION

Psychosomatic medicine is well on the way to becoming a singular specialty. It now has its coterie of practitioners, its specialty publications, its journals, its monographs, and its historical treatises. True, it is still lacking an international society and a specialty board. But if things move as rapidly and in the same direction during the next 10 years as they have in the past 25, we may expect in the not-too-distant future, both a world-wide society and a specialty board. These are eventualities which I, for one, do not envisage with pleasure or satisfaction.

—*Galdston, 1955, p. 441*

Reactions are usually strongest with the newness of an idea, whether supportive or oppositional. After a while, the concept exists quietly on its own or gradually dies a slow death. In de Mandeville's (1711) treatise on hypochondriasis and hysteria, the physician Philoperio tells his patient Mifomedon about fads in medicine:

> An Hypothesis when once it is established a little time becomes like a Sovereign, and receives the same homage and respect from its Vassals, as if it was Truth itself. No Hypothesis ever became famous before it had pleased a great part of the learned World, and ever since *Paradise* Mankind has had the same strength of Thought: the rest depends all upon Experience; wherefore as long as that increases [*sic*], and our fickleness continues, it is impossible that ever a System or Opinion should be generally received, or last forever.
>
> *(pp. 113–114)*

After a span of turbulent times, especially fueled by the panic of defunded services, the idea for a stronger representation of C-L services and its potential acceptance as a subspecialty had "pleased a great part of the learned World." The alarm began to spread more intensely with cessation of NIMH funding in the mid-1980s. In his presidential address to members of the Academy of Psychosomatic Medicine, William Webb (1987) asked how their organization should respond to impending "turf wars, interprofessional rivalries, conceptual disputes, competing journals, and various organizations" (Webb, 1988, p. 148). The robust quest for subspecialization may well have begun there, followed by a sequence of discussions, controversies, arguments, dissensions, and rivalries.

If we recognize that we have been traveling a road punctuated with uncertain milestones and signposts, arriving at this point is not a destination but merely another place to pause and contemplate where and what we have come from and where we might be going. All entities, whether human individuals or organizations, as they grow and mature, go through periods of *sturm und drang*. In humans, it is called growth or development; in organizations, it is called "politics" or "disaffection."

The road to specialization has been winding and at times jarring, with occasional potholes along the way. General hospital psychiatry, C-L psychiatry, and psychosomatic medicine all have in some manner or other sought to achieve greater rapprochement between medicine and psychiatry. As anticipated by Galdston, there is *indeed* an international organization in the International College of Psychosomatic Medicine (begun in 1971) and now a "board" with designation of psychosomatic medicine as the seventh psychiatric specialty. This chapter retraces the journey as it considers in some detail the complexities of the quest for specialty recognition and looks at changes in psychosomatic medicine (as C-L psychiatry) that have catalyzed this quest.

"I am persuaded," Galdston (1955) wrote,

> that the historical function of the psychosomatic movement is not to add another to our Babel of specialties but, rather, to vitalize the whole of medicine, with the holistic and ecological viewpoint. When that has been achieved, the psychosomatic movement will have fulfilled its mission and it will have been absorbed into medicine [and the notion of a separate psychosomatic specialty will be unnecessary—added by au.].
>
> *(p. 449–450)*

Of interest is that Galdston's (1958) subsequent writings addressed the life and death of specialties.

While psychosomatic medicine is hardly a new idea, reactions to its reemergence are as intense as they were years ago. The subject episodically emerges and retreats like the figures on a Black Forest weather clock. Galdston's comments have an eerily familiar sound. At the time of his writing, psychosomatic medicine was flourishing in both lay and professional circles. As psychosomatic medicine blossomed between the 1920s and 1940s, advocates proclaimed that it would become the "new medicine." Galdston, a physician/psychiatrist/psychoanalyst was doubtful about the relevance of specificity between personality patterns and definitive "psychosomatic disorders," concerned that it was the wrong idea about etiology of disease; it would fragment medicine and take it in an undesirable direction, away from a holistic or ecological approach, in what Galdston preferred to call "Social Medicine" (p. 448).

Similar concerns were broadcast in opposition to more recent efforts to seek specialization for the discipline. "Stakeholders" promptly voiced their positions. Articles appeared espousing controversial points (Blumenfield, 1988; Muskin, 1988). Application for subspecialty recognition is an arduous process, not one that everyone in the field was eager to embark on. Because psychosomatic medicine is not as readily identifiable as, for example, gastroenterology, infectious disease, parasitology, and other medical disciplines, the topic itself lacks ideological clarity and boundaries and does not lend itself readily to definition. The continual suggestion for name changes over the years has not been helpful (Schwenk, 1999; Thompson, 1993). In a single issue of *Psychosomatics*, for example, the proposal is put forward to designate C-L psychiatry as "Medical Psychiatry," a seeming defensive redundancy since psychiatry has always been "medical." Besides "psychosomatic medicine" and "C-L psychiatry," we have "general hospital psychiatry," "behavioral medicine," "neuropsychiatry," "med-surg psychiatry," "psychosocial psychiatry," "psychobiological psychiatry," and a variety of others proposed over the years, reflecting considerable uncertainty about the identity of the field.

The American Psychosomatic Society (APS), long uneasy with its name, developed the Committee on Name Change (Lane, 1999) and invited an extensive survey of suggestions for a name change, ultimately finding favor mostly with what it already had. And different countries have their own history and practice of naming, so that in the United Kingdom, for example, psychiatry has long been referred to as "medical psychology," and schools of psychosomatic medicine have generally been either free-standing, autonomous disciplines or allied with internal medicine rather than psychiatry.

History does indeed have a way of repeating itself. As we contemplate the future of the field, questions abound as to whether designating psychosomatic medicine as a specialty aligned with psychiatry (rather than with medicine, for example, or an independent domain) fulfills its considered mission. Dubos (1968) wrote, "A new kind of knowledge is needed to unravel the nature of the cohesive forces that maintain man in an integrated state, physically, psychologically and socially, and enable him to relate to his surroundings" (p. 244). Very simply stated, this worldview is what humanity has sought in one manner or another, beginning with interest in the relationship of mind to body and of the whole to the universe. A most recent iteration of the search is the oft-recycled concept of the biopsychosocial approach (Engel, 1977) with all its possibilities and imperfections (Benning, 2015; Ghaemi, 2009; Kontos, 2011). Most recent ripples in the field seem less rooted in a "new knowledge" than in economic and political forces that have reshaped all of medicine and with it, psychiatry and its components. Controversy ensued over the reason a name with such an ambiguous history would be resurrected anew.

Dueling Societies?

In the early years of psychosomatic medicine, two organizations were founded to "unravel the nature of cohesive forces that maintain man in an integrated state" (Dubos, 1968, p. 244). In 1942, the American Psychosomatic Society (first called American Society for Research in Psychosomatic Problems) was established by Dunbar, Alexander, Carl Binger, Edward Weiss, I. Arthur Mirsky, Dana Atchley, Stanley Cobb, and three nonphysicians (Margaret Mead and two psychologists dedicated to research). Dunbar herself only reluctantly accepted the term "psychosomatic"; of interest, according to historian Shorter (1992), Dunbar "situated the diagnosis and treatment of [psychosomatic and somatoform disorders] in departments of internal medicine" (p. 261).

Twelve years later, the Academy of Psychosomatic Medicine was founded by a small group of disaffected physicians, only three of whom were psychiatrists, with a much broader focus on clinical issues of immediate interest to practitioners of all branches of medicine, not exclusively psychiatrists. Wilfrid Dorfman founded the journal *Psychosomatics* in 1960, describing its purpose as fundamentally a defensive move against the tendency of specialties to pay excessive attention to detail, with an undesirable "decrease in attention to the total person." Coincidentally, this was, in part, the rationale for the entire *reformist* psychosomatic movement against medicine's increasing technologization of the 1920s and 1930s. The two organizations (APS and APM) would figure prominently in sometimes acrimonious negotiations around the topic of specialization. In some sense, from the very beginnings, their two diverse missions foretold the tensions that would occur later. From sequential presidencies of both these organizations, Tom Wise (1995), consummate politically sensitive clinician, would eventually present his APS presidential address as the *Tale of Two Societies*, to assess their respective contributions and repercussions to the journey along the pathway to specialization. Acknowledging their shared but disparate interests and missions, Wise embraced the hope for a collaborative future as pursuit of subspecialization moved forward. Subsequent events will be discussed more extensively below.

To Specialize or Not to Specialize

Keeping in mind that ideas evolve in the context of the times and cultures in which they emerge, we can allow that prominent psychiatrists who, on earlier occasion, considered C-L decidedly not a specialty (e.g., Schwab, 1968; Lipowski,

1986; Galdston, 1955, 1958; Alexander, 1950; Dunbar, 1935; Seguin, 1970; Binger, 1960) later became supportive, active participants in constructing the application for specialty status.

Very early in the seeding of American psychosomatic medicine, Weiss and English (1943) published the first textbook on the subject. In it, they wrote:

> Psychosomatic is a relatively new term, but it describes an approach to med-
> icine as old as the art of healing itself. It is *not a specialty* but rather a point
> of view which applies to all aspects of medicine and surgery. . . . When the
> integration [physiology and psychology] is complete, we may not have to
> use the term, for good medicine will be psychosomatic.
>
> *(p. 3; emphasis by au.)*

In 1960, one of the founders of the journal *Psychosomatic Medicine*, Carl Binger (1960), wrote:

> Psychosomatic medicine is *not a specialty*. The proper future of psychoso-
> matic medicine is its disappearance, with replacement by a true holistic or
> comprehensive medicine. This is a far distant goal. For the present, psy-
> chosomatic medicine is necessary, both for purposes of special research and
> especially for the education of practicing physicians and surgeons as well as
> younger students.
>
> *(pp. 249–250; emphasis by au.)*

Embedded in these comments are faint echoes of liaison psychiatry.

Describing the field of consultation psychiatry in the first handbook of consultation psychiatry, John Schwab (1968) offhandedly comments that psychiatrists
early on avoided consultation because of poor reimbursement; later, "expanded
private and government insurance plans" began to attract at least part-time interest. Psychiatrists with an interest in establishing private practice began to see
consulting as a way to build up a referral network, not so much as a full-time
career. The handbook devotes two or three sentences to how a fee for service
should be negotiated. Schwab wrote:

> I believe that this flurry of interest in psychiatric consultation *should not gen-*
> *erate a subspecialty*; the term is only descriptive of psychiatric activities with
> patients who complain of somatic distress or seek the help of physicians, sur-
> geons, or general hospitals for treatment. The consulting psychiatrist should
> be a specialist only in the sense that he is dedicated to comprehensive medi-
> cine, with a view of man as a creature of biology, a social being, and a part
> of his culture.
>
> *(p. viii; emphasis by au.)*

Psychosomatic medicine, Schwab states, grew as a reaction to specialization in medicine (p. 3). Schwab's incisive comments carried the weight of wisdom and probably slowed the inevitability of subspecialty status of the field.

Even Franz Alexander (1950), the venerated psychosomatic researcher, speaks regularly in his book *Psychosomatic Medicine* of an "approach," a "multidisciplinary procedure in which psychiatrists collaborate with experts in the different branches of medicine" (again, hints of liaison) (p. 13). His intent throughout appears to be instruction of medical practitioners of all disciplines to become aware that "every bodily process is directly or indirectly influenced by psychological stimuli because the whole organism constitutes a unit with all of its parts interconnected" (p. 12). "Modern scientific medical psychology is but an attempt to place medical art, the psychological effect of the physician upon the patient, on a scientific basis and to make it an integral part of therapy" (p. 18), with "recognition that this new approach . . . could *no longer be restricted to the field of psychiatry*" (p. 43; emphasis by au.). And of the term "psychosomatic," Alexander states that it "has been subjected to much criticism, chiefly because it seems to imply a dichotomy between mind and body. This dichotomy is precisely what the psychosomatic point of view tries to avoid." He adds that "most terms referring to a complex subject matter are ambiguous" (p. 49).

Echoing Alexander's definition and the statement of the APS of the "psychosomatic approach, Eugene Meyer (1959)—an active psychiatric consultant at Johns Hopkins, describing psychosomatic medicine as "a field of such broad and indefinite scope" (p. 298)—wrote:

> [P]sychosomatic medicine is a way of approaching problems of health and disease . . . to apply the best and most modern psychodynamic understanding of human personality function in all phases of medical practice, diagnosis, therapy and research. . . . It is emphasized that psychosomatic medicine is *not a specialty in medicine* but rather an elaboration of medical theory and practice which takes into account the role of psychological processes in the form and functions of the body in health and disease.
>
> *(p. 298; emphasis by au.)*

There must have been some resistant premonitory sense in these pioneers that, indeed, they were embarking on a course that could certainly one day be controversial and even lead to psychosomatic medicine or C-L psychiatry being considered a specialty.

Less than 20 years later, Tom Hackett (1978) wrote of oppositional developments in the field:

> The term 'psychosomatic' leaves a bad taste in the mouths of physicians. It reminds them of the 1930s, 1940s and 1950s when various psychosomatic

schools espoused doctrines linking specific psychological profiles with diseases designated as psychosomatic. Compounding this misunderstanding has been the term's abuse by the general public, who regard anything psychosomatic as either imaginary or nervous in origin.

(pp. 5–6)

At the time of writing, with this in mind, Hackett implied that "consultation-liaison" was a more palatable and acceptable designation of what the psychiatric consultant did. Those enthusiastic pioneers who had predicted a great future for the field of psychosomatic medicine were already experiencing a backlash to its impact!

Little more than a decade later, commenting on a growing desire for subspecialty recognition, McKegney and colleagues (1991) questioned the appropriateness of regarding C-L psychiatry a subspecialty; they argued that C-L had application not to a special category of patient but rather to *all* "special" aspects of psychiatry and medicine, more like a "supraspecialty" in its general applicability.

The Growth of C-L Psychiatry

After the slow start noted by Schwab (1968), interest in C-L psychiatry in the 1960s was beginning to percolate, with increasing numbers of trainees being drawn to the field, perhaps catalyzed by Schwab's and Lipowski's compelling writings on the subject. In response to this growing interest, enthusiasm began to stimulate more organizational presence of the field. Organizations like the Association for Academic Psychiatry (AAP), the American Psychosomatic Society (APS), and the Academy of Psychosomatic Medicine (APM) all showed growing interest. The AAP, successor to the federally supported Early Career Psychiatrist program, under Carol Nadelson's AAP presidency (1970s), established its first "Special Interest" section in C-L psychiatry to accommodate the growing numbers of AAP members expressing interest, and it appointed me chair of that section. The section established several task forces: funding (Guggenheim); research (Houpt & McKegney); training guidelines (Cohen-Cole).

The journal *Psychiatry in Medicine* (Lipsitt, Bibring, Blumgart & Cope, 1970), devoted largely to C-L topics, was launched to accommodate escalating numbers of articles on C-L topics. The journal's prefatory note included in its objectives that

our sights should be set on a broader definition of illness, which acknowledges the psychosocial aspects of all illness, the relationship of doctor and patient to the illness and to each other, and the relevance of the total system which sees body, mind, family and society as parts of a greater whole.

(p. 1)

Suggestions for the informal gathering of regional C-L groups were voiced, and a survey of interest for "nationalization" of the field appeared in *Psychiatric News* in 1974. The small notice brought hundreds of responses, many with letters describing their experience, their programs, and their plans for future development. The robust outpouring of interested psychiatrists was a reflection of a perceived isolation, a kind of "homelessness" and "hunger" for affiliation with C-L entities. In addition, it also brought welcome news of solidly functioning programs such as that of the Mayo Clinic; for example, a letter from M. J. Martin (1974) described the "heavy involvement of the Mayo Clinic in consultative psychiatry." He described how 15 adult psychiatrists spent half their time doing consultative work, with 4,500 outpatient and 1,500 inpatient consults the previous year. Martin confessed that he had just seen his five thousandth outpatient consultation!

Most letters expressed outright eagerness for a national group. One psychiatrist group, calling itself the New York Society for Liaison Psychiatry, convened in Jay Lefer's (1976) office to plan regular meetings. They later circulated a newsletter (November 1, 1976) plumbing local interest, carrying the following notation:

> In an issue of *Psychiatry News*, Don Lipsitt suggested the formation of a national organization with chapters for Liaison Psychiatrists to serve needs not being adequately met by any organization then existing. . . . A group of New York liaison psychiatrists liking the idea began to meet and has since held monthly meetings. . . . We have now reached the stage where we feel it is desirable to enlarge in size and develop a more formal structure.
>
> *(p. 1)*

The new group solicited members not only from New York but from surrounding areas of New Jersey, Westchester and Long Island, and southern Connecticut. It planned to develop discussion groups and programs on cancer units, adolescent med-surg units, hemodialysis units, primary care education, C-L research, funding, insurance, ethics, and other topics of relevance and interest to their C-L colleagues.

Inaugural officers included Robert Steinmuller, Jay Lefer, MaryAnn Cohen, Larry Goldblatt, and David Weisselberger, in addition to a board of directors consisting of Charles Barbanel, Jerry Finkel, Donald Kornfeld, Norman B. Levy, David Preven, Ray Rako, and Franz Reichsman. An advisory board was appointed consisting of James Eaton, Don Lipsitt, Edward Sachar, James Strain, and Milton Viederman. Recognizing the value of the "team" approach to C-L activity, a diversity of mental health professionals was invited to membership. Smaller, less formal, groups of C-L psychiatrists formed in Philadelphia, Boston, and other regions of the country. In Boston, an ad hoc group of newly appointed chairs of psychiatry in community hospitals (John Reichard, Don Lipsitt, Jerry Wacks, John Merrifield, Arthur Berg) met to strategize establishment of C-L programs in their respective institutions.

In every instance, the bugaboo of progress emerged: fiscal barriers! In contrast to the abbreviated fee-charging advice in Schwab's 1968 book, less than 15 years later Finkel's (1983) book on current trends and new perspectives in C-L psychiatry carried a 24-page chapter on the economic woes of the field (Levitan, 1983). Liaison psychiatrists were beginning to express serious concern about prospects for their future.

Dawning of a New Age

Free-market approaches to reimburseability of C-L service had been a failure, and those intent on lowering the cost of health care looked at psychiatric care as a place to save money. Psychologists and social workers were the preferred providers of insurance companies. Leaders of the C-L field were abuzz with concerns about the actual threat to viability of the discipline. Consensus began to build that although pioneers like Schwab had forcefully argued that the field should not become a specialty, even those who had originally agreed were now persuaded that specialization status could rescue the field. A new age had dawned!

Whether C-L psychiatry should be designated a distinct subspecialty of psychiatry had long been debated, but not until the cessation of NIMH funding in the 1980s was it addressed with such intensity and even furor. Practitioners in the field had been content to "let sleeping dogs lie" until issues of reimbursement for service arose. For many years, patient and physician access to psychiatric consultation was accepted in some hospitals as "part of the room rate," perhaps a kind of "loss leader" to cast it in marketplace terms. It was provided as an ancillary service to attending physicians of a hospital's staff, and administrators—who generally knew (or cared) little about what departments of psychiatry did—began to take notice when greater scrutiny of budgetary matters really mattered. As additions or deletions of staff in each department depended on ability to pay for themselves, questions of supportability began to concern department chairs, and an energized search ensued for ways to enhance reimburseability for service.

Psychiatry in the general hospital was never known for its ability to pay for itself and was thus always at risk of budgetary cuts when the fiscal squeeze impacted the institution. In quasi-panic, a kind of Brownian motion characterized the search for ways to economize without jeopardizing services. Sometimes the very structure of a department was forced by "guidelines" imposed by insurance companies, defining what services they considered reimbursable and what service was "medically necessary." Since C-L activities were generally misunderstood by insurers, they were unlikely to be paid for. And when "consultations" of all types were reimbursed at all, only one (of any medical discipline) in a day would be covered, resulting in competition over which service would "get to the patient first." A younger generation of physicians seemed to develop a tolerance for this kind of "game playing," but older physicians unaccustomed to such aspects of practice were thoroughly outraged over seemingly dictatorial standards.

Insurance companies insisted that C-L services must "prove" their efficacy if they were to be recompensed, although no such requirement was imposed on other medical or surgical services. Nevertheless, the message was broadcast that payment would rest on research; it would have to demonstrate the value of C-L services in enhancing medical and surgical services and to simultaneously generate cost-saving interventions. In the meantime, many creative ideas circulated to assure payment for psychiatric consultations; specific coding and diagnosis was one (cf. chapter 8 above, "A 'Lack of Means' ").

Throughout the 1970s, longtime C-L psychiatrist members of the APS were facing an uphill struggle to establish a viable C-L component in the society's annual programs. The fate of psychosomatic medicine had always been a concern of its founders, and now, in 1970, the ripple effect of disaffections in the field were being felt by the oldest American psychosomatic organization. Peter Regan (1970) wrote of the difficulties experienced in "striving to serve as a link pin between the giant separatist enclaves of medicine" (pp. 1298–1299). Whatever the intensity of the concern at the time, Peter Knapp (1971), one of the society's most dedicated researchers, asked whether "the psychosomatic movement has fulfilled itself and is now in its dodo-age, rapidly becoming extinct." Knapp commented on the "considerable fluidity of the boundaries" of psychosomatic medicine necessitating the periodic need to "inquire about the nature of its identity [and] . . . if the prediction is correct that changing medicine will find its way back to its psychosomatic roots, members of the Psychosomatic Society should be present at the meeting" (p. 363). McKegney (1974), one of its younger members, editorialized about how the field was attempting to ensure the link to the "giant separatist enclaves" of general medicine, family medicine, primary care, and comprehensive medicine (p. 373).

The very fluidity of boundaries and identity admitted by Knapp and others may have incited Freyhan (1976), at the third international conference of the International College of Psychosomatic Medicine in Rome (1975), to ask whether psychosomatic (*sic*) was obsolete (p. 381). In his reappraisal of the field, he concluded that "psychosomatic medicine as an interdisciplinary approach remains viable and necessary for medical practice and for research [but] there is no longer any place for simplistic models" (p. 385).

No Place for C-L?

The American Psychosomatic Society's membership consisted predominantly of clinical psychiatrists, but program planners dedicated to research reports reluctantly set aside time and space for workshops and lectures on C-L topics. Energetic overtures were made by Chase Kimball, Jim Strain, and Ed Sachar to establish sustainable C-L topics in the context of mostly research-focused programs; meetings were slotted either into very early or very late times, a source of constant grumbling by those who slept late or enjoyed their evenings out. Strain, Kimball, and Garant (a C-L nurse) managed a 7:00 a.m. workshop on "The teaching of liaison medicine and psychiatry" attended by 100 members: Participants included Jim Eaton, John Cleghorn (from McMaster University), Fred Guggenheim, Pat McKegney, Don Oken, Al Silverman, and Don Lipsitt at the 1976 annual meeting of the society, but the occasional successful "annual" program was often a one-time occurrence.

In 1976, in correspondence I had with Kimball, I had written:

> Perhaps your workshops have made some impact on the Society and have lubricated the way toward a fuller development of an increasing interest around the country in liaison psychiatry, but I feel there are still factions at work which may very well have a dampening effect on progress in this area.
>
> *(April 15, 1976).*

Kimball's response alludes to

> Herb Weiner's commentary re: the continual (if not increasing) fractionation that develops in academia between the essential researcher (often bench or laboratory) as opposed to the clinical investigator and teacher-clinician. My own feeling has been that both [APS and APM] need the other and that the APS has been a natural forum for it, but only if APS encourages and provides a forum for the convening of teacher-clinicians during the formal APS meetings and the presentation of some educational activities in the pages of *Psychosomatic Medicine*.
>
> *(June 18, 1976)*

Kimball also expressed his opposition to development of "yet another organization," with concerns about "splintering" and "dilution" of the "rigor of research." Kimball was an invaluable advocate for high-quality C-L programs, and his premature death was a great loss. The robust advocacy for recognition of C-L activities appeared to generate increased resistance on the part of the governing officials to allot prominent time slots to C-L presentations. Two cultures seemed to coexist (uneasily) in the society, one of the clinical, practical, activity-prone C-L clinicians and the other of the more sanguine, patient, thoughtful (largely Ph.D.) physiologic and psychosomatic researchers (reminiscent of Alexander's concerns). The tensions between the two were worthy of a sociological study, reflected in one of the longest chapters in Dorothy Levenson's (1994) book on the society's history, to which interested readers are referred for greater detail.

The struggle for increased recognition by C-L psychiatrists often found its way into presidential addresses of the society, with at least one expressing concern that observers of the society's mission and function would perceive C-L psychiatry as "all there is" to psychosomatic medicine (Graham, 1969; B. Engel, 1986).

Very gradually, disgruntled members of APS began to drift over to membership in APM, further distressing the official officers of the former. With a diverse membership of mental health professionals interested in psychosomatic medicine, APM had a record of practice-oriented programs liberally interspersed with topics of relevance to C-L psychiatrists; it also had a younger, clinically oriented membership than the society. An APS membership survey in 1995 showed the largest percentage of members declaring interest in behavioral medicine and C-L psychiatry, although by 1995 both categories had dropped in numbers from 1987, behavioral medicine from 42% to 30% and consultation-liaison psychiatry from 46% to 27%, a serious decrement in membership.

The society hobbled along with its bimodal orientation. Strong feelings erupted. When, as a resident, I was invited by Mort Reiser, editor of the society's journal, to present my idea about a journal for C-L topics, I was overwhelmed with vituperative comments about board members of the new journal and, except for one or two council members, totally negative views about such a journal. One very senior psychosomatic researcher blurted out, "We don't need another memorial to [name omitted]." For the first time, I became aware of the intensity of such competition and the calumny that august professional organizations were capable of. In later years, I was not so surprised when, in a group discussion about organizational memberships being "cannibalized" by the more persuasive organization, one member of an advisory panel bellowed, "Who cares about them?" Webb's remarks about increasing competitiveness seemed apropos.

Responding to the need for increased recognition of C-L psychiatry, several organizations were expanding their interest. The need actually spawned a new organization, the American Association of General Hospital Psychiatrists, founded by Joseph English, Gerald Flamm, Stuart Kiell, Andrew Slaby, and others to address growing interest in psychiatry's role in the general hospital. Over a decade, with dwindling numbers and activities engaged in by other well-established organizations, this one expired.

The section on C-L psychiatry of AAP, with its strong base of dedicated psychiatric teachers, many of whom actively engaged in liaison activities, held a special meeting at its annual gathering in 1978 in New Orleans, attended by 70 interested members. Reasons for growing interest were described: low level of program development in training centers; increasing publication of C-L topics; research; primary care movement; and funding concerns. Proposed functions of the section were outlined: representation of regional liaison groups in the section; liaison with other organizations like APS, American Academy of Family Practice, APA, and others; a clearinghouse service for C-L topics through newsletters, job postings, program announcements, and the like; cross-fertilization with psychologists and other behavioral scientists interested in C-L issues; mutual support for isolated groups and individuals with common interests; recommend curriculum guidelines for C-L training; demonstrate to medical schools and hospitals the possible cost-effectiveness of good liaison programs; develop methodologies for evaluating programs; promote funding and reimbursement mechanisms for liaison services (January 17, 1978, minutes).

Fueling the excitement was a memo (February 28, 1979) from Mel Sabshin, medical director of APA, announcing endorsement by APA's Board of Trustees of two new policy statements regarding C-L psychiatry. These policies grew out of the APA Committee on C-L Psychiatry and Primary Care Education, the Council on Medical Education and Career Development, and the Institute of Medicine's (IOM) report on developments in primary care. The policies were as follows: (1) "Basic medical student education should include some experience in consultation/liaison psychiatry . . . [and] students should be taught psychiatry by consultation/liaison psychiatrists in primary care settings . . . formally affili- ated with the primary care program and should possess basic skills in general medicine." (2) "All psychiatric residency programs should include significant supervised experience in which the resident functions as a consultation/liaison psychiatrist in an ambulatory care setting, particularly in primary care . . . [pro- viding] a foundation for more extensive consultation/liaison experiences during or following completion of training" (February 28, 1979).

With expanding interest and proliferation of literature on C-L psychiatry's broader application in medical settings, another journal was warranted. I founded *General Hospital Psychiatry* in 1979. Noting its focal point of the general hospital, the journal's introduction states,

> The general hospital is a sociocultural matrix through which psychiatry can fulfill its functions. Psychiatry can promote an integrated holistic approach to health and illness, with the general hospital and its extensions serving as workshop, laboratory, institution of continuing education, and therapeutic center.
>
> *(Lipsitt, 1979, p. 2)*

Anachronistically, and only worthy of a Dilbert cartoon, the APA Assembly and Board of Trustees decided to "sunset" the C-L committee as the primary orga- nization searched for ways to economize in a fiscally stringent environment. This committee had one of the highest budgets. Nevertheless, a strong letter (Lipsitt, 1980) from the committee to Leigh Roberts, chair of the Ad Hoc Commit- tee to Study Councils and Components, persuasively urged the committee to "avoid discarding the baby with the bath." The letter noted the organizational inconsistency of publicly espousing the need for increased numbers of psychiatrist educators while internally burying and making less visible this important focus by plans to eliminate the only agency within APA with major interests and activities in consultation-liaison matters and evolving programs in primary care. Plans for the committee's demise were scrapped, and the sun was up again!

Inevitable Specialization

By the late 1980s, efforts of the revitalized APA C-L committee had succeeded in having C-L training officially added to residency requirements. Interest in the AAP section grew, with annual meetings and task force reports each year gradually absorbed into the plan to seek subspecialty recognition.

Objectives of the AAP section overlapped markedly with those of other concerned organizations. Collaboration was clearly advisable to provide strength in numbers and lobbying power. The forces appeared to be lining up for the inevitable pursuit of subspecialization status.

Amidst the miasma of organizational turmoil, an article appeared in the journal *Hospitals* (Keeran, Pasnau & Richardson, 1981), appealing to hospital administrator and organizational staff readers to take note of the "explosion" of "medical-behavioral" needs of their institutions. The great increase in patients entering hospitals with psychiatric or emotional conditions highlighted how, lest they expose themselves to deficiencies of health care quality and liability,

> staff must recognize the importance of behavioral approaches in medicine and provide appropriate services to meet psychosocial needs of all patients . . . [and] hospital administrators must be aware of the political, organizational, and operational ramifications of these developments.
>
> *(p. 56)*

Whether this forceful admonition sharpened appreciation of the intended audience to the value of C-L services in their institutions is not clear, but for concerned psychiatrists the article reinforced their growing awareness that "these problems require well-thought-out public relations programs and positive action" (p. 59).

The imperative call for action was heeded by several prominent C-L psychiatrists. What follows is a rather tedious account of the process by which application for subspecialization came about, a bit akin to observing sausage or congressional legislation being made.

References

Alexander, F. (1950). *Psychosomatic Medicine*. New York, NY: W.W. Norton & Co.

Benning, T.B. (2015). Limitations of the biopsychosocial model in psychiatry. *Advances in Medical Education and Practice, 6*, 347–352.

Binger, C. (1960). Response to question from Y. Ikemi. *Psychosomatic Medicine, 22*, 249–250.

Blumenfield, M. (1988). Subspecialization in psychiatry is a necessity. *Psychosomatics, 29*, 153–154.

De Mandeville, B. (1711). *Treatise of the Hypochondriack and Hysterick Passions*. London, UK: Dryden Leach.

Dubos, R. (1968). *So Human an Animal*. New York, NY: Scribner's.

Dunbar, H.F. (1935). *Emotions and Bodily Change: A Survey of Literature on Psychosomatic Interrelationships*. New York, NY: Columbia University Press.

Engel, B.T. (1986). Psychosomatic medicine, behavioral medicine, just plain medicine. *Psychosomatic Medicine, 48,* 466–479.

Engel, G.L. (1977). The need for a new medical model: A challenge for biomedicine. *Science, 196,* 129–136.

Finkel, J.B. (1983). *Consultation-Liaison Psychiatry: Current Trends and New Perspectives.* New York, NY: Grune & Stratton.

Freyhan, F. (1976). Is psychosomatic obsolete? A psychiatric reappraisal. *Comprehensive Psychiatry, 17,* 381–386.

Galdston, I. (1955). Psychosomatic medicine: Past, present, and future. *Archives of Neurology and Psychiatry, 74,* 441–450.

Galdston, I. (1958). The birth and death of specialties. *Journal of the American Medical Association. 167,* 2056–2061.

Ghaemi, S.N. (2009). *The Rise and Fall of the Biopsychosocial Model.* Baltimore, MD: Johns Hopkins University Press.

Graham, D.T. (1969). Psychosomatic medicine needs a new start (Editorial). *Hospital Practice, 4,* 1–2.

Hackett, T.P. (1978). Beginnings: Liaison psychiatry in a general hospital. In T.P. Hackett & N.H. Cassem (Eds.). *Massachusetts General Hospital Handbook of General Hospital Psychiatry.* (pp. 1–13). St. Louis, MO: C.V. Mosby.

Keeran, C.V., Jr., Pasnau, R.O., & Richardson, M. (1981). Medical-behavioral "explosion" affects hospital operation, policy. *Hospitals, 55,* 56–59.

Kimball, C.P. (1976). Letter to D.R. Lipsitt, June 18, 1976.

Knapp, P. (1971). Revolution, relevance and psychosomatic medicine: Where the light is not. *Psychosomatic Medicine, 33,* 363–374.

Kontos, N. (2011). Perspective: Biomedicine—Menace or straw man? Reexamining the biopsychosocial argument. *Academic Medicine, 86,* 509–515.

Lane, R.D. (1999). APS name change. *American Psychosomatic Newsletter, 10,* 7.

Lefer, J. (1976). New York society for liaison psychiatry. *Newsletter,* November 1, 1976.

Levenson, D. (1994). *Mind, Body, and Medicine: A History of the American Psychosomatic Society.* Philadelphia, PA: Williams & Wilkins.

Levitan, S.J. (1983). Evaluation of consultation-liaison psychiatry: Better health at lower cost? In J.B. Finkel (Ed.). *Consultation-Liaison Psychiatry: Current Trends and New Perspectives.* (pp. 25–49). New York, NY: Grune & Stratton.

Lipowski, Z.J. (1986). Consultation-liaison psychiatry: The first half century. *General Hospital Psychiatry, 8,* 305–315.

Lipsitt, D.R. (1976). Letter to C. Kimball, April 15, 1976.

Lipsitt, D.R. (1979). Psychiatry and the general hospital: An editorial. *General Hospital Psychiatry: Psychiatry, Medicine and Primary Care, 1,* 1–2.

Lipsitt, D.R. (1980). Letter to L.M. Roberts, October 30, 1980.

Lipsitt, D.R., Bibring, G.L., Blumgart, H.L., & Cope, O. (1970). Editors' prefatory note: A statement of purpose. *Psychiatry in Medicine, 1,* 1–2.

Martin, M.J. (1974). Letter to D.R. Lipsitt, June 18, 1974.

McKegney, F.P. (1974). Psychosomatic medicine and primary care medicine: Can there be a meeting? (Editorial). *Psychosomatic Medicine, 36,* 373–376.

McKegney, F.P., O'Dowd, M.A., Schwartz, C.E., & Marks, R.M. (1991). A fallacy of subspecialization in psychiatry. Consultation-liaison is a supraspecialty. *Psychosomatics, 32,* 343–346.

Meyer, E. (1959). The psychosomatic concept: Use and abuse. *Journal of Chronic Disease, 9,* 298–314.

Muskin, P. (1988). Subspecialization in psychiatry may fragment the profession. *Psychosomatics, 29,* 155–156.

Regan, P.R. (1970). Psychosomatic medicine—Future directions. *American Journal of Psychiatry, 126,* 1298–1299.

Schwab, J.J. (1968). *Handbook of Consultation Psychiatry.* New York, NY: Appleton-Century-Crofts.

Schwenk, T.L. (1999). The tyranny of names in mental health care. *Journal of the American Board of Family Practice, 12,* 99–101.

Seguin, C.A. (1970). *Introduction to Psychosomatic Medicine.* Madison, CT: International Universities Press.

Shorter, E. (1992). *From Paralysis to Fatigue: A History of Psychosomatic Illness in the Modern Era.* New York, NY: Free Press.

Thompson, T.L., 2nd. (1993). Should we shift the name of "consultation-liaison" to "medical-surgical" psychiatry, "psychiatry in medicine and surgery," or some other term? *Psychosomatics, 34,* 259–264.

Webb, W.L., Jr. (1987). Ethical aspects of the continuum of care concept. *Psychiatric Hospitals, 18,* 147–151.

Webb, W.L., Jr. (1988). Presidential address: A new challenge for the Academy of Psychosomatic Medicine. *Psychosomatics, 29,* 148–152.

Weiss, E., & English, O.S. (1943). *Psychosomatic Medicine.* Philadelphia, PA: W.B. Saunders.

Wise, T.N. (1995). A tale of two societies. *Psychosomatic Medicine, 57,* 303–309.

10

SPECIALIZATION AT LAST

Hopeful Remedy

There are only two or three human stories, and they go on repeating themselves as fiercely as if they had never happened before.
            —*Willa Cather, 1913,* O Pioneers, *Part II, Chapter 4*

Introduction

Specialization at last! After a long stumbling journey, consultation-liaison psychiatry has reached not the end of the road but an important milestone. Alas, the specialty is to be called psychosomatic medicine. Over the decades, both C-L and PM have had their identity problems, with both names and missions of their respective entities changing more often than that of any other discipline in medicine. This chapter will discuss how structure and organization ponderously articulate with the official declaration of the seventh specialty of psychiatry (not medicine) to fly the banner of psychosomatic medicine.

David T. Graham, professor of medicine at the University of Wisconsin Medical School, had been a long-standing member of the American Psychosomatic Society (APS), with a strong commitment to research in that field. In 1969, he wrote an editorial in the journal *Hospital Practice* entitled "Psychosomatic medicine needs a new start."

It begins:'

> In two decades [i.e., since 1949] "psychosomatic medicine" has become a household word, a cocktail hour conversation piece for the *au courant*, a convenient diagnostic wastebasket. If its backers had had promotional, rather

than scientific goals for it, the campaign could be considered a rousing success. However, for many who invested high scientific hopes, it has been a disappointment.

(p. 1)

Massive misstatement of the psychosomatic concept by laymen, he added, "has at least the excuse of being misinformed" (p. 1). He proceeds with an explication of the vulnerability of the concept to confusion, the misguided endeavor to treat mind and body as though they are separate entities. He does not give up entirely on the utility of the concept, stating that

> one current trend gives some promise of providing a new start for psychosomatic medicine. Emphasis on comprehensive care, on the social setting of health and disease, and on family practice may well revive professional and scientific interest in it. . . . One supposes that the growth of this recognition will lead to more intensive scientific study of stimulus-response relationships . . . stimuli that are, implicitly or explicitly, chiefly dealt with in psychosomatic medicine.
>
> *(p. 2)*

The confusions, he states, "must be cleared away before any real progress can be made" (p. 2).

Is the recognition of psychosomatic medicine as psychiatry's seventh specialty the "new start" that Graham wished for, or is it a resurrection of the old confusions, misstatements, and pitfalls that he deplored in 1969? Have old confusions indeed been cleared away?

At least since the 1960s, as we have seen, it had long been advised by professionals in the field that psychosomatic medicine should not become a specialty. Yet by late 1960s, it was no longer possible to deny the move in exactly that direction, in psychiatry, not medicine. All organizations with an active interest in C-L psychiatry felt the pinch of fiscal stringencies; whatever other motivations to seek specialty status were proposed, funding was the premier concern. With Rockefeller and Macy Foundation largesse a thing of the distant past and support by NIMH funding about to cease, creative ideas were urgently needed. This chapter follows C-L's "yellow brick road" in the quest for specialty status.

C-L Vulnerability

Besides imminent defunding of federal programs, other irritants were nipping at the heels of C-L psychiatry as well. Psychologists were lobbying for a larger part of the medical-psychiatric pie. With a surge in interest in "health psychology," there had already been intense lobbying for prescribing privileges, with some small success in a few states. Also, a weakening of C-L psychiatry's "medicalized" orientation was threatened with an ill-conceived proposal to eliminate medical internship for future psychiatrists (Romano, 1970). Those advocating for subspecialization felt that it was essential to preserve the medical identity of C-L psychiatry and psychiatry in general. An absence of standardized training and practice was being singled out as reason for being snubbed by insurance companies, grant funders, and even department chairmen; insurance companies were preferentially reimbursing services by social workers and psychologists rather than the "higher-cost" psychiatrists. The Community Mental Health movement was employing largely nonpsychiatrist staff, tending to further demedicalize the mental health profession. The whole field of psychiatry was said to be struggling through an "identity crisis," with APA workshops addressing the theme "What is a psychiatrist?"

Geriatric psychiatry, with which C-L psychiatry had much in common, having already sought and secured specialized status, heartened C-L psychiatrists who saw this as a hopeful sign and model for their own objectives.

Brook Lodge I

With a sense of urgency, the suggestion was made to Robert Pasnau, an esteemed, experienced C-L psychiatrist, with the right "connections," that he convene a group of C-L leaders for serious discussion of the status of the discipline and the prospects for specialization. Well-published, with educational credentials and strong APA ties (president, 1986–1987), Pasnau seemed the right person at the right time to convene such a group. The Upjohn Company lent its peaceful and commodious educational conference center, Brook Lodge in Augusta, Michigan, for a first meeting. Twenty-two invited, self-paying C-L psychiatrists met there on November 30, 1981.

Rapid consensus was achieved about the urgency of group survival. Discussions covered a proposal to form a national society of liaison psychiatrists as a forceful action and lobbying group, coalescing what had otherwise been isolated overtures to date. The group focused on identifying interested organizations and individual practitioners, current interface with government, opportunities for multisite research, standards for teaching and training in liaison psychiatry, and plans for future strategies. Participants became acquainted with each other's biases both for and against, some much stronger than others. They clearly were not of a single mind, but, in two days of lively conversation and debate, all subscribed to the fundamental goal of the conference "to develop a comprehensive national strategy for addressing the negative tide that endangers the continued vitality and development of our field" (Brook Lodge Conference summary). The concept of a national organization, however, was tabled pending further exploration.

Revived APA Interest

There were expressions of disappointment over the years for what appeared to be a low level of support for C-L psychiatry. However, in the late 1970s and early 1980s, it had begun to show more interest as the "primary care movement" was evolving. One of its many components was the Committee on Psychiatry and Primary Care. Organizational deliberations and action do not always make sense, and for reasons of economic restructuralization, just at that time, as previously mentioned, the Committee on Psychiatry and Primary Care had been targeted, by an ad hoc committee on restructuring, for "sunsetting" because of its comparatively large budget, although it was fairly promptly restored.

With new attention by APA officials, the committee was renamed the Committee on C-L Psychiatry and Primary Care Education (CCLPPCE) and designated the "common pathway" for all matters related to C-L psychiatry (September 23, 1981). Added to its portfolio was the mandate to incorporate aspects of the emerging field of "behavioral medicine," especially as it related to primary care.

Now cast in its expanded role of "broker" for all APA matters related to primary care, the committee, just two months before the Brook Lodge meeting, "endorsed the global charge to develop policy and monitor the role of consultation-liaison psychiatry as it relates to psychiatry and primary medical care and education" and said "the APA should support the strengthening of consultation-liaison psychiatry in the primary care setting" (Meeting minutes, September 23, 1981, Jimmie Holland, chair). The committee "felt it could be utilized as a 'political arm' when needed, seeing itself as 'on call' to mobilize resources as, for example, in relation to recent cutbacks in funding" (Committee minutes). With these changes taking place just prior to the Brook Lodge gathering, the new committee definition would obviously be a source of tension as the idea of specialization unfolded.

The first meeting of the renamed committee was six months following Brook Lodge in Toronto (May 19, 1982, acting chair, Don Lipsitt). In addition to regular committee members, James Eaton (chief of NIMH's Psychiatry Education Branch) and APA Deputy Director Carolyn Robinowitz were in attendance. Proceedings of the Brook Lodge conference were thoroughly reviewed, the committee declaring that "the additional development of yet another agency in the form of a C-L task force at this time would possibly dilute the mandate of the CCLPPCE just at a time when it was becoming more task oriented and stabilized" (Minutes, May 19, 1982).

Members noted that "mechanisms exist through the Office of Education, the Educators Development Project for Psychiatric Education, the Council on Medical Education and Career Development, and the Committee on Psychiatry and Primary Care Education . . . to provide adequate representation for the many societies, and organizations and individuals with an interest in the development of C-L programs" (May 19 minutes). Recommendation was therefore made to bolster existing structure and function of the APA to address these vital issues and, somewhat redundant to the Brook Lodge actions, to establish a "working group to examine funding, research, and education and to compile a roster of resource people representing other interested groups" (May 19 minutes). In addition, it proposed that council assign consultants who can work directly with the CCLPPCE in these areas. Committee recommendations were funding (Guggenheim, Detre & Feighner); research (McKegney & Kornfeld); and education (Cohen-Cole & Strain), with Eaton as general consultant. All suggested consultants, except Feighner and Detre had attended the Brook Lodge conference. If the Brook Lodge conference had done nothing else, it energized the APA committee and mobilized it to action. The big surprise was that the APA, previously having shown little interest in C–L psychiatry, now was catalyzed to secure control of the proceedings. Whatever the minutes recorded, everyone recognized "the elephant in the room" of a desire for specialization of C–L psychiatry.

Between the years 1982 and 1986, the Committee on C–L Psychiatry worked on its "assignments" during its annual meetings. At the committee's meeting on September 22, 1983 (Tom Wise, chair), three action items were presented to the Council on Medical Education and Graduate Education for consideration: (1) a request that training in C–L psychiatry be required by the Residency Committee for all psychiatrists; (2) a request that an official Task Force on C–L funding be established; and (3) request for approval of a collaborative descriptive statement of the definition, purpose, and skills of C–L psychiatry jointly edited by APA and the American Hospital Association section on general hospital psychiatry. All action items were thoroughly discussed but rejected, with council request that all be more fully developed, especially in conjunction with other APA councils and components.

Also during this time, levels of C–L interest in district branches (DB) of the APA were explored. A survey of interest revealed that very few DBs had formal committees devoted to the topic, but most expressed interest in attending an invitational meeting to benefit from the committee's input and guidance. In the meantime, meetings with the Residency Review Committee later achieved acceptance of recommendations for official inclusion of C–L training for the first time in psychiatric residency. And Cohen-Cole, Haggerty, and Raft (1982) of the Association for Academic Psychiatry teamed with the committee to propose objectives in C–L training for psychiatry residents. Liaison activities to Academies of Pediatrics and Family Physicians and American College of Physicians were a continuing endeavor. The Task Force on Cost-Effectiveness of C–L psychiatry chaired by Fred Guggenheim diligently collected data on the ways various C–L services funded their programs and presented a vast array of these at committee meetings in 1984 and 1985. A cost-effectiveness workshop was held jointly with NIMH in 1984 where researchers were able to meet with a C–L consultant and a health care economist to review presubmission grant proposals.

As organizations with significant C–L interests became aware of transformative events, worry began bubbling up over direction and control. In July 1987,

Bernard Frankel, C-L section leader of the Association for Academic Psychiatry, sent a letter to all members, beginning with, "As you know, the topic of subspecialization is stirring up a lot of controversy and debate these days," soliciting input from association members. In as balanced a way as possible, he outlined the pros and cons. Pros: Since specialization is "inevitable," we should "take greater control of how it is accomplished"; that "a unique body of knowledge exists, with specific textbooks and journals"; "that there exist national organizations wholly or to a significant degree devoted to this subspecialty"; "fellowships in this subspecialty exist"; "our ability to survive economically in an increasingly competitive environment will be greatly enhanced." On the negative side, he listed the following: "[F]ragmentation will lead to decreased quality and satisfaction in clinical care (similar to criticism in medicine)"; "likely to be a deleterious effect on psychiatric residency training from disturbance of the dynamic equilibrium currently existing among subspecialty interests in many training programs and being subject to the Board establishment of C-L training standards"; "reimbursement and referrals ought to reflect the fact that among non-psychiatric physicians and mental health professionals, psychiatrists are uniquely qualified to treat medically ill patients with psychiatric disorders and should not be dependent on board certification as subspecialists." Responses were invited to be sent to Troy Thompson, chair of the APA Committee on C-L Psychiatry (also a member of AAP and APM, and a prime advocate of specialization [Thompson, 1993]).

Between 1981 and 1989, time was devoted to working out tensions and resistances among affected organizations. The APA Committee on C-L Psychiatry and Primary Care Education seemed largely to ignore the issue of specialization although successive chairs of that committee were APM members. The energies of annual committee meetings were spent defining the identity, skills, training, and experience of the C-L psychiatrist as well as the committee's various liaisons with family practice, internal medicine, and pediatric programs. With slow progress being made during this period, however, much "backroom" activity proceeded through the offices of the Academy of Psychosomatic Medicine (APM) and its representatives. APM had already amended its name to include the words "Official C-L Organization" and had excluded all those from membership who were not psychiatrists, in a sense compromising the definition of C-L psychiatry as a "team" endeavor. The APA C-L committee was, in many ways, most troublesome as it attempted to clarify the future role of the APA and its various councils and components in what was being nurtured as the specialization process.

At the annual meeting of the APA May 9, 1989, in San Francisco, the Committee on C-L Psychiatry and Primary Care Education was informed by its chair, Troy Thompson, that the academy had organized a task force ("Consortium") composed of a number of psychiatric organizations, to meet two or three times during the next year to "attempt to coordinate the efforts of the C-L organizations." Charles Ford of the academy had been chosen to coordinate and chair the task force, with the "explanation" that "his primary proposal is that the APM become the umbrella organization for C-L" (Minutes, May 9, 1989). Apparently the APM had become impatient waiting for movement by the committee; the APA ad hoc Committee on Subspecialization reported that "the issue is not urgent and should be studied carefully, . . . that we do have some time before taking further action [on "added qualifications"]." Nevertheless, out of this conflictual situation at this meeting, the recommendation was made that Fawzy and Pasnau once again convene a group of C-L psychiatrists—this time about 40—for Brook Lodge II, now eight years after Brook Lodge I (Fawzy, at the 1988 meeting, had already collected names of potential invitees and had recommended a "repeat of the national C-L retreat"). The implicit message of these mixed directives seemed to mark the trending exclusion of the APA committee, with APM's assumption of responsibility for the move toward specialization. A restating of the APA committee's charge followed:

> That the Council on Medical Education and Career Development recommend to the Joint Reference Committee and Board of Trustees that the charge of the Committee be changed to read: "The Committee will focus on the interface between psychiatry and other medical disciplines, monitor and assist in the development of the fields of consultation/liaison psychiatry, behavioral medicine and medical psychiatry, including clinical, educational, research, and administrative activities in these fields that relate to psychiatry. The Committee will address and promote the teaching of consultation/ liaison psychiatry in psychiatry residency programs and of psychiatry to non–psychiatric physicians and to monitor the psychiatric content to [sic] primary care education and other health care professionals as appropriate to improve their recognition of psychiatric disorders and for them to develop skills in when and how to consult and refer to psychiatrists. The Committee will develop liaisons (and serve as resource) as appropriate and as coordinated through the APA liaison committee between the APA and other medical educational organizations."
>
> (Minutes of May 9, 1989, submitted by Troy Thompson, chair)

With this redefinition of the committee's function, Ford could now send a memo to the APA stating that the C-L committee was "more invested in relationships with family practice organizations rather than C-L activities" and therefore not suited as a coordinating resource for subspecialization activities. Earlier council recommendations that the committee play a major role were nullified.

During this interim, C-L members of APS were slowly migrating to APM, with noticeable decrease in the former and increase in the latter. C-L psychiatrists in APS were becoming restless and perhaps agitated. Significant numbers of C-L psychiatrists with membership in the American Psychosomatic Society felt they were accorded little time in annual programs and were inadequately represented in the pages of the journal *Psychosomatic Medicine*.

Clearly, the APA Committee on C-L Psychiatry, meeting at most only once or twice a year, had not dealt directly with the subspecialization issue. In whatever way APM had arrived at its role of "umbrella" organization for C-L psychiatry, it now had the numbers, the motivation, and the support to move ahead with greater alacrity on the matter of subspecialty recognition. Regardless of the feelings of interested organizations about the process, one had to be impressed with the finesse with which APM had maneuvered into this activist position!

A consortium of representatives from organizational "stakeholders" agreed to schedule postconference meetings for further discussion and action (and toward that aim, five task forces were proposed: C-L Fellowship Training [Bernard Frankel, chair]; Standards for Consultation Psychiatry [Fawzy Fawzy, chair]; C-L Research [G. Richard Smith & James Levenson, chairs; later, James Strain]; C-L Funding [Fred Guggenheim, chair]; and Liaison Networking [Don Lipsitt, chair]). Charles Ford, whose strong positive position was that APS should be the mantle of all that evolved, would serve as chair of the consortium. Several of those attending were members of more than one association, representing, besides APM, the American Psychosomatic Society (APS), Association for Academic Psychiatry (AAP), American Association of General Hospital Psychiatry (AAGHP), the APA Committee on C-L Psychiatry and Primary Care Education (CCLPPCE), and New York Society for Liaison Psychiatry (NYSLP). The Steering Committee was established with a two-year mandate to plan future deliberative meetings, either free-standing or in conjunction with annual meetings of representative organizations. Members of the Steering Committee were Mary Ann Cohen and Peter Wilson of the NYSLP; Barney Dlin, John Hayes, and Charles Ford of the APM; Gregory Fritz of the American Academy of Child and Adolescent Psychiatry; Troy Thompson of the APA's CCLPPCE; Bernard Frankel of the AA; and Don Lipsitt of the APS.

The APA's Council on Medical Education and Career Development held a summer retreat in 1989, attended by Robert Pasnau, suggesting that "the C-L Committee could become the coordinating group between a new C-L Consortium and the APA." The council briefly considered and rejected the establishment of a new council with "task forces within the Council to look at issues such as accreditation, certification, liaison with appropriate organizations, research issues, funding, and service delivery." The council registered concern that the consortium was acting "outside the APA," viewed by the council as "in fact a crisis." Chair of the CCLPPCE at the time was Tom Wise, also an active member of both APS and APM.

Curiously, a letter from Pasnau had already gone out in *March* 1989, inviting participants to Brook Lodge II. Representatives were invited from APM, APS, APA, AAP, AAGHP, American Academy of Child and Adolescent Psychiatry, American Association of Directors of Psychiatric Residency Training (AADPRT), and New York Society for Liaison Psychiatry. Invitees were informed that reports of consortium task forces that had been meeting in 1988 and 1989 would be discussed. This meeting would differ from the previous one not only in numbers of invitees but also with invited official representation from APA by Medical Director Melvin Sabshin and Deputy Director Carolyn Robinowitz. The invitation read, "It is the goal of this meeting to discuss the challenges of the 1990s and to make recommendations that will have equally important consequences for the coming decade."

Two or three meetings were held by the consortium, often with different representatives, and sometimes with rancorous repercussions. Other C-L-interested organizations such as the American Society for Psychosomatic Obstetrics and Gynecology (ASPOG) and the American Association of Directors of Psychiatric Residency Training (AADPRT) were added to the group.

To attempt to stem the migratory tide of members to APM, the APS had called a special retreat in September 1987 to review its status and revisit its mission to

> promote and advance the scientific understanding of the interrelationships among biological, psychological, behavioral and social factors in human health and disease, and the integration of the fields of science that separately examine each, and to foster the application of this understanding to education and improved health care.
>
> *(Meeting announcement)*

Cognizant of the disgruntlement of the more clinically oriented members, the council nonetheless was committed to its basic research orientation. It reiterated that

> the understanding to be provided by psychosomatic research is an essential ingredient for the comprehensive understanding of human disease in terms that will lessen the burden of human suffering. The promotion of these goals and their assimilation into medical teaching and practice are the central missions of the Society.
>
> *(Minutes, September, 1987)*

There would be no dilution of these values for the sake of preserving membership numbers! No mention is made of one discipline over another, of specialization or of psychiatry, including C-L psychiatry.

The reality of the situation was that, even with psychosomatic medicine flourishing in research and publication, C-L programs were languishing, with uncertain times ahead. C-L programs throughout the country had not increased in at least a decade (Schubert & McKegney, 1976), some even vanishing; patients from medical and surgical wards were not being referred for psychiatric consultation in numbers that were anticipated (Wallen, Pincus, Goldman & Marcus, 1987); residents training in psychiatry were being exposed to less C-L experience (Tilley & Silverman, 1982), and improvement in economic circumstances were not being forecast. Lipowski (1986) noted that C-L psychiatrists engaged vigorously in "controversies . . . over the objectives they should strive for and the strategies chosen to achieve them" (p. 312). Practitioners of C-L psychiatry became painfully aware that the comfortable years of Rockefeller, Macy, and NIMH support had blinded them to certain political, economic, conceptual, and organizational necessities that could affect the viability of their field of activity.

Brook Lodge II

This was the context in which Brook Lodge II, with increased representation, was expected to essentially reboot earlier enthusiasm and momentum of Brook Lodge I. And, indeed, through the good auspices and support of honorary chairperson Robert Pasnau and the Education Division of Upjohn Pharmaceuticals, 41 participants gathered in Augusta, Michigan, for another round of talks, June 22–24, 1989, this time much more focused on the issue of subspecialization.

The attendance of Mel Sabshin and Carolyn Robinowitz lent a much more "official" cast to deliberations. Task force reports were read and reflected a fairly consistent positive note of urgency for the pursuit of subspecialty approval. The Network Report summarized a survey of 135 C-L psychiatrists regarding attitudes toward specialization, with two-thirds supporting and one-third opposing. The same proportion endorsed standardized guidelines for the field and would also join a single national organization for C-L psychiatry if it existed. The report ended with a reading of the APA's ad hoc Committee on Liaisons and the Assembly Committee on Planning: The joint committees were

> looking for ways to avoid fragmentation; to maintain the loyalty and interest of psychiatrists with special interests and practices within the APA, so that the Association can continue to speak for psychiatry . . . [with] some overlapping membership among components and the ad hoc Committee on Specialization to ensure exchange of information and to avoid duplication of effort.
>
> *(p. 6, Report of Networking/Liaison Task Force)*

Sabshin brought a leveling element to ensuing discussion with a thoughtful low-key review of possible undesirable fallout: Would specialty recognition have a splintering or fragmenting effect on the field of psychiatry as a whole? How might a C-L psychiatrist function compared to a well-trained psychiatric consultation nurse? What could a C-L psychiatrist do any different from what an experienced general psychiatrist could do? Would non-C-L psychiatrists be disenfranchised as viable consultants? (Proceedings of the National Conference on Consultation-Liaison Psychiatry, p. 3).

Carolyn Robinowitz added that although the APA had had a long-standing ambivalence toward C-L psychiatry, the Committee on C-L Psychiatry had existed for some 15 years and had accomplished much. Nevertheless, her impression was that "added qualifications" rather than full-board specialization would "strengthen the field as a whole by promoting greater expertise, exploration and knowledge and that APA could support certain C-L psychiatry interests by, for example, developing a financial guide for C-L program directors (Proceedings, p. 3).

The resolution of the 1989 second Brook Lodge meeting raised the feelings of some so feverishly that the APA C-L committee devoted its entire fall meeting (September 14, 1989, Tom Wise, chair) to reviewing the conference results. It had been resolved (1) that we designate C-L psychiatry a subspecialty, (2) that we continue the consortium for a minimum of two years, and (3) that during that period, we develop (a) a short-range plan to provide operational rules, fiscal support, and a structural organization, and (b) long-range strategies leading toward accreditation, certification, and funding.

Fawzy was made chair of the Task Force on Certification in APM, as Wise and Noyes implemented strategies for moving forward. The decision was made through the consortium to submit application to the American Board of Psychiatry and Neurology (ABPN) requesting specialized status, primarily under the auspices of APM. In preparation for "greasing the skids" for submission of an application for "added qualifications," consortium chair Ford (June 29, 1990) requested of APA president Benedek that an ad hoc commission on subspecialization be convened under APA auspices, while acknowledging the existence of a C-L committee under the APA umbrella; however, he stated, "[I]t is not the appropriate entity to consider the issue of subspecialization because its task has been reorganized to focus on primary care education," and "its need to report to the Council of Graduate Education would preclude the rapid responses required for these pressing subspecialty issues." It was apparently not known that submission would later involve a slow migration through many more councils, components, committees, Assembly, Board of Trustees, ABPN, Joint Reference Committee, and others before a response would be forthcoming. Around the same time, Ford submitted a letter to Gerald Flamm, speaker of the assembly, from the C-L "caucus" requesting "official observer status in the Assembly to have a voice without a vote" in their deliberations.

Dots Connected

The dots now seemed to be connected. Gradually, the thinking of leaders in the field was that C-L would benefit from recognition as a *legitimate* specialty, with establishment of fellowships and more stature as a discipline with a history, a corpus of research and literature. In the years between 1981 and 1990, while plans were being formulated to seek subspecialty status, at least six presidents of APA had identified themselves strongly with C-L psychiatry (John Talbot, 1984–1985; Carol Nadelson, 1985–1986; Robert Pasnau, 1986–1987; Paul Fink, 1988–1989; Herbert Pardes, 1989–1990; and Steven Sharfstein, 1995–1996), an "inside" coincidence that would seem to promise sympathetic APA response; Michelle Riba's

(2004–2005) presidential theme would in time celebrate the successful final application for specialty designation. To reaffirm the interest of C-L psychiatrists in research and as though to imprint its bona fides, the consortium, with other organizations like AAP, sponsored a "First" C-L Research Forum, preceding the annual APA May meeting in New York City in 1990.

Try, Try Again

After two or three meetings of the consortium, there was general, if at times halting, agreement that the arduous task of submitting application for subspecialty approval should begin. Russell Noyes undertook to marshal this endeavor, with input from the consortium Steering Committee.

Following the model of geriatric psychiatry's application, a first venture into the application process occurred in June 1990. Documents were sent directly to the ABPN with a copy to APA president Benedek, but apparently without much processing through other "stakeholders." The application for "added qualifications" in C-L psychiatry was submitted to APA's ad hoc Committee on Specialization, chaired by James Trench. Purpose of the proposal described several objectives:

> 1) to improve psychiatric care of medically ill patients; 2) to standardize fellowship training in consultation-liaison (C-L) psychiatry; 3) to raise the level of expertise among psychiatrists working with the medically ill; 4) to improve the utilization of consultation-liaison services; 5) to encourage research and teaching in consultation-liaison psychiatry; and 6) to recognize the added qualifications of specially trained psychiatrists. (Application #1, June, 1990).

The text of the application amplified these objectives and included supportive reference to books, journals, articles, fellowships, and model curriculum for trainees. After long deliberation, the application was rejected as being devoid of a "special patient population."

At the annual Components Meeting of the CCLPPCE on September 13, 1990, Tom Wise, chair of the committee, reported the discouraging response from ABPN that they were "not interested in having C-L become a subspecialty with formal added qualifications," and were questioning "whether C-L psychiatry is really a part of general psychiatry or whether boundaries of this discipline were not sufficiently clear to merit such added qualifications."

Undaunted, the consortium, now absorbed by the APM, pushed forward. Wise met with James Trench, the chair of the ad hoc Commission on Specialization, to discuss next steps. Trench offered not merely condolences but suggestions on revision of the documents to be resubmitted, but with muted expectation of the results.

The January 1991 issue of *General Hospital Psychiatry* carried a thoughtful editorial by Robinowitz and Nadelson (1991) in support of specialization, emphasizing that "[o]ne of the most persuasive reasons for the formal recognition of C-L as a subspecialty is that it would foster the development of uniform standards of program accreditation and individual qualifications," and adding that "there is currently no mechanism to set standards for or evaluate the quality of fellowship training" (p. 3). Their conclusion was that "Consultation-Liaison Psychiatry has matured to a valued and valid subspecialty research and practice area" and that "formal recognition of the area along with careful planning will be beneficial to our patients, the public, and the field" (p. 3).

Russell Noyes undertook the arduous task of reworking the application and incorporating Trench's suggestions as well as input solicited from allied organizations. On February 21, 1991, a revised document was submitted to the Commission on Subspecialization, again requesting "added qualifications" for C-L psychiatry. This time, the application's introduction referred to the "crisis" prompting the application and referred more descriptively to the consortium and its work with multiple organizations. Endorsements of APA's CCLPPCE and Council on Medical Education and Career Development were added. On this occasion, C-L psychiatry was defined as "rest[ing] on a knowledge base that has grown and expanded since the founding of psychosomatic medicine in 1939." Other material differed little from the original application. After a lengthy review process, the proposal was once again denied.

By January 1992, with yet further revisions, the proposal was again resubmitted, again requesting "added qualifications." Introductory material on this occasion stressed the emergence of C-L psychiatry systematically from the introduction of psychobiology by Adolf Meyer early in the twentieth century. The application was organized around fulfillment of the criteria for specialization: defining the patient group; scientific foundation of the field; subspecialist knowledge and skills; content of the educational curriculum; advanced training in the subspecialty; need for the subspecialty; available staff resources; effect of the subspecialty on psychiatry; participation of subspecialists in psychiatric education; and capacity for research.

The review "cycle" was outlined by APA staff member Jeanne Robb: beginning with the Joint Reference Committee and Assembly Executive Committee in February, then working its way through the Board of Trustees, the full assembly, area councils, additional assembly, and board meetings in the fall, as well as the Council on Medical Education and Career Development, the Committee on C-L Psychiatry and other committees dealing with psychiatric education, expecting to complete the process by December 1992. When finally reviewed, the ABPN unfortunately again rebuffed the effort on two counts: (1) The Accreditation Council for Graduate Medical Education (ACGME) had declared a moratorium on new medical specialties (lifted later in 1992), and (2) ABPN was concerned that C-L psychiatry was defined by a procedure ("consultation") common to *all* psychiatrists and a particular site of care (general hospital), rather than being focused on a (specific) patient population. (And Ford had hoped to bypass the APA Committee on C-L Psychiatry to hasten the process!)

Tom Wise straddled the awkward position of having been chair of the APA Committee on C-L Psychiatry and Primary Care Education immediately following Brook Lodge II, and he had also held sequential presidencies of APM and APS, so that he was in a strategic position to suffer the slings and arrows of all but also to engage in a bit of shuttle diplomacy. Exemplary psychiatrist and astute politician/conciliator, in closing out his 1993–1994 term with APS, Wise (1995) culminated his service with a presidential speech on *A Tale of Two Societies*, intended to review and reduce tensions between the two organizations. However, a persuasive appeal for collaborative enterprise did not abort the inexorable movement toward change.

By 2001, it was back to the drawing board. In this instance, application was being requested for specialization in "psychosomatic medicine," and the patient population targeted was described as the "complex medically ill." With input from all quarters, including international endorsement from the International Organization for Consultation-Liaison Psychiatry and the European Society for Consultation-Liaison Psychiatry and Psychosomatics, application this time included sponsorship by the Association for Medicine and Psychiatry, a relatively young organization dedicated to an integrated model of care, addressing combined residencies of psychiatry and medicine and pediatrics. Application carried the statement "Recognition of a subspecialty field of Psychosomatic Medicine was endorsed by the American Psychiatric Association (APA) by action of its Board of Trustees in July of 2001." In September 2001, the new application was submitted, put through a similar long review process, and, by March 2003, rewarded with approval by the American Board of Medical Specialties (ABMS), the ABPN, the APA, the American Medical Association (AMA), and the American Council of General Medical Education (ACGME). For most, great rejoicing abounded; the APM was designated the organization to develop guidelines for fellowship training and administering of qualifying examination. Others exclaimed surprise that accreditation was for "psychosomatic medicine," not "consultation-liaison psychiatry."

Over 20 years in the making, the road to specialization had indeed been long and bumpy. Now the difficult work would begin, setting up mechanisms for evaluating programs, establishing fellowships, and developing guidelines for residency training. Psychosomatic medicine, once considered all but defunct, was resurrected! The next chapter will assess this tortuous achievement.

References

American Psychiatric Association. (1981). Committee on Consultation-Liaison Psychiatry and Primary Care Education. Minutes, September 23, 1981.

American Psychiatric Association. (1982). Committee on Consultation-Liaison Psychiatry and Primary Care Education. Minutes, May 19, 1982.

American Psychiatric Association. (1983). Committee on Consultation-Liaison Psychiatry and Primary Care Education. Minutes, September 22, 1983.

American Psychiatric Association. (1989a). Committee on Consultation-Liaison Psychiatry and Primary Care Education. Minutes, May 9, 1989.

American Psychiatric Association. (1989b). Committee on Consultation-Liaison Psychiatry and Primary Care Education. Minutes, September 14, 1989.

Cather, W. (1913). *O Pioneers.* (Part II, Chapter 4). Boston, MA: Houghton Mifflin.

Cohen-Cole, S.A., Haggerty, J., & Raft, D. (1982). Objectives for residents in consultation psychiatry: Recommendations of a task force. *Psychosomatics, 23,* 699–703.

Ford, C.V. (1990). Letter to APA president T. Benedek, June 29.

Graham, D. (1969). Psychosomatic medicine needs a new start. *Hospital Practice, 4,* 1–2.

Lipowski, Z.J. (1986). Consultation-liaison psychiatry: The first half-century. *General Hospital Psychiatry, 8,* 305–315.

Pasnau, R.O. (1989). Letter of invitation. March 1989.

Robinowitz, C.B., & Nadelson, C.C. (1991). Consultation-liaison psychiatry as a subspecialty (Editorial). *General Hospital Psychiatry, 13,* 1–3.

Romano, J. (1970). The elimination of the internship: An act of regression. *American Journal of Psychiatry, 126,* 1565–1575.

Schubert, D.S., & McKegney, F.P. (1976). Psychiatric consultation education—1976. *Archives of General Psychiatry, 33,* 1271–1273.

Thompson, T.L., 2nd. (1993). Some advantages of consultation-liaison (medical-surgical) psychiatry becoming and added qualification subspecialty. *Psychosomatics, 34,* 343–349.

Tilley, D.H., & Silverman, J.J. (1982). Survey of consultation-liaison psychiatry program characteristics and functions. *General Hospital Psychiatry, 4,* 265–270.

Wallen, J., Pincus, H.A., Goldman, H.H., & Marcus, S.E. (1987). Psychiatric consultations in short-term general hospitals. *Archives of General Psychiatry, 44,* 163–168.

Wise, T.N. (1995). A tale of two societies. *Psychosomatic Medicine, 57,* 303–309.

SECTION IV

Post-Specialization

Preamble: *Specialization at last! After a long stumbling journey, consultation-liaison psychiatry has reached not the end of the road but an important milestone. Alas, the specialty is to be called psychosomatic medicine. Over the decades, both C-L and PM have had their identity problems, with both names and missions of their respective entities changing more often than that of any other discipline in medicine. This section will discuss how structure and organization articulate with the official declaration of the seventh specialty of psychiatry (not medicine) to fly the banner of psychosomatic medicine.*

11

SPECIALIZATION

Boon or Bane?

Much literary criticism comes from people for whom extreme specialization is a cover for either grave cerebral inadequacy or terminal laziness, the latter being a much cherished aspect of academic freedom.

—*John Kenneth Galbraith,* The Age of Uncertainty, *1977*

Introduction: After Specialization, What?

Once achieved, organizations must design structures for their survival. Vigilance is essential to monitor and preserve the values, mission, interest, and vitality of its constituents. They must have the sturdiness, creativity, and relevance to resist animosity, competition, and political and economic harassment. History is punctuated with a graveyard of "movements," "organizations," "religions," "governments," and such that have failed to maintain their viability. Now that C-L psychiatry has traversed a bumpy road as psychosomatic medicine and achieved its designated status, the future will assess how it will maintain its own promise. This chapter asks whether naming this clinical specialty "psychosomatic medicine" adds clarity and other desirable attributes to the field or simply muddies the picture; a limited prophesy is offered.

Twelve years have passed since psychosomatic medicine was approved as the seventh subspecialty of psychiatry. While this is a blink of the eye in historical time, it may give us a moment's pause to ask what, for better or worse, we have wrought.

Looking back, in 1863, an esteemed professor stands before a graduating class of medical students and, in dramatic oratory and impeccable logic, implores them to heed the importance of "the psychic element of man—the mind, the soul, the spirit—or, by *what other name soever it may be designated* [emphasis by au.]" that they most certainly will encounter in medical practice.

These words were uttered by Pliny Earle (1863), a medical reformist and the first to be named professor of medical psychology at the Berkshire Medical Institute in Northampton, Massachusetts. The lecture was given at Bloomingdale Hospital, where George Henry (1929–1930) later would elaborate his ideas about liaison psychiatry and Gregory Zilboorg (1941) would write his voluminous book on *A History of Medical Psychology* with Henry's assistance.

To highlight his protestation about the "psychological ignorance" of most physicians, Earle (1863) makes the point that "medical psychology" is essential in every medical school; supporting his argument, he quotes a report of the National Medical Association stating as much. The extract reads, in part:

> Until a general provision is secured for the education of all students in medical psychology, no physician who has not had special qualifications, both by study and practice in this department, should consent to give testimony in cases of alleged insanity, unless after consultation and concurrence with an acknowledged expert.
>
> *(p. 278)*

The proposed need for specialized expert knowledge in this area presages the "liaison" function of psychiatrists who can help their uninformed colleagues to be helpful to their patients. Even the physician naïve in medical psychology can be helped to realize that

> [i]f medicine is, as the ethical codes allege it to be, a truly benevolent and charitable profession, he [the physician, can] . . . by friendly advice, by prudent counsel, by an occasional word of monitorial caution among his employers . . . exert a salutary influence in suppressing those causes, in lessening their influence and preventing the full development of insanity when in its incipient stages. The immediate causes are operating everywhere and no physician should be ignorant of them.
>
> *(p. 270)*

Most physicians of the time, Pliny asserted, felt that they were born with innate understanding of the mind and therefore not needful of expert instruction (p. 271). This tendency to decline consultation would later be described as "resistance" (Greenhill, 1977).

Almost 150 years after Earle's exhortation, psychiatrists and others continue the struggle to define the field (see, for example, Dimsdale, 1991; Greenhill, 1980, 1981; Guthrie, 2006; Houpt, 1987; Lloyd, 1980; Lloyd & Mayou, 2003; Lipowski, 1983, 1986; Mayou, 2001; Oken, 1983; Pasnau, 1988; Schubert, 1983; Smith, 2003; Strain, 1983), "soever it may be designated," as the psychological dimension of medicine; the need for expert knowledge in the field continues to be recognized, although not always clear what it should be called or who best to administer it. For the present, the chosen designation is "psychosomatic medicine," the imprimatur given by the authorities that determine such matters, and psychiatrists are deemed the experts. Much debate, controversy, discussion, and opposition occurred prior to the naming, and much will follow.

It Shall Be Known by Its Name

With specialization comes a guise of certainty, of definition, of stability in an otherwise uncertain world (Lipsitt, 2003). From beginnings in America, the word was only half-heartedly applied to the innovative work of a few researchers interested in mind-body relations. As we have noted, eminent experts have repeatedly "cautioned" that it not be considered a "specialty" but that ideally it "belongs" to all of medicine. Stanley Cobb (1952), for example, began his career as a neuropathologist, then was founding director in 1934 of the Massachusetts General Hospital's Psychiatry Department at the urging and support of Alan Gregg; throughout his career, he insisted that "the line between 'physical' and 'mental' is entirely arbitrary" (p. 115).

Cobb was a founding father of psychosomatic medicine, on the original editorial board of *Psychosomatic Medicine*; embraced a multidisciplinary department, including psychoanalysts; and launched a robust consultative service in his hospital. Increasingly in his continuing career, he voiced adamant opposition, if not antagonism, to the splitting of the profession into its component parts—neurology vs. psychiatry, psychiatry vs. medicine, psychoanalysis vs. medicine, psychosomatics vs. psychiatry, emotions vs. intellect, or psyche vs. soma. In a memorial speech for Jacob Finesinger, a revered member of his department, he said, speaking of such splits,

> Most of the barriers . . . are personal and emotional . . . built up by us as defenses against our feelings of inadequacy. We seem to specialize because of what we do *not* know. Specialization can be a retreat into a corner where one learns more and more about less and less; one can protect himself from the effort of broad correlation by devaluating [*sic*] the work of others. . . . In the practice of all branches of medicine, psychological factors will be considered important as a matter of course. In a few years perhaps we will cease to hear anything about psychosomatic medicine. Like many other branches of investigation it will have served its purpose and be taken back into its Mother Medicine to lose its identity for the common good.
>
> *(1959, p. 304; emphasis original)*

Were Cobb alive today, he might be surprised, if not disappointed! Even Eric Wittkower (1977), the first president of the International College of Psychosomatic Medicine, had expressed the hope that "the psychosomatic approach would be absorbed by medicine" and boldly exclaimed that [psychosomatic medicine] "is perhaps the only field of research and study in medicine dedicated to its own dissolution" (p. 11).

From its earliest beginnings, psychosomatic medicine has been a rather ineffable entity, difficult to define, objectionable by some, overdrawn by others, at various times an attitude, at others an approach, an attitude, a perception, a theory, a movement, a philosophy, at times affiliated with internal medicine, at others with psychiatry, indebted to psychoanalysis and other fields of study.

When Johann Christian Reil named psychiatry (originally *psychiaterie* in 1808), it was his intention that it embrace the principle of continuity of psyche and soma, and of inseparability of psychiatry and medicine, in which "one can see the whole; an affection of the one process of life, which sometimes accentuates this and sometimes that side" (Marneros, 2008, p. 1). From psychiatry's beginnings, it was the medical discipline concerned largely with psychopharmacology, such as existed at the time, and psychotherapy, as it was developing. Diagnosis, treatment, and management of mental illness were regarded part of all branches of medicine. Only a decade later, this characterization of medicine was called "psychosomatic" by the German physician Heinroth (1818), later (ca. 1926) called "*psychosomatic medicine*" by Felix Deutsch (1959).

Charitably, we might say that specialty designation has given more credence, respect, acknowledgement, and credibility to the fact that psyche and soma do coexist and indeed belong in that wedded state, although early writers skeptically continued to maintain them apart through the hyphen (Winnicott, 1954, 1966). Unfortunately, confirming and emphasizing that psychosomatic medicine is a *psychiatric* specialty rather than an aspect of all medicine may represent a step backward. The early wellsprings of psychosomatic medicine were in fact from general medicine, then from psychoanalysts who had their introduction to psychosomatics in Germany and Vienna where it was not defined as a psychiatric discipline (and Freud never used the term). Early members of the American Psychosomatic Society (APS) were a heterogeneous mix of internists, psychiatrists, obstetricians, pediatricians, psychologists, and others, all with a proclaimed interest in a holistic, comprehensive medicine. The beginnings of the Academy of Psychosomatic Medicine (APM) in 1954 were similar, except with a much more "practice-oriented" bent. In a highly democratized setting, all claimed propriety to psychosomatic medicine.

But now, at least in the United States, psychosomatic medicine has been proclaimed by the reviewers to "belong" to psychiatry, elaborated as the practice of psychiatric consultation to the "complex medically ill." (It is not clear who the many officials were who signed off on approval of the name of this specialty or how many of them had experience in either C-L or psychosomatic medicine.) C-L psychiatry is identified as an "aspect" of that specialty, yet by accreditation it is proclaimed different than psychosomatic medicine. The designation "C-L psychiatry" now commonly appears in parentheses to "explain" its relevance to psychosomatic medicine.

The Company They Keep

The phrase is often repeated that C-L psychiatry is the "clinical arm" of psycho-somatic medicine, a kind of robotic appendage of the putative mothership, or just another interchangeable name for psychosomatic medicine. However, clinical experience and even the literature of both fields suggest that this relationship may not be as depicted (Lipsitt, 2001). Contrary to popular parlance, it would appear that C-L psychiatry did not spring from psychosomatic medicine, but rather just the reverse. The first "handbook" of consultation psychiatry (Schwab, 1968) contains 472 references, only 26 of which are to the premier psychosomatic journal *Psychosomatic Medicine*.

Flanders Dunbar, herself a pioneer of the field, was a psychiatric consultant before she was a psychosomatician. She hesitated long, before founding a journal (1939) and a society (1942) of that name, to call the field psychosomatics. Her epic, meticulously assembled book of over 2,200 examples of the application of psychological awareness to medical situations from 1910 to 1933 was entitled simply *Emotions and Bodily Changes* (1935). She carried out her early work mostly in departments of internal medicine (Shorter, 1992, p. 261).

Consequent to this event, Dunbar's book uneasily set the stage for subsequent evolutionary steps of a field "soever it may be designated," in this case "psychosomatic medicine." Whatever Dunbar's hesitation, the name stuck, perhaps the most salubrious at the time and influenced by German usage. Uncomfortably tolerated by its adherents, it was vigorously debated for at least the next four decades, with frequent suggestions along the way for name changes, as previously noted.

As the special interest group of psychiatrists accrued experience in consulting to medical/surgical colleagues, sequential presidential addresses of the psychosomatic societies questioned the relationship of C-L psychiatry to psychosomatic medicine (Engel, 1986; Graham, 1979). Similarly, some have proclaimed that C-L psychiatry sprang from general hospital psychiatry. Again, this is a historically specious characterization since C-L psychiatry existed prior to a surge in general hospital psychiatry. Indeed, C-L activity was practiced in institutions where no psychiatry departments existed at all! (Dale & Wright, 1962; Glasscote & Gudeman, 1983; Lipsitt, 1984; Schulberg, 1963). Later development of inpatient units created a haven for onsite psychiatrists, thus expanding consultative availability, not necessarily an enhancement when consultants had to fragment their clinical responsibilities among multiple services (Schulberg, 1963).

In the year that APS was founded, Ebaugh and Rymer (1942) published a book on teaching psychiatry in medical education. A fundamental principle of psychiatric teaching, they claimed, was

> the close relationship of psychiatry to medicine in general. . . . [P]sychiatry has a vastly broader scope than mental disease . . . a very real part to play in all branches of medicine. . . . [S]o important is this relatively new aspect

of medicine that we believe it cannot fail in time to permeate the whole medical curriculum and the outlook of the entire medical profession toward disease. Psychosomatic medicine is going to be the focus of emphasis in psychiatry and we must constantly stress the importance of emotional factors in disease.

(Bunker, 1944, p. 504)

This had been the stated objective of psychosomatic medicine from its very beginning (Bunker, 1944, p. 504, quoting Ebaugh & Stryker), with repetitive expressions of disappointment at its failure to attain that objective. More than 60 years later, the new specialty of psychosomatic medicine appears to claim the same objectives (Saravay, Steinberg, Solomon & Hong, 1984)!

In the decades following the founding of APS, "psychosomatic" was generally associated with *research*, less with clinical activity. Application by lay public and even medical professionals saw the term used inappropriately, usually pejoratively (for example, "supratentorial" by referring physicians or "out to lunch" by the public). "Psychosomatic" leaves many puzzled, uncertain, or even—as noted in a recent review of the word in the lay public—offended (Stone, Colyer, Feltbower, Carson & Sharpe, 2004). An experienced C-L psychiatrist has written in the British journal *The Lancet*, "Today the word psychosomatic remains etymologically impeccable, but practically useless, since in popular usage psychosomatic is all psyche and no soma" (Wessely, 2011, p. 182).

Pasnau (1982), assessing the "crossroads" of C-L psychiatry and psychosomatic medicine, explained why the concept of psychosomatic medicine had been discarded:

1) If only certain illnesses were psychosomatic, it implied that others were not; 2) the concept perpetuates the dualism between mind and body and hence, paradoxically, violates the psychosomatic approach, which incorporates the unity of biopsychosocial functions; 3) the concept postulates a psychogenic etiology, which leads to the assumption that psychological intervention or psychotherapy is needed to cure the illness; 4) *clinical use of the term psychosomatic alienates patients, often implying that the physician believes them to be mentally ill, malingering, or (worse) hopeless cases.*

(p. 991; emphasis by au.)

With C-L more clearly associated with clinical activity and "psychosomatic" most often, in informed circles, identified with research, the alignment of membership in APS into separate enclaves reinforced this distinction. The split was even more accentuated as those with clinical interests migrated to APM, with its more dedicated clinical focus (see Levenson, 1994, entire Chapter 10).

Clinical experience and even the literature of both fields suggest that the relationship of C-L to psychosomatic medicine may not be as intertwined as depicted.

If indeed they are closely related, one would expect their respective literatures to reflect that interdigitation. My own curiosity resulted in an examination of the literatures of both fields. If the disciplines are related, would this examination reveal evidence of "cross-pollination"?

To test this hypothesis, I (Lipsitt, 2001) reviewed extensive lists of core C-L publications to determine their reliance on citations to *Psychosomatic Medicine* (PM), considered the premier psychosomatic journal launched about the same time as "liaison psychiatry" (Billings, 1939). C-L psychiatry, general hospital psychiatry, and psychosomatic medicine all developed along parallel tracks in the 1930s (Lipsitt, 2000).

Comparing literatures from C-L psychiatry and psychosomatic medicine from the 1930s through 2000, findings are cataloged in Table 11.1.

TABLE 11.1 Percentage of Psychosomatic Medicine Citations in Reference Lists of C-L Literature

Basic lists
APM application (APM, 1992) 4.00%
AAP (Mohl & Cohen-Cole, 1985) 0.65%
Strain et al. (1999) 0.00–27.40%

Research reviews
McKegney and Beckhardt (1982) 3.30%
Cohen-Cole, Haggerty, and Raft (1982) 5.10%

Textbooks
Comprehensive text
Enelow (1980) 8.40%
McKegney (1985) 11.10%
Popkin (1995) 2.40%

American handbooks
Greenhill (1981) 10.30%
Schwab (1968) 5.50%

Articles
Schwab (1985, 1989) 4.30–4.60%
Oken (1983) 12.60%
Romano (1961) 0.00%
Lipowski
   General principles (1967a) 7.40%
   Clinical aspects (1967b) 4.30%
   Theoretical aspects (1968) 21.00%
   Review of first half century (1986) 6.50%

Adapted from D. R. Lipsitt. (2001). Consultation-liaison psychiatry and psychosomatic medicine: The company they keep. *Psychosomatic Medicine*, 63, 896–909. Printed with permission by Wolters Kluwer Health, Inc.)

The organizational papers of Lipowski (1967a, b, 1968) (actually published in PM), cite only 4.30% from PM for clinical issues, 7.40% for general principles, and, as might be expected, a high of 21% for theoretical issues. Schwab's handbook of consultation psychiatry (1968) draws only 5.50% of its references from PM. And Greenhill's extensive review of C-L psychiatry in the *American Handbook of Psychiatry* (1981) derives 10.30% of its citations from PM. Of perhaps even greater interest is that the first application for "added qualifications" in C-L psychiatry cited only 4.00% of its extensive reference list from PM, 7 of 177 references (with a later submission showing 5 of 96 references to PM or 5.2%). It is not included in the study, but review as of this writing of subsequent change of application from "added qualifications" in C-L psychiatry to "subspecialization" of psychosomatic medicine surprisingly does little better, even omitting from its list of relevant (historical) references Alexander's (1950) definitive text on *Psychosomatic Medicine*, Dunbar's (1935) foundational book on emotions and bodily changes, or Weiss and English's (1943) first American textbook of *Psychosomatic Medicine*. The reverse is revealing as well, in that PM cited hardly any articles appearing in the C-L literature. My survey did not include references to psychosomatic medicine from sources other than *Psychosomatic Medicine*, since this journal developed *pari passu* with C-L psychiatry, while others had different timelines. These findings beg this question: How much does C-L psychiatry depend on psychosomatic medicine for its base?

C-L Psychiatry Does Not Equal Psychosomatic Medicine

If C-L psychiatry is indeed the "clinical arm" of psychosomatic medicine, how do the quotidian skills and activities of a consulting psychiatrist draw on psychosomatic research, with which the term has most universally been associated?

In 1987, Robert Pasnau, president of APA, gave an address titled *Consultation-Liaison Psychiatry: Progress, Problems and Prospects* (1988). It alludes to C-L psychiatry as an emerging subspecialty for which "added qualifications" will be requested. The article never uses the word "psychosomatic" except in the reference list (4 of 18). Pasnau identifies "six key elements for consultation-liaison psychiatry practice" as follows: 1) establish close collaboration with referring physicians; 2) emphasize prevention; 3) establish good relationships with patients; 4) help patients to understand and deal with major problems; 5) involve entire health care team in treatment planning; and 6) emphasize humanism and concern for the dignity of the patient (Pasnau, 1988, p. 12). It is my assumption that none of these key elements rely on the corpus of psychosomatic research or knowledge. The author adds "significant categories for future consultation-liaison psychiatry research: 1) diagnosis; 2) disease mechanisms; 3) biological treatment; 4) health services; and 5) psychosocial treatments for medical disorders" (p. 13). While some of these domains (especially items 2 and 3) may conceivably rely on psychosomatic research, the point could be argued that they could just as heavily draw on other disciplines for supportive data (e.g., sociology, anthropology, epidemiology).

We will see, in fact, how much of what a C-L psychiatrist does has little to do with psychosomatics, perhaps more with psychoanalysis, interviewing, and psychotherapy. In recent years, clinical application of psychopharmacology, of little concern to psychosomaticians except in psychophysiological research, is a large part of the C-L psychiatrist's skills. Even anxiety, depression, grief, and bereavement have been only minimally part of psychosomatic medicine's repertoire. And, although early psychosomatic researchers were also practicing physicians and psychoanalysts, today they are largely Ph.D.s working in physiology and neuroscience laboratories.

Case Examples

The following abbreviated case descriptions represent a sampling of patients seen in consultation on a C-L service:

> Case One: The consultant was asked to see a 48-year-old woman readmitted after surgery and chemotherapy for breast cancer because of pains in her arms and difficulty breathing, without clear etiology. The patient was interviewed at the bedside. She had been tearful at times, and she had had angry interactions with the staff. After introductions and a review of her surgical history, hospitalization, and family history, she quickly turned to a description of her anger at doctors for not keeping her informed, about their disagreement over her diagnosis and treatment, and especially about a doctor who said of her emotional reaction "we have to stop this nonsense." Family history included a father who died at 49 of a heart attack and a sister who had open-heart surgery for heart disease. She spoke of how guilty she felt being away from work and also how upset she was to have to wear a wig. She said she felt she was not in control of her life, having to depend on others more than usual. The psychiatrist discussed with the resident the patient's compulsive and hysterical traits, her sadness at her losses, her fear of heart disease (like father and sister), and a need to be fully informed of everything planned for her. While the interview was more extensive, basic information was quickly available to respond to the request for consultation.
>
> Case Two: A 29-year-old single woman working as a nursing home aide was brought to the emergency room by her mother, found to have overdosed on alcohol and diazepam (Valium). History revealed that a recent change of nursing home assignment had severed contacts with good friends and that she had also broken up with a boyfriend with whom she was living; she was now forced to return to living with a mother with whom she had a "tense relationship." Although she had been seeing a "counselor" for the past six months, she was told by him that she was "doing extremely well." She said, "He's going to kill me" (when he

learns of her behavior). Her attempt included use of both mother's and therapist's pills. The consultant addressed the several losses endured by this emotionally immature, impulsive woman and her fear of now losing her therapist "because of how well she was doing." Consultant's recommendations included discussion with mother, removal of "suicide sitter," and contact with "counselor" to urge continuing therapy. Discussion with patient centered around helping her to understand the "pain" of losses and ways to cope more effectively with them. Discussion with hospital staff included comment that patient's work in nursing homes with "elderly women" was perhaps an adaptive way to learn better how to interact with "mother."

Case Three: A 65-year-old man recently retired from his job as an electronics engineer was admitted to hospital with foot pain, a leg ulcer, and generalized vasculitis. The patient's surgeon reluctantly acquiesced to psychiatric consultation on the urging of a nurse who noted the patient's description of shame associated to "spontaneous crying without apparent reason." Absent a diagnosis of pseudobulbar palsy, previous history included surgeries for gallbladder disease and noncancerous prostatectomy. In the interview, he was very pleasant, articulate, and intelligent, but expressed feelings of helplessness with a "bad leg" and the decreased mobility it had caused him. He recalled a friend with Parkinson's disease whose hands had been tied in bed to prevent dislodging a catheter and told his wife never to let that happen to him. He seemed slow to speak of his prostate surgery, said he was unsure why he had it, and said that he had experienced erectile dysfunction for 15 years before the surgery. His sexual function he said was "zilch." When asked about his crying, he said he thought he was "just a fruitcake." He was asked by the consultant if he thought that talking about his prostatectomy had anything to do with his concerns about his leg; he thought it "far-fetched" but began to cry and said, "You see, there it goes again, out of nowhere." It was restated to him that maybe uncertainties about his leg were reviving old uncertainties about his prostate and fears of being "disabled" by both. While he tended to dismiss this "far-out" idea, he appeared much relieved and said, "Maybe I should see a psychiatrist," but was assured that it would only be a necessity if he wanted to explore some of these ideas, not because he was "a fruit cake." Staff was instructed about the man's enforced passivity, feeling "unmanly," and possibly being "afraid of losing his leg" but unable to describe his emotions for fear of being labeled a "fruit cake." Some discussion ensued with staff about the relationship of personality style to response to illness.

It would be difficult to ascertain how the fundamentals of "psychosomatic medicine" played a role in any of these cases, except as aspects of "the psychosomatic approach" might be embedded in the consultant's clinical style, or how "stress" may influence illness. For the most part, practitioners in the field refer to their practice as "consultation-liaison," rather than "psychosomatic."

To further examine the question of psychosomatic medicine's relation to C-L practice, I have cataloged some of the "cases" from my own experience for which input from psychiatric consultation had been sought: for example, impulse control, cognitive problems, consent, death and dying, "sundowning" (delirium), overdose, suicidal impulse or attempt, pain (chest and other), reaction to burn, hospitalization, surgery, grief reaction, hyperventilation, panic, postoperative delirium, weakness and fatigue, medication side effects, psychotropic drug prescription, dialysis, transplant surgery, cosmetic surgery, anniversary reaction, seizure activity, multiple sclerosis, personality disorder, doctor-patient relationships, perceptual distortion, "behavior change," ward/staff tensions, and so on. Additionally, guidelines established by APM (Bronheim et al., 1998) include other indications for psychiatric consultation in the following: agitation/anger, coping problem, eating disorder, child abuse, postpartum changes, preoperative assessment, sleep disorder, malingering, "transfer," hypochondriasis, ethical issues, and so on. Much of psychosomatic research has been in the area of cardiovascular disorders, and familiarity with such studies can enhance the C-L psychiatrist's knowledge when specific organs are in question, but otherwise consultation rarely relies on psychosomatic research for effective intervention.

Supporting this position, a review of 2,000 referrals for psychiatric consultation (Lipowski & Wolston, 1981) lists the "most common reasons for referral" as follows: "help with diagnosis; advice on patient management; past psychiatric history; request for transfer to a psychiatric unit; staff-patient conflict; and issues regarding competence to refuse treatment." Diagnostic problems included the following: psychiatric presentation of a physical illness; somatic presentation of a psychiatric illness; suicide attempt; noncompliance with medical treatment. Seventy percent of diagnoses included adjustment disorder with depressive mood and organic mental syndromes, especially delirium, and a 70–80% incidence of comorbidity. As many as 20–30% of referrals revealed no psychiatric diagnosis at all or presented with somatization or suicide attempt (p. 130). Again, reliance on "psychosomatic medicine" or research would appear elusive.

While addressing any of these issues may involve allegiance to a "psychosomatic approach," it may be difficult to identify the role of psychosomatic research in any of them. C-L psychiatry and psychosomatic medicine share common interests in the intricacies of mind-body-brain relationships; their missions overlap, but psychosomatic medicine with its research focus does not appear paramount in the daily work of the psychiatric consultant; in fact, knowledge of internal medicine and neurology may be of greater import.

Both C-L psychiatry and psychosomatic medicine are committed to an integrated approach to health care that acknowledges the relevance of biological, psychological, and social factors. But such interests are not unique to them.

Currently, there is general interest in holistic, integrated, collaborative, or comprehensive health care in a variety of disciplines (Wise, 2000).

Milton Rosenbaum—former chairman and professor of psychiatry at Albert Einstein Medical Center in the Bronx, New York, an early Rockefeller Foundation fellow, and a longtime member of the American Psychosomatic Society—began his career as a psychoanalytically trained physician researcher on the forefront of the psychosomatic movement. Into his 90s, he was consulting to patients at the University of Arizona. With Teresita McCarty, they wrote (1994):

> In our experience, we see relatively few patients who have what were considered classical psychosomatic disorders. The majority of our cases relate to suicide attempts, delirium, complicated medical disorders with psychiatric symptoms, classic psychiatric illness, substance abuse, burn, head injuries, and competence evaluations. In a recent review of our consultation requests only 2% were for "psychosomatic" problems.
>
> *(p. 573)*

They attribute the decline to

> lack of or loss of interest in psychosomatic medicine by C-L psychiatrists, changes in the patient population in university teaching, reduction in the length of hospital stay, introduction of diagnosis-related groups, and the increasing cost of hospitalization and medical care.
>
> *(p. 573)*

Explaining current practice, they state:

> We are in the business of triage and psychopharmacology, not psychosomatic medicine. . . . "[L]iaison" has faded since early 1980s and C-L should more properly concentrate on delivering "high quality consultation services," and less on trying to become acceptable friends with other services.
>
> *(p. 573)*

The differences in "our" (C-L psychiatrists) culture and demands, personal training, and lifestyles from those of other services require that we accept their situation without trying to change it, they advise. Much of what may have been included in liaison—talk with family members, with nursing staff, with previous and current physicians and hospitals—is still provided.

While we cannot plumb the intricacies of the decision-making process to switch application for specialty status from C-L psychiatry to psychosomatic medicine, it is apparent that the confusion surrounding the term and the turbulent past of the field was not a deterrent. Practice of C-L psychiatry today is much easier to define; the word "consultation" is more readily recognized than the word "psychosomatic" or the broad field of psychosomatic medicine. When depart-ments advertise for additional staff, they generally list their positions as C-L, not psychosomatic (or both). Most consultation services continue to refer to them-selves as C-L services. According to Wise, "[T]he consultation psychiatrist does not view himself as psychosomaticist" (Wise, 2000, p. 182).

The same year that psychosomatic medicine was declared a subspecialty, Pincus (2003) wrote an article questioning whether the future of behavioral health and primary care was "drowning in the mainstream or left on the bank." Discussed are "powerful conceptual models" (e.g., Engel's [1977] biopsychosocial model) and treatment frameworks (e.g., behavioral medicine/health psychology and consultation-liaison psychiatry) as useful integrative models, but no men-tion is made of psychosomatics. Pincus attests to his "discomfort" in using the poorly defined term "behavioral health," with its inclusion of "mental health disorders, substance abuse conditions and a broad range of psychosocial problems as well as behavioral aspects of general medical conditions" (p. 1), while omitting psychosomatic medicine entirely. He lists the various adjectives used to relate to behavioral health components in primary care: "mental, behavioral, emotional, social, psychological, psychosocial, biopsychosocial, addictive/substance-related, cognitive, stress-related, maladaptive, brain, and nervous." The list does not include "psychosomatic." Definitional problems, he states, are complicated because "bio-logical, psychological, behavioral and socioenvironmental interventions are all relevant" (p. 2). Again, no mention of psychosomatics! Is this merely an egregious oversight, or does it suggest that the term is irrelevant in speaking of how C-L psychiatrists endeavor to promote a more integrative health care approach that helps primary care physicians increase their awareness of "behavioral factors" in their daily work?

Avoiding the need and challenge to make difficult distinctions, a consensus statement of European and American C-L groups stated, "For purposes of this document the terms 'Psychosomatic Medicine' (PM) and 'Consultation-Liaison Psychiatry' (CLP) are considered interchangeable" (Leentjens, Rundell, Wolcott, Guthrie, Kathol & Diefenbacher, 2011, p. 487). The paper states that, for devel-opment of guidelines, "use was made of the results of scientific research when possible," yet no references to *Psychosomatic Medicine* are included! (p. 491).

The choice of "psychosomatic medicine" rather than C-L psychiatry for spe-cialty status is especially curious given how many experts in the field have declared its failures or even demise. Taylor (1987) describes:

> In a presidential address to the APS in 1960, Eric Wittkower gloomily pre-dicted an end to this epoch of psychosomatic medicine. He anticipated that the field would soon become dominated by physiologists, neurobiologists, and biochemists. As this began to happen, many psychoanalytically trained physicians joined their more biologically oriented medical colleagues and became psychophysiological researchers. Others shifted their investigative

focus from the intrapsychic worlds of their patients to the life setting in which the disease process commenced.

(p. 2)

Assessing Psychosomatic Medicine's Future

Life and the world are forever changing. It is too early to assess the effects of designating the work of the C-L psychiatrist as "psychosomatic medicine." Given the slowness with which progress occurs, a decade is insufficient to assess adequately changes in funding mechanisms, numbers of fellows, referral rates, training guidelines, and styles of practice. What can we say about events since accreditation? What about increases in reimbursement for services? What of fellowships: increase or decrease? What about referral rates; have they improved? Research grants? Relations or collaborations with other organizations and nonpsychiatrist colleagues? Membership? Has there been any increase in students choosing psychiatry? There are many researchable questions to pursue. Should the "interface"—a term most likely first introduced in C-L by Schwab and Clemmons (1966)—be redefined?

Even small system changes can have large ripple effects. As an example, the introduction of hospitalists into the medical system has changed the relation of patients to their own doctors, thus affecting one aspect of effective liaison. And the rapidity with which patients are discharged from hospital affects the consultant's interaction with patients. In the United States, liaison has all but disappeared (Cavanaugh & Milne, 1995; Saravay, 1995) while in Europe and the United Kingdom interest is growing (Guthrie, 2006; Huyse, Herzog, Malt & Lobo, 1996; Mayou, 2001; Sollner & Creed, 2007).

There is no question that C-L services have drastically changed. Early influences were psychoanalytically oriented, with greater kinship with psychosomatic medicine, but this has changed considerably. The debate over the value of "liaison" has perhaps had much to do with the change, and some services have even dropped the term. Any likelihood of "comprehensive" ongoing care will have to occur in ambulatory settings such as "medical homes" or "accountable care organizations" (Gonzalez 1993; Katon & Unutzer, 2011; Meyer, Peteet & Joseph, 2009).

To the extent that C-L psychiatry and psychosomatic medicine share common roots, the seeds have propagated widely, now having flowered in epidemiology, sociology, psychology, anthropology, genetics, radiology, behavioral science, neuroscience, communication, phenomenology, ethics, philosophy, forensics, and other disciplines. With a doctrine of multicausality and a pragmatic or pluralistic approach to the great complexities of modern medicine and health care, C-L psychiatrists are interested in the effect of conflict and stress on disease, a systems view of illness, the influence of occupation and job loss, psychological sequelae of family relations, object loss, separation, bereavement, doctor-patient relationships, environmental factors, personality structure, and more. Research in these topics, in whatever discipline it occurs, will continue to interest and inform the C-L psychiatrist, however affecting medical practice.

All of this litany is not to minimize the value of psychosomatic medicine. Its success may, in fact, be measured by the extent to which it has permeated much of our lives, personally, academically, and clinically. But it seems unlikely that it defines the major activity and scientific base of the C-L psychiatrist. The future field of academic interest must perforce cover more than a single subject or journal. The basic readings of the field may include those of anthropology, sociology, economics, and politics in addition to medicine.

My travel along this road is one small snapshot of how C-L psychiatry and psychosomatic medicine may relate; others will certainly have different viewpoints. As Saravay (2008) stated in the opening remarks of his APM presidential address, "The new name of our subspecialty, 'Psychosomatic Medicine,' challenges our field to rethink its identity and to rethink how [it] may affect who we are and what we do" (p. 3).

Predictions

Going forward, the field will have many opportunities to rethink the change. Differences and similarities of C-L psychiatry and psychosomatic medicine will reflect a variety of thoughtful assessments. On the virtual eve of accreditation of psychosomatic medicine, Kornfeld (2002), in his Hackett Award presentation, outlined the many contributions of C-L psychiatry to medicine. The review by Ali, Ernst, Pacheco, and Fricchione (2006) asks how far we have come in C-L psychiatry and presents a hopeful future for psychosomatic medicine; they nevertheless report a survey in which one-third of 25 fellowship directors "felt that the quality of education would not necessarily improve with accreditation" (p. 221).

The same questions that were raised by Pasnau (1982) for C-L psychiatry of the 1980s can be applied to psychosomatic medicine of the 2000s. Considering the many internal and external pressures on C-L psychiatry, Pasnau, wrote, it (C-L)

> can expect to sputter along without firm financial support from departments of psychiatry and general hospitals. Questions remained whether liaison would be dropped and the practice would revert to a consultation-only model. Would behavioral medicine supplant the role of C-L psychiatry? . . . If it [C-L psychiatry] meets the research, fiscal, and political challenges, finds a way to make peace with psychologists and other behavioral scientists, develops a close collaboration with nursing, continues to enjoy the support of the departments of psychiatry, and transforms the consultation model into a more comprehensive consultation-liaison model, the future for liaison psychiatry will be bright indeed.
>
> (p. 995)

Almost a decade later, Jeffrey Houpt (1989), a former C-L psychiatrist and medical school dean emeritus, likewise tried to predict the future of C-L psychiatry. While he considered C-L psychiatry a logical choice for consideration as a subspecialty. . ." (p. 53) he anticipated that the C-L psychiatrist would become more of a medical and neurological expert as well as psychiatrist, that liaison would be essentially nonexistent and that more non-medical health providers would be involved in interventions that did not require the "integrating abilities of the psychiatrist. Stoudemire and Fogel (1988) anticipate an entire transformation of the field into a new model of "medical psychiatry" (p. 207).

The changes we have experienced and will continue to do so were not unexpected. As committed as he was to searching for specific etiologies of psychosomatic disorder, Alexander—like Freud—entertained the expectation that other scientific discoveries might supplant their theories. In *Psychosomatic Medicine* (1950), Alexander writes:

> The question may be raised, then, as to whether the psychosomatic approach should be considered as a transitory method which will be abandoned as soon as we are able by improved electroencephalography and other physiological techniques to study those brain processes which today yield only to psychological methods.
>
> *(p. 50)*

Alexander nevertheless believed that some brain processes related to interpersonal relationships may continue to resist explanation in any other than psychological or sociological terms (p. 51). According to Alexander, much would be known about the anatomy and physiology of the brain, but not about thought or ideas; as Seymour Kety, a leading American neuroscientist and former director of NIMH, said, one day we will know everything there is to know about *memory*, but probably never about *memories*. The field is set for the neuroscientists!

C-L psychiatrists have developed a new appreciation of the importance of relevant research. And the field is alive with innovation. British, European, and Asian interest has expanded with unusual cross-cultural multinational collaboration, especially focused on liaison aspects of treatment of patients with complex comorbidities; whether addressed as C-L psychiatry or psychosomatic medicine, they have contributed valued insights to dimensions of the field (Freudenreich et al., 2015; Grassi et al., 2015; Huyse & Steifel, 2007; Huyse et al., 1996; Kishi et al., 2007; Steifel, 2006).

And psychology, which long ago was more fused with philosophy than medicine, has been growing closer to medicine, so that what has previously been a competitive relationship will find greater compatibility and common objectives in health care.

Recitative

This book describes the foundations not simply of what C-L *is* but also of what C-L is *becoming*, for no one can accurately predict what the future holds, what consequences will result from "next steps" in the evolution of the many complexities that make up our world, both individual and ecological. Our most precise knowledge lies in what has gone before, what our historical foundations are, even as poorly as we might comprehend them. We await the future with curiosity and hope. Would psychobiology going forward be more promising than psychosomatic medicine going back?

References

Academy of Psychosomatic Medicine. (1992). *Application for Certification for Added Qualifications in Consultation-Liaison Psychiatry.* Chicago, IL: Academy of Psychosomatic Medicine (unpublished document).

Alexander, F. (1950). *Psychosomatic Medicine.* New York, NY: W.W. Norton & Co.

Ali, S, Ernst, C., Pacheco, M., & Fricchione, G. (2006). Consultation-liaison psychiatry: How far have we come? *Current Psychiatry Reports, 8,* 215–225.

Billings, E.G. (1939). Liaison psychiatry and intern instruction. *Journal of American Medical Colleges, 14,* 375–385.

Bronheim, H.E., Fulop, G., Kunkel, E.J., Muskin, P.R., Schindler, B.A., Yates, W.R., . . . Stoudemire, A. (1998). The academy of psychosomatic medicine practice guidelines for psychiatric consultation in the general medical setting. The academy of psychosomatic medicine. *Psychosomatics, 39,* S8–S30.

Bunker, H.A. (1944). American psychiatry as a specialty. In J.K. Hall, G. Zilboorg, & H.A. Bunker (Eds.). *American Psychiatry 1844–1944.* (pp. 479–505). New York, NY: Columbia University Press.

Cavanaugh, S., & Milne, J. (1995). Recent changes in consultation-liaison psychiatry: A blueprint for the future. *Psychosomatics, 36,* 95–102.

Cobb, S. (1952). *Foundations of Neuropsychiatry.* (5th edition). Baltimore, MD: Williams & Wilkins.

Cobb, S. (1959). Jacob Ellis Finesinger. 1902–1959. *Journal of Nervous and Mental Disease, 129,* 415–416.

Cohen-Cole, S., Haggerty, J., & Raft, D. (1982). Objectives for residents in consultation psychiatry: Recommendations of a task force. *Psychosomatics, 23,* 699–703.

Dale, P.W., & Wright, H.S. (1962). The care of psychiatric patients in a general hospital without special facilities. *American Journal of Psychiatry, 118,* 930–932.

Deutsch, F. (1959). *On the Mysterious Leap from the Mind to the Body. A Study on the Theory of Conversion.* New York, NY: International Universities Press.

Dimsdale, J.E. (1991). Challenges, problems, and opportunities in consultation-liaison psychiatry research. *Psychiatric Medicine, 9,* 641–648.

Dunbar, H.F. (1935). *Emotions and Bodily Changes: A Survey of Literature on Psychosomatic Interrelationships, 1910–1033.* New York, NY: Columbia University Press.

Earle, P. (1863). Psychologic medicine: Its importance as a part of the medical curriculum. *American Journal of Insanity, 24,* 257–280.

Ebaugh, F.G., & Rymer, C.A. (1942). *Psychiatry in Medical Education.* New York, NY: The Commonwealth Fund.

Enelow, A.J. (1980). Consultation-liaison psychiatry. In A.M. Freedman, H.I. Kaplan, & B.I Sadock (Eds.). *Comprehensive Textbook of Psychiatry.* (5th edition, pp. 1980–1985). Baltimore, MD: Williams & Wilkins.

Engel, B.T. (1986). Psychosomatic medicine, behavioral medicine, just plain medicine. *Psychosomatic Medicine, 48,* 466–479.

Engel, G.L. (1977). The need for a new medical model: A challenge for biomedicine. *Science, 196,* 129–136.

Freudenreich, O., Huffman, J.C., Sharpe, M., Beach, S.R., Celano, C.M., Chwastiak, L.A., . . . Stern, T.A. (2015). Updates in psychosomatic medicine: 2014. *Psychosomatics, 56,* 445–469.

Galbraith, J.K. (1977). The age of uncertainty. *BBC Television Series.*

Glasscote, R.M., & Gudeman, J. (1983). *The Use of Psychiatry in Smaller General Hospitals.* Washington, DC: American Psychiatric Press.

Gonzalez, J.J. (1993). Outpatient consultation-liaison psychiatry: An unfulfilled promise? *General Hospital Psychiatry, 15,* 360–362.

Graham, D.T. (1979). What place in medicine for psychosomatic medicine? *Psychosomatic Medicine, 41,* 357–367.

Grassi, L., Mitchell, A.J., Otani, M. Caruso, R., Nanni, M.G., Hachuzuka, M., . . . Riba, M. (2015). Consultation-liaison psychiatry in the general hospital: The experience of UK, Italy, and Japan. *Current Psychiatry Report, 17,* 44.

Greenhill, M.H. (1977). The development of liaison programs. In G. Usdin, (Ed.). *Psychiatric Medicine.* (pp. 115–191). New York, NY: Brunner/Mazel.

Greenhill, M.H. (1980). Liaison psychiatry as therapy. *Currents in Psychiatric Therapy, 19,* 123–128.

Greenhill, M.H. (1981). Liaison psychiatry. In S. Arieti, (Ed.). *American Handbook of Psychiatry.* (Vol. 7, 2nd edition, pp. 672–702). New York, NY: Basic Books.

Guthrie, E. (2006). Psychological treatments in liaison psychiatry: The evidence base. *Clinical Medicine, 6,* 544–547.

Heinroth, J.C.A. (1818). *Lehrbuch der storungen des seelenlebens oder der seelenstorung und ihrer behandlung—aus rationaler sicht.* Leipzig, GER: Vogel.

Henry, G.W. (1929–1930). Some modern aspects of psychiatry in a general hospital practice. *American Journal of Psychiatry, 9,* 481–499.

Houpt, J.L. (1987). Products of consultation-liaison psychiatry. *General Hospital Psychiatry, 9,* 350–353.

Houpt, J.L. (1989). The future of consultation-liaison psychiatry as a subspecialty. In J. Yager (Ed.). *The Future of Psychiatry as a Specialty.* (pp. 47–55). Washington, DC: American Psychiatric Publishing.

Huyse, F.J., Herzog, T., Malt, U.F., & Lobo, A. (1996). The European consultation-liaison workgroup (ECLW) collaborative study. I. General outline. *General Hospital Psychiatry, 18,* 44–55.

Huyse, F.J., & Steifel, F.C. (2007). Controversies in consultation-liaison psychiatry. *Psychosomatic Research, 62,* 257–258.

Katon, W., & Unutzer, J. (2011). Consultation psychiatry in the medical home and accountable care organizations: Achieving the triple aim. *General Hospital Psychiatry, 33,* 305–310.

Kishi, Y., Meller, W.H., Kato, M., Thurber, S., Swigart, S.E., Okuyama, T., . . . Aoki, T. (2007). A comparison of psychiatric consultation-liaison services between hospitals in the United States and Japan. *Psychosomatics, 48,* 517–522.

Kornfeld, D.S. (2002). Consultation-liaison psychiatry: Contributions to medical practice. *American Journal of Psychiatry, 159,* 1964–1972.

Leentjens, A.F., Rundell, J.R., Wolcott, D.L., Guthrie, E., Kathol, R., & Diefenbacher, A. (2011). Psychosomatic medicine and consultation-liaison psychiatry: Scope of practice, processes, and competencies for psychiatrists working in the field of C-L psychiatry and psychosomatics. A consensus statement of the European association of consultation-liaison psychiatry and psychosomatics (EACLPP) and the academy of psychosomatic medicine (APM). *Journal of Psychosomatic Research, 70,* 486–491.

Levenson, D. (1994). *Mind, Body, and Medicine: A History of the American Psychosomatic Society.* Philadelphia, PA: Williams & Wilkins.

Lipowski, Z.J. (1967a). Review of consultation psychiatry and psychosomatic medicine. I. General principles. *Psychosomatic Medicine, 29,* 153–171.

Lipowski, Z.J. (1967b). Review of consultation psychiatry and psychosomatic medicine. II. Clinical aspects. *Psychosomatic Medicine, 29,* 201–224.

Lipowski, Z.J. (1968). Review of consultation psychiatry and psychosomatic medicine. III. Theoretical aspects. *Psychosomatic Medicine, 30,* 399–422.

Lipowski, Z.J. (1983). Current trends in consultation-liaison psychiatry. *Canadian Journal of Psychiatry, 28,* 329–338.

Lipowksi, Z.J. (1986). Consultation-liaison psychiatry. The first half-century. *General Hospital Psychiatry, 8,* 305–315.

Lipowski, Z.J., & Wolston, E.J. (1981). Liaison psychiatry: Referral patterns and their stability over time. *American Journal of Psychiatry, 138,* 1608–1611.

Lipsitt, D.R. (1984). Not by beds alone. Presentation at 137th Annual Meeting of the American Psychiatric Association. Los Angeles, CA: May 5–11.

Lipsitt, D.R. (2000). Psyche and soma: Struggles to close the gap. In R.W. Menninger & J.C. Nemiah (Eds.). *American Psychiatry After World War II (1944–1994).* (pp. 152–186). Washington, DC: American Psychiatric Press.

Lipsitt, D.R. (2001). Consultation-liaison psychiatry and psychosomatic medicine: The company they keep. *Psychosomatic Medicine, 63,* 896–909.

Lipsitt, D.R. (2003). Psychiatry and the general hospital in an age of uncertainty. *World Psychiatry, 2,* 87–92.

Lloyd, G.G. (1980). Liaison psychiatry from a British perspective. *General Hospital Psychiatry, 2,* 46–51.

Lloyd, G.G., & Mayou, R.A. (2003). Liaison psychiatry or psychological medicine? *British Journal of Psychiatry, 183,* 5–7.

Marneros, A. (2008). Psychiatry's 200th birthday. *British Journal of Psychiatry, 143,* 1–3.

Mayou, R. (2001). Liaison psychiatry. *British Journal of Psychiatry, 179,* 273–275.

McKegney, F.P. (1985). Consultation-liaison psychiatry. In H.I. Kaplan & B.J. Sadock (Eds.). *Comprehensive Textbook of Psychiatry.* (4th edition, pp. 1219–1223). Baltimore, MD: Williams & Wilkins.

McKegney, F.P., & Beckhardt, R.M. (1982). Evaluative research in consultation-liaison psychiatry. Review of the literature: 1970–1981. *General Hospital Psychiatry, 4,* 197–218.

Meyer, F., Peteet, J., & Joseph, R. (2009). Models of care for co-occurring mental and medical disorders. *Harvard Review of Psychiatry, 17,* 353–360.

Mohl, P.C., & Cohen-Cole, S.A. (1985). Basic readings in consultation psychiatry. *Psychosomatics, 26, 431*–440.

Oken, D. (1983). Liaison psychiatry (liaison medicine). *Advances in Psychosomatic Medicine, 11,* 23–51.

Pasnau, R.O. (1982). Consultation-liaison at the crossroads: In search of a definition for the 1980s. *Hospital and Community Psychiatry, 33,* 939–995.

Pasnau, R.O. (1987). Psychiatry in medicine: Medicine in psychiatry. *American Journal of Psychiatry, 144,* 975–980.

Pasnau, R.O. (1988). Consultation-liaison psychiatry: Progress, problems and prospects. *Psychosomatics, 29,* 4–15.

Pincus, H.A. (2003). The future of behavioral health and primary care: Drowning in the mainstream or left on the banks? *Psychosomatics, 44,* 1–11.

Popkin, M.K. (1995). Consultation-liaison psychiatry. In H.I. Kaplan & B.I. Sadock (Eds.). *Comprehensive Textbook of Psychiatry.* (6th edition, pp. 1592–1605). Baltimore, MD: Williams & Wilkins.

Reil, J. (1808). *Rhapsodieen uber die anwendung der psychischen curmethode auf geisteszeruttungen.* Halle, GER: Curt.

Romano, J. (1961). Basic contributions to medicine by research in psychiatry. *Journal of the American Medical Association, 178,* 1147–1150.

Rosenbaum, M., & McCarty, T. (1994). The relationship of psychosomatic medicine to consultation-liaison psychiatry. *Psychosomatics, 35,* 569–573.

Saravay, S.M. (1995). Academic consultation-liaison service. The problems and the promise. *Psychosomatics, 36,* 91–94.

Saravay, S.M. (2008). Presidential address: Academy of psychosomatic medicine, Tucson, AZ, November 2006. *Psychosomatics, 49,* 3–7.

Saravay, S.M., Steinberg, H., Solomon, S.P., & Hong, G.K. (1984). A confirmation of NIMH training objectives for consultation-liaison residents. *American Journal of Psychiatry, 141,* 1437–1440.

Schubert, D.S. (1983). Practical distinctions between consultative psychiatry and liaison medicine. *Advances in Psychosomatic Medicine, 11,* 77–87.

Schulberg, H.C. (1963). Psychiatric units in general hospitals: Boon or bane? *American Journal of Psychiatry, 120,* 30–36.

Schwab, J.J. (1968). *Handbook of Psychiatric Consultation.* New York, NY: Appleton-Century-Crofts.

Schwab, J.J. (1985). Psychosomatic medicine: Its past and present. *Psychosomatics, 26,* 83–93.

Schwab, J.J. (1989). Consultation-liaison psychiatry: A historical overview. *Psychosomatics, 30,* 245–254.

Schwab, J.J., & Clemmons, R.S. (1966). Psychiatric consultations. The interface between psychiatry and medicine. *Archives of General Psychiatry, 14,* 504–508.

Shorter, E. (1992). *From Paralysis to Fatigue. A History of Psychosomatic Medicine in the Modern Era.* New York, NY: Free Press.

Smith, G.C. (2003). The future of consultation-liaison psychiatry. *Australia and New Zealand Journal of Psychiatry, 37,* 150–159.

Sollner, W.W., & Creed, F. (2007). European guidelines for training in consultation-liaison psychiatry and psychosomatic medicine. Report of the EACLLP workgroup on training in consultation-liaison psychiatry and psychosomatics. *Journal of Psychiatric Research, 62,* 501–509.

Steifel, F.C., (2006). Reflections and perspectives. *Medical Clinics of North America, 90,* 759–760.

Stone, J., Colyer, M., Feltbower, S., Carson, A., & Sharpe, M. (2004). "Psychosomatic": A systematic review of its meaning in newspaper articles. *Psychosomatics, 45,* 287–290.

Stoudemire, A., & Fogel, B. (1988). The emergence of medical psychiatry: A provocative viewpoint. *Psychosomatics, 29,* 207–213.

Strain, J.J. (1983). Liaison psychiatry and its dilemmas. *General Hospital Psychiatry, 5,* 209–212.

Strain, J.J., Campos-Rodenos, R., Carvalho, S., Diefenbacher, A., Malt, U.F., Smith, G., . . . Strain, J.J. (1999). Further evaluation of a literature database: The international use of a common software structure and methodology for the establishment of national consultation/liaison databases. B. Consultation-liaison psychiatry database. *General Hospital Psychiatry, 21,* 438–502.

Taylor, G.J. (1987). *Psychosomatic Medicine and Contemporary Psychoanalysis.* Madison, CT: International Universities Press.

Weiss, E., & English, O.S. (1943). *Psychosomatic Medicine.* Philadelphia, PA: W.B. Saunders.

Wessely, S. (2011). On the soma side of the street. (Book review of *Integrated Care of the Complex Medically Ill). The Lancet, 369,* 181–182.

Winnicott, D.W. (1954). Mind and its relation to the psyche-soma. *British Journal of Medical Psychology, 27,* 201–209.

Winnicott, D.W. (1966). Psycho-somatic illness in its positive and negative aspects. *International Journal of Psychoanalysis, 47,* 510–516.

Wise, T.N. (2000). Consultation-liaison psychiatry and psychosomatics: Strange bedfellows. *Psychotherapy and Psychosomatics, 69,* 181–183.

Wittkower, E.D. (1960). Twenty years of North American psychosomatic medicine (presidential address). *Psychosomatic Medicine, 22,* 308–315.

Wittkower, E.D. (1977). Historical perspective of contemporary psychosomatic medicine. In Z.J. Lipowski, D.R. Lipsitt, & P.C. Whybrow (Eds.). *Psychosomatic Medicine: Current Trends and Clinical Applications.* (pp. 3–13). New York, NY: Oxford University Press.

Zilboorg, G. (with Henry, G.W.). (1941). *A History of Medical Psychology.* New York, NY: W.W. Norton.

Appendix One
DRAMATIS PERSONAE

Our revels now are ended. These our actors,
As I foretold you, were all spirits. . . . We are such stuff
As dreams are made on, and our little life is rounded with a sleep.

Shakespeare, The Tempest, Act 4, Scene 1

In the early stages of a discipline's development, it is fairly easy to identify "pioneers," major contributors to its very existence. Not often do geniuses like Freud, Cannon, Selye, or Pavlov come along, just as music rarely enjoys a Mozart, Beethoven, Brahms, Bach, or Hayden. The foregoing text alludes to a large number of significant "players" (for example Cobb, Lindemann, Bibring, Deutsch, Alexander, Eaton), but, as interested others are drawn to the field, their increased numbers alone sometimes obscure their additional contributions to the discipline. Seminal figures like George Engel, Chase Patterson Kimball, Morton Reiser, and Patrick McKegney, whose work is well known, will not be recorded here. This section is an effort to acknowledge a few of those individuals who have added significantly to the field of C-L psychiatry. Such an effort is risky for it is certain to omit any number who should be recognized, but limitations of space, time, and knowledge are extenuating factors. For omissions and oversights, I extend my sincere apologies. The following is a review of some of the individuals with whom I have had personal or literary acquaintance. In addition, a reproduction of the list of Hackett awardees is suggestive of an approximation of the many C-L psychiatrists who have lent their interest and effort to advancement of the field.

Z. J. ("Bish") Lipowski

In the literature of C-L psychiatry, perhaps no single name is more cited than that of Zbigniew Lipowski, a psychiatrist born in Poland and who emigrated to the United States via London and Canada in 1955. His story is worth telling.

Imagine what it must be like, as a youngster, to witness the daily execution of one's friends, family, and classmates, for no discernible rhyme or reason. For a horrifying two months in 1944, the people of Poland, having been threatened by the Nazis since their invasion in 1939, rose up defiantly against great military odds to battle their occupiers. Anticipating support from the advancing Russian Army, the Polish General "Bor" Komoroski was able to rally an oppositional force, the Polish Home Army, persuading them that the "time was right." With some modest success against the Germans in Vinynus, Lublin, and Lvov, Polish fighters were heartened and confidently pushed on to Warsaw with similar expectations. Support never came from the Russians, since Stalin had differences of opinion with Roosevelt and Churchill about what should happen with Poland, and help from the Allies was modest and ill planned. The Freedom Fighters of Warsaw, in spite of their determination, were doomed from the start. Death and destruction surrounded them, their ultimate survival depending on slogging through sewers only to face obliteration at their exit. Young boys and girls saw their parents executed as they held hands. Surviving was indeterminate and random. Those who survived nonetheless felt it was better to go down fighting than to die on their knees, and they took solace from having been part of perhaps one of the bravest, most defiant episodes of World War II. After two months of minor successes, with fierce fighting, constant bombing, and shelling and daily executions, greatly out-militarized by the Germans, the remaining Poles sought a ceasefire. By early October, 85% of the city had been destroyed, 200,000 were dead, and no help came from either the Russians or the Western Allies; the Uprising was over.

Zbigniew Lipowski was one of those who survived. The underground cell of which he was a member was exterminated. Close friends were executed in the city square. The evidence and stench of death were everywhere. Finally, he and other survivors were packed off on a train to "nowhere" from which he escaped and made his way to Cracow, where the Germans were too busy fending off the Russians to be very concerned about a few Poles. Attributing his survival to luck and determination to "make something of my life," he enrolled in Cracow University to study medicine, a strong interest since reading Kretschmer's *Physique and Character* when he was 17. He was an avid reader, partly a habit instilled at an early age, but now a welcome "escape" from the "disturbing reality" as he put it. In his own words, his "new interest was strengthened by my personal experience of extreme stress brought about by constant threat of death, and by hunger, cold, and other deprivations." These assaults on both body and mind were indelibly imprinted evidence of the inseparability of mind and body and inevitably forged young Lipowski's conviction that this, were he to survive, would be his area of study.

Although admitted to medicine at Cracow University, he found living in now-Stalinist Poland unbearable and managed, in 1946, to escape to London where he studied English and obtained a place in medicine at Dublin College of the National University of Ireland. Upon completion of medical studies in seven years, he became a house physician in a neurological hospital and began applying to

North American institutions for postgraduate study of psychiatry. He was thrilled to be accepted by McGill University and, after four years of intense study, was awarded a diploma in psychiatry with distinction in 1959. The die was cast!

Lipowski knew that he wanted to pursue psychosomatic medicine and asked his department chief if he could develop a psychiatric consultation service at the Royal Victoria Hospital, part of Allan Memorial Institute. Unfamiliar with that aspect of psychiatry, his chief advised him to locate a place where proper training for such an endeavor could be obtained. Applying to several training sites in the United States, he received the most attractive offer from Dr. Erich Lindemann, chief of psychiatry at Massachusetts General Hospital (MGH). Bish, as he has been known, was one of the first two fellows in consultation psychiatry at MGH, working closely with Drs. Avery Weisman and his young assistant, Thomas Hackett, running a consultation service for the hospital. The MGH staff was heavily populated with psychoanalysts, of which Avery was one but Tom was not. Tom, a newcomer to the MGH, told Bish how his appointment had been questionable because he was not analytically trained. As two individuals with a history of not being acceptable to the "system," Bish and Tom hit it off admirably and remained lifelong friends. Bish found Tom lively, energetic, warm, and humorous; this must have been a remarkable antidote to the cold, deathly, hostile experience of his adolescence. With Tom's Irish heritage, Bish's conversations of his Dublin experience further bonded the two. In spite of what was a most intellectually stimulating year of experience, "full of humour and laughter," Bish declined an offer to remain on staff at MGH and returned to Montreal to fulfill his wish to establish a consultation service at Royal Victoria Hospital, the first in Canada. There he remained for the next 11 years, immersed in consultation-liaison psychiatry, psychosomatic medicine, and extensive writing of and teaching of the same.

Bish was always wary of excessive authoritarianism, and, when he found politics in Quebec too oppressive, he moved with his family to the United States, where he was recruited to direct a psychiatric consultation service at Dartmouth Medical College. He could never be pinned down about any theoretical orientation, which he insisted was his experience of having too much of the fanaticism of both Germany and Russia. Unbeknownst to many about Bish is his three-year personal psychoanalysis, spoken of little by him. He was respectful of the field, admired his psychoanalyst, but steered clear of subscribing to what he saw as psychoanalytic dogma. Applied eclecticism, personal observation, and meaningful relationship—with interest in art, nature, music, and philosophy—coalesced to make him an ideal psychiatric consultant.

To his psychoanalytic experience, he attributes the breaking of a writing block, and testimony to that success is his prolific outpouring, especially during the 1980s, of meaningful writings on C-L psychiatry and psychosomatic medicine, with evidence of scholarly pursuit of intriguing, sometimes remote, aspects of the field. Bish demonstrated masterful skill in writing and editing in a language that was not his own.

By 1983, with a desire for a more European-like ambience, Bish returned to Canada, this time to Toronto to assume the position of professor of consultation-liaison psychiatry. But his coincident assignment to an inpatient service was not of his liking, and, for the ensuing years, he felt he had made a wrong move. Nevertheless, he found pleasure in his continued writing, including a book on delirium eight years before his death. This he had long ago promised to write, motivation derived from his own experience of a delirious illness as a child.

Throughout his life, Bish had a great respect for matters of the intellect. He had been a rather shy lonely kid growing up. His parents had sent him away to boarding school at a young age, where he felt out of place and depressed about being separated from his family. He took refuge in books, claiming to have read 160 books in one year, especially novels, as well as texts on philosophy, art, and culture. He retained this intellectual curiosity throughout his life, even through the terrible war years. And later, during his academic career, he would spend pleasurable hours in libraries, scouring old texts for interesting historical anecdotes about psychiatry and psychosomatic medicine. Such is the interesting piece about a Polish princess "cured" of melancholia by Benjamin Franklin during his stay in London (Lipowski, 1984a). The episode, discovered by Lipowski in an obscure unpublished Polish manuscript, provides the stage to discuss brief therapy, transference cure, and music therapy as well as the characteristics of a "good psychotherapist" demonstrated by Franklin's charisma, warmth, interest, and empathy, not to mention his facility with his "harmonica." Another interesting, perhaps even autobiographical essay (Lipowski, 1970), was based on a psychological hypothesis by a lesser French philosopher, Jean Buridan, who postulated that an animal placed between two equally appealing food sources would be so conflicted about the choice that it would die of starvation. This simplistic (and wrong) hypothesis was Lipowski's jumping-off point to discuss pathological conflict and that posed by the overload of stimuli from an affluent society on its people. Bish's transition from war-torn Poland to the more affluent North American continent may well have posed similar conflictual responses!

Bish was an astute observer and chronicler of the evolution of C-L psychiatry. From his earliest much-cited trilogy of papers (Lipowski, 1967a, 1967b, 1968) detailing, for the first time, the organization of extant knowledge of the field in 1966–1967, his papers portray a virtual timeline of the field's development. Papers on "Current trends in consultation-liaison psychiatry" (1983a), "consultation-liaison psychiatry: The first half century" (1986), and "Consultation-liaison psychiatry at century's end" (1992) bookend the entire field. This last paper seemed to be "rushing" the end of the century, perhaps premonitory of his impending death in 1997.

Intercurrent papers on integration of psychiatry and medicine (1983b), meaning of the word and history of psychosomatic medicine (1984b), the impact of somatization on the whole of medicine (1988), the role of teams in C-L practice (1981), and psychiatry's role in organic medicine (1978, 1987) punctuated his output. Hardly a serious paper on these topics exists that does not cite at least one of Lipowski's works.

Although Bish had achieved full academic status in the institutions he served, colleagues believed he might have assumed positions of greater authority and impact had it not been for his opposition to abuses of power and structure, echoes of earlier experiences. He was reluctant to join professional organizations and was intolerant of those in the field who proselytized or shamelessly aggrandized themselves. He was less than enthusiastic, in his final professional position, of assignment to an inpatient unit, but, as had happened in Warsaw, he adapted to circumstances he found himself in, even publishing papers on the inpatient experience.

Evidence that good instincts are not easily quelled by bad experience is apparent in Bish's persistent appreciation of gratifying things in life. He cherished a farm he bought in Quebec and loved nature and animals and the freedom they exuded. He owned parakeets, and I once observed him kiss one of these creatures in a touching display of affection. He was an informed appreciator of art, music, and other products of culture. On a visit to our home, he once dropped to his knees to examine an oriental rug, much to the embarrassment of his wife.

Bish's demise at the early age of 73 was a great loss to the field. But his considerable contributions to C-L psychiatry and psychosomatic medicine are a lasting invaluable legacy. This scholarly, modest, appreciative man, whose facility with the written and spoken English language exceeded that of many natives, continues to influence and, in some measure, direct the course of C-L psychiatry today.

Much of the vicissitudes of C-L psychiatry is to be culled from Lipowski's many publications (1974b, 1978, 1981, 1983a, 1983b, 1984b, 1987, 1988). The important trilogy published in *Psychosomatic Medicine* in 1967–1968 gave organizational structure and status to the emerging field. A compulsive scholarship and need to solidify his formative experience at the newly established consultation service of the Massachusetts General Hospital gave rise to thoughtful exegesis of the history, concepts, and application of principles of consultation psychiatry.

A catalog of Lipowski's writings chronicles the history and important milestones of C-L in papers that laid the foundation for both general hospital consultation psychiatry and psychosomatic medicine. From the outset he noted the difficulty of distinguishing between domains of consultation psychiatry and "the ill-defined area of psychosomatic medicine" with activities "developing vigorously in two directions," one addressing psychophysiological research and the other "consultation or liaison psychiatry." Of note is Lipowski's equating of "consultation" and "liaison," for the first time, to be further elaborated and defined in future publications. In his fellowship experience with consultation at MGH, he had observed that "the tendency to avoid the word 'psychosomatic' in this context is striking and no doubt related to its ambiguous meaning" (1967a, p. 154). He attributed this to the expectation that a psychiatric consultant "would become a victim of misinterpretation of his function and be considered an expert in the limited area of so-called psychosomatic disorders, with resulting limitation of his scope of work and usefulness" (p. 154). This dilemma has persisted throughout C-L psychiatry's staggering march to specialization.

Lipowski's description of the ideal consultation may appear almost quaint, looked at through the retrospectroscope of contemporary practice that is so controlled by economic strictures. In Lipowski's world of the early 1960s, he saw the consultant as a participant observer in an "operational group" of which the patient was the center. The group included physicians, nurses, social workers, and others in the "social field" surrounding the patient, the psychiatrist with a psychodynamic "detached" orientation, applying his or her knowledge and practical suggestions to identifying and modifying sources of stress to ameliorate the situation for the patient.

In a perfect world, elements of this orientation persist, but the fiscal realities of contemporary practice would restrict opportunities to apply these principles.

In the first of his three papers, Lipowski offers a conceptual framework of a typical consultation that has general applicability to a broad range of circumstances. His practical conception is that every consultation should be considered from three basic elements: the nature of the request for consultation; a phase of information gathering; and communication of findings, opinions, and advice to significant parties. While praising the contribution of Meyer and Mendelson (1961) to an understanding of process as influenced by transference and countertransference issues, Lipowski declares his conceptualization to have "more general validity and practical usefulness [and to be] less abstract and more descriptive" (p. 161). This declaration may be a subtle hint at Lipowski's drift away from the psychodynamic orientation of his mentors at MGH toward a more descriptive, "practical" approach to the process of consultation.

On the other hand, Lipowski is laudatory of the "practically useful facet of diagnosis" that makes use of personality style, a psychoanalytically oriented medical psychology, that is "a special contribution of a group of psychiatrists under the leadership of Bibring at the Beth Israel Hospital in Boston" (1967a, p. 164). This, he writes, "is application of psychodynamics to concrete medical problems at its best" (p. 165). As a relative newcomer to the field of consultation psychiatry, Lipowski may have been in the throes of formulating his own approach to the field. His training under Avery Weisman and Tom Hackett most likely offered a diversity of approaches to consultation. Weisman, a psychoanalyst, selected the young resident Hackett as his assistant, to "balance the ticket" so to speak. Together, in 1956, with Lindemann's instruction, they established the Consultation Service. And both functioned in a department chaired since 1954 by psychoanalytically oriented Erich Lindemann, a department heavily populated at the time by psychoanalysts in the Boston community. Whatever the case, Lipowski's review of the important literature at the time is matched only by that of Schwab, whose handbook of consultation psychiatry appeared at the same time as Lipowski's seminal papers.

At this early phase of Lipowski's own career, he anticipates the need for specialized training in consultation psychiatry, based on his observation that even after four years of "unusually comprehensive undergraduate training in psychiatry," most young doctors were unable to apply their knowledge appropriately to the task of consulting in medical settings. Distinguishing consultation psychiatry from inpatient psychiatry, with which it had already developed *pari passu* over a period of two decades, Lipowski conceptualized consultation psychiatry as a "branch of *preventive psychiatry*" and as "the practice and teaching of *psychosomatic medicine* as a science of and approach to human life phenomena which attempts to bring together the organismic and the psychosocial modes of abstraction" (1967a, p. 168; emphasis original). In such pronouncement, he sets the stage for future discourse on both the practical and humanistic aspects of the field as well as its potential for closing the gap between psyche and soma.

By the 1970s, with considerable development of C-L services in general hospitals, Lipowski was enthusiastically predicting that the C-L model "is likely to prevail in psychiatry [as a whole] in the coming years" (1974a, p. 623). Similar enthusiasm had been expressed for decades by psychosomaticians. Neither group has realized its expectations, perhaps because a narrow focus has obscured the proponents from monumental changes throughout medicine in subsequent decades. Lipowski appears by this time to have solidified his notion that the growth of C-L was largely due to the proliferation of inpatient psychiatric units, but many programs developed even in the absence of such units or hospitals that had no psychiatry departments at all. It seems clear that C-L psychiatry had a trajectory of its own!

C-L psychiatry is not associated with any particular theory but rather has a pluralistic approach to patient care. A definition proposed by Lipowski is comprehensive and succinct in its simplicity. C-L psychiatry, he states, "has derived conceptually from an old tradition in human thought, one that advocates a view of man as a body-mind complex in dynamic interaction with the social and non-human environments" (1974a, p. 625).

Psychosomatic medicine between 1930 and 1955 created great enthusiasm surrounding its apparent application to medical practice. Much of the excitement followed on the research of Franz Alexander and his psychoanalytic colleagues. It promised much but ultimately, as so often happens with high expectations, ended in considerable disappointment. Lipowski's review of psychosomatic history's rise and fall . . . and then rise again in the decade of the 1970s reveals a virtually hypomanic declaration of "spectacular comeback," marking "the twilight of the golden age of reductionism, of an intolerant and narrow approach to the study and treatment of disease from a purely biological, psychological, or social viewpoint" (1977, p. 233).

John J. Schwab

John Schwab is perhaps best known by early C-L psychiatrists for the first "handbook" of psychiatric consultation, published in 1968, when "psychiatric consultation has come of age" (p. vii). He began writing in 1966 and had acknowledged early contributions to the field of Lipowski as well as Mendel and Solomon (1968), the latter already espousing the need for liaison services and special training for psychiatric residents who would engage in this process. The handbook was an especially rich source of information about the burgeoning field, addressing not only the fundamentals, techniques, and procedures of C-L psychiatry but also its relevance to diagnosis and management in medicine and surgery as well as pediatrics and the community at large. Since the book emerged before there was Internet, it provided the most complete bibliography of the literature of the field extant at the time. With a detailed account of the organization, structure, and function of a C-L service (program), it was/is indeed a builder's guide for anyone embarking on the development of such a program.

John's dedication to research is evident from his postdoctoral studies in physiology (an M.S. in physiology from University of Illinois in 1949) and postgraduate studies in epidemiology at Duke and University of Florida. Funded studies on the epidemiological roots of mental illness and chairmanship of the NIMH Center for Epidemiological Studies review committee reflect this unique psychiatric interest and competence. He had also served as president of the American Association of Social Psychiatry. His broad interests in the impact of culture and community on mental illness included a study of depression in the Amish culture. Of somewhat amusing interest is that even before psychiatric training, Schwab had listed in his CV that he served as internist and "psychosomaticist" at the Holzer Clinic in Gallipolis, Ohio, from 1954 to 1959, *after which* he first entered psychiatric residency at the University of Florida Hospital, making clear the nature of his career objectives.

With residencies in both medicine and psychiatry, followed by a NIMH Career Teaching Award in 1962, Schwab rapidly advanced in his academic teaching career to professor of psychiatry *and medicine*, director of the C-L program, and director of residency training at University of Florida until 1974, at which time he joined the faculty at University of Louisville School of Medicine (where he had received his M.D. degree in 1946) as chairman of the Department of Psychiatry and Behavioral Sciences and as associate director of clinical psychopharmacology research until his retirement in 1993. He built a very strong department that was highly esteemed throughout the country.

John's perspective on the value of consultation on patients in medical settings is expressed succinctly in this sentence: "[The psychiatric consultant] will be better equipped for his job when he enlarges his knowledge of people and their distress by recalling his medical education and by seeing man in a social perspective" (Schwab, 1968, p. vii). In this statement, we see John's commitment to a comprehensive model of health care, also reflected in his unusually broad interests in social medicine, epidemiology, physiology, and psychopharmacology.

His interest, energy, advocacy, and productivity in the field of C-L psychiatry is evident in his edited or co-edited 9 books, 11 monographs, and over 250 articles.

Personally, in John's presence, one was immediately aware of his reverence and optimism for our humanity.

Maurice H. Greenhill

While Greenhill's name is not one that trips readily off the tongues of C-L psychiatrists, and his psychiatric interests were not confined only to that discipline, his incisive writings on the topic have been of foundational relevance. I did not have personal acquaintance with him but feel that his few writings on C-L psychiatry have had a formative impact on the field. Reading his work, one has a distinct impression of a dedicated and knowledgeable psychiatrist with a keen eye to what is valuable and what is dross. His account of the difficulties encountered in attempts to "reach" nonpsychiatrists is the best I have seen. He counsels wisely the novice psychiatrist consultant attempting to teach others what he or she knows about patient care. His activist approach to all he surveyed carried over to civic matters, revealed in his encounters with the mayor of New York City on crime rates in parts of the city (see, for example, R.W. Snyder, 2014).

Greenhill's (1977) exegesis on the development of liaison programs is arguably the most extensive and insightful there is. He recounts how while at Duke (1947–1952) he conducted a survey of experiences in the teaching of psychosomatic medicine to the hospital's staff, finding it "surprising that only a handful of reports exist on structured curricula" toward that objective. He reports on his efforts to train 100 interns and residents in Duke's Department of Medicine. Results of his efforts with colleague Kilgore appeared in *Psychosomatic Medicine* in 1950, perhaps one of the earliest reported such efforts (Greenhill & Kilgore, 1950). In this paper are reported techniques of dealing with resistance over a period of five years by maintaining a specific program structure endorsed and supported by the chief of medicine, described as an essential ingredient (pp. 153–154). Realistically addressing the challenge, Greenhill states, "Until we have the knowledge, let us not expect of the physician that he can be part psychiatrist" (p. 179). In the meantime, he writes, "[L]et us design programs in which psychiatry is more direct and decisive in the care of the sick and dying. . . . Social forces have now given us that opportunity and the timing is right to grasp it" (p. 179). He may have been prescient in this remark: "The integral model [of] psychiatry is considered to be the generic operation of patient care and to the functions of the hospital" (p. 180). In spite of his critical remarks, Greenhill remains optimistic for the future of (C-L) psychiatry as he concludes that "tomorrow is today as far as general hospital psychiatry is concerned, and in the scattered and frenetic searches of psychiatry for its place in the sun, it may well be that the model of the general hospital psychiatrist will prevail" (p. 182).

Greenhill was strongly committed to the psychiatrist's resources as a teacher (Greenhill & Kilgore, 1950; Greenhill, Fitzpatrick & Berblinger, 1950). He had begun his own 40-year teaching career at Harvard in 1939, moving to Duke for several years before becoming chair of psychiatry at Albert Einstein College of Medicine in the late 1950s. He died in 1981 at the age of 71.

Robert O. Pasnau

With long-standing interests in medicine, music, and philosophy, Pasnau was destined to drift toward the comprehensive field of consultation-liaison psychiatry. Natural talent as a teacher and a comfortable social grace also suited him for the politics of the profession. In 1985, he was voted president-elect of the American Psychiatric Association and in the year of his presidency chose for the annual meeting the theme of "Psychiatry in Medicine," as it had embodied his career-long interest. He moderated (a term well chosen for the events) both Brook Lodge conferences with grace and fairness, pivotal events on the road to specialization. Recognizing the place of C-L psychiatry in medicine, he was editor of one of the earliest compendiums of C-L topics (Pasnau, 1975), including his own chapter detailing experiences as liaison psychiatrist to obstetric-gynecological services; in the early days of C-L, he was the "go-to" person in that field. As with so many who have entered the field of C-L psychiatry, he avows in the introduction to his text that the reason for "editing this book was my growing concern for the health of people and my fear that in spite of years of experience and knowledge, most physicians remain in the dark about the interaction of mental and physical health" (1975, p. ix). Both Lipowski and Schwab contributed important chapters, and the book became a model for several that appeared later illustrating how psychiatry could enhance virtually every other medical discipline. In fact, just three years later, with colleagues and mentees, he co-edited another volume (Faguet, Fawzy, Wellisch & Pasnau, 1978) described by Lipowski as a "practically useful and valuable book" (foreword), containing encounters of psychiatry at the interface with special situations in medicine. The editors' introduction explains that individual chapters were selected to "demonstrate 1) the multidisciplinary character of the new liaison psychiatry, 2) the community and family orientation of the treatment methodologies, and 3) the liaison psychiatrist's unique role in serving the traditional physician's functions of personal, comprehensive, and continuous care through the course of the patient's illness" (introduction).

Thomas P. Hackett

Tom Hackett was a major force in C-L psychiatry before his untimely death at age 59. At an early age, Tom had been mentored in Cincinnati by Gustav Eckstein (1970), professor of Physiology and author of the epic volume *The Body Has a Head*. He became an assistant instructor in physiology prior to medical school. In the medical school in Cincinnati, he most likely was influenced to some extent by the teachings of Maurice Levine, the psychiatrist who had mentored trainees like Milton Rosenbaum, John Romano, George Engel, and Morton Reiser. By 1955, at Massachusetts General Hospital (MGH), he had inherited the rudiments of C-L psychiatry from the department founded by Stanley Cobb. Then under the tutelage of Avery Weisman, staff psychiatrist/psychoanalyst, the two of them developed the C-L service. From that experience came two seminal publications on the consultation process (Hackett & Weisman, 1960a, b), emphasizing psychodynamic aspects of the process.

With T. P. Hackett and Cassem (1978), he co-edited the first edition of the MGH *Handbook of General Psychiatry*, with the introductory chapter by Hackett (1978) titled "Beginnings: Liaison psychiatry in a general hospital" (pp. 1–14), changed in subsequent issues to "Beginnings: Psychosomatic medicine and consultation psychiatry in the general hospital," to reflect Hackett's expressed doubts about the value of liaison practice. His original chapter refers to his first fellow as "the doughty and venerable scholar, Z.J. Lipowski" (p. 1), with whom he formed a lifelong friendship and whose "encyclopedic guide to the published information on this psychiatric subspecialty" he strongly commended to his students (p. 1). Already in 1978 he noted that the American Psychosomatic Society, "which has many strong links to consultation-liaison work, rarely gave more than a nod of acknowledgment to presentations or panels discussing this aspect of psychiatry" (p. 1). Referring to the confusion of terminology applied to the discipline, he states, "[W]hatever it is called, psychiatry in the general hospital has many facets" (p. 6), which he addressed throughout his career in his usual "down-to-earth" practical style. With Weisman, Cassem, and other colleagues, he introduced important clinical observations of "black patch psychosis" (after eye surgery [Weisman & Hackett 1958]), importance of supporting denial in post-myocardial infarction (Olin & Hackett, 1964), and predilection to death (important to assess prior to surgery [Weisman & Hackett, 1961]). He had become president of the Academy of Psychosomatic Medicine just a few months before his death. Perpetuating support of the discipline and its practitioners, his wife Eleanor and colleagues established the Thomas P. Hackett Award to recognize individuals in the field "demonstrating distinctive achievements in consultation-liaison/ psychosomatic training, research, clinical practice and leadership." The list is reproduced here to acknowledge significance of this award, to recognize the many contributors to the advancement of C-L psychiatry, and to compensate for my lack of time and resources to amplify the contributions of each recipient: Edwin H. Cassem, 1989; W. Alwyn Lishman, 1990; Zbigniew J. Lipowski, 1991; Avery D. Weisman, 1992; Norman B. Levy, 1993, founder of psychonephrology; Jimmie C. Holland, 1994, founder of psychooncology; Donald S. Kornfeld, 1995; George B. Murray, 1996; Alan Stoudemire, 1997; James S. Eaton, Jr., 1998; Thomas N. Wise, 1999; Don R. Lipsitt, 2000; Michael K. Popkin, 2001; James J. Strain, 2002; Wayne J. Katon, 2003; Joel E. Dimsdale, 2004; Richard Mayou, 2005; Russell Noyes, Jr., 2006; Fritz Huyse, 2007; Theodore A. Stern, 2008; Francis Creed, 2009;

Donna E. Stewart, 2010; William S. Breitbart, 2011; James R. Rundell, 2012; James L. Levenson, 2013 and Lewis M. Cohen, 2014.

James J. Strain

Strain's contributions to C-L psychiatry have been many and extensive. The small book he co-authored with James J. Strain and Stanley Grossman (1975) characterized a thoughtful detailed definition of liaison psychiatry in its relatively early stage of development. The book provided case examples of the "ombudsman" function of the psychiatrist at Montefiore Hospital, where stalwarts of psychosomatic medicine Morton Reiser, Herbert Weiner, and Edward Sachar taught and engaged in research. The book emphasizes the importance of the supporting role of both the chief of medicine (Hammerman) and the hospital administrator (Cherkasky). An important epilogue by Cherkasky offers a candid expression of both the benefits and challenges of liaison psychiatry from an administrator's point of view, of great value to anyone directing a C-L service. When Strain moved to New York's Mount Sinai Hospital, he directed a highly esteemed C-L service in which many of the country's C-L psychiatrists trained. Strain's interest in teaching, consultation effectiveness, and outcome of training led to innovative software development to document C-L activities and training experiences of C-L fellows (with colleagues Hammer and Lyons, a program called MICRO-CARES (Hammer, Lyons & Strain, 1984), distributed to many university settings in the United States and abroad, facilitated multi-institutional as well as multicultural studies, a new frontier in the scope of C-L psychiatry). Hundreds of publications and international presentations have given Strain a kind of ambassadorial role in the field, which continues to this day.

Milton Viederman

Viederman's effectiveness as a C-L psychiatrist influenced many trainees at Cornell Medical College to appreciate the usefulness in C-L work of the "life narrative" as a mechanism of psychotherapeutic brief encounters with patients. Incorporating elements of both Felix Deutsch's anamnestic interviewing technique and Adolf Meyer's life history, the "life narrative" reflected back to the patient applied psychoanalytic intervention techniques in a Bibring-like way with demonstrable effectiveness (Viederman, 1983).

Thomas N. Wise

Tom Wise, a graduate of the Johns Hopkins psychiatry program, has been a virtual renaissance man of the field, in every aspect of the C-L discipline. He has edited a journal, published untold numbers of volumes on various topics in C-L psychiatry, and been president of every organization whose major focus has been

C-L or psychosomatic medicine. As chairman of his department and professor of psychiatry, he has been a role model and mentor to many future C-L psychiatrists. He is, in a word, the consultant's consultant. It is no coincidence that he is widely represented in this text on the specialization process.

Other contemporary practitioners who have made major contributions include Tom Webster, Carolyn Robinowitz, Stephen Saravay, Maurice Steinberg, Fred Guggenheim, Hoyle Leigh, Steven A. Cole, Jon Streltzer, Stephan Levitan, Jerry Finkel, Michael Blumenfield, Michael Wise, Arthur Barsky, Peter Reich, Malcolm Rogers, Robert Pasnau, Michelle Riba, Linda Worley, Philip Muskin, Malkah Notman, Robert Joseph, Donald Meyer, Roger Kathol, Douglas Drossman, Kurt Kroenke, Donna Stewart, Fawzy Fawzy, Donald Kornfeld, and David Spiegel. In addition, European and Asian colleagues include Takashi Hosaka, Graeme Smith, Else Guthrie, Geoffrey Lloyd, Richard Mayou, Francis Creed, Vladan Starcevic, Tatjana Sivik, Fritz Huyse, Chiharu Kubo, Simon Wessely, and Marco Rigatelli. I have focused on those who have had international activity in C-L psychiatry and apologize for unintentional oversights.

References

Eckstein, G. (1970). *The Body Has a Head*. New York, NY: Harper & Row.

Faguet, R.A., Fawzy, F.I., Wellisch, D.K., & Pasnau, R.O. (Eds.). (1978). *Contemporary Models in Liaison Psychiatry*. New York, NY: Spectrum Publications.

Greenhill, M.H. (1977). The development of liaison programs. In G. Usdin (Ed.). *Psychiatric Medicine*. (pp. 115–191). New York, NY: Brunner/Mazel.

Greenhill, M.H., Fitzpatrick, W.N., & Berblinger, K.W. (1950). Recent developments in teaching of comprehensive medicine. *North Carolina Medical Journal, 11,* 615–619.

Greenhill, M.H., & Kilgore, S.R. (1950). Principles of methodology in teaching the psychiatric approach to medical house officers. *Psychosomatic Medicine, 12,* 38–48.

Hackett, T.P. (1978). Beginnings: Liaison psychiatry in a general hospital. In T.P. Hackett & N.H. Cassem (Eds.). *Massachusetts General Hospital Handbook of General Hospital Psychiatry*. (pp. 1–14). St. Louis, MO: Mosby.

Hackett, T.P., & Cassem, N.H. (Eds.). (1978). *Massachusetts General Hospital Handbook of General Hospital Psychiatry*. St. Louis, MO: Mosby.

Hackett, T.P., & Weisman, A.D. (1960a). Psychiatric management of operative syndromes. I. The therapeutic consultation and the effect of noninterpretive intervention. *Psychosomatic Medicine, 22 ,*267–282.

Hackett, T.P., & Weisman, A.D. (1960b). Psychiatric management of operative syndromes. II. Psychodynamic factors in formulation and management. *Psychosomatic Medicine, 22,* 356–372.

Hammer, J.S., Lyons, J.S., & Strain, J.J. (1984). Micro-Cares: An information management system for psychosocial services in hospital settings. *Proceedings of the Annual Symposium on Computer Applications to Medical Care.* November 7, pp. 234–237.

Lipowski, Z.J. (1967a). Review of consultation psychiatry and psychosomatic medicine. I. General principles. *Psychosomatic Medicine, 29,* 153–171.

Lipowski, Z.J. (1967b). Review of consultation psychiatry and psychosomatic medicine. II. Clinical aspects. *Psychosomatic Medicine, 29,* 201–224.

Lipowski, Z.J. (1968). Review of consultation psychiatry and psychosomatic medicine. III. Theoretical issues. *Psychosomatic Medicine, 30,* 395–421.

Lipowski, Z.J. (1970). The conflict of Buridan's ass or some dilemmas of affluence: The theory of attractive stimulus overload. *American Journal of Psychiatry, 127,* 273–279.

Lipowski, Z.J. (1974a). Consultation-liaison psychiatry: An overview. *American Journal of Psychiatry, 131,* 623–630.

Lipowski, Z.J. (1974b). Sensory overloads, information overloads and behavior. *Psychotherapy and Psychosomatics, 23,* 264–271.

Lipowski, Z.J. (1977). Psychosomatic medicine in the seventies: An overview. *American Journal of Psychiatry, 134,* 233–244.

Lipowski, Z.J. (1978). Organic brain syndromes: A reformulation. *Comprehensive Psychiatry, 19,* 309–322.

Lipowski, Z.J. (1981). Liaison psychiatry, liaison nursing and behavioral medicine. *Comprehensive Psychiatry, 22,* 554–561.

Lipowski, Z.J. (1983a). Current trends in consultation-liaison psychiatry. *Canadian Journal of Psychiatry, 28,* 329–338.

Lipowski, Z.J. (1983b). Integration versus reductionism in psychiatry. *Integrative Psychiatry, 1,* 60–64.

Lipowski, Z.J. (1984a). Benjamin Franklin as a psychotherapist: A forerunner of brief psychotherapy. *Perspectives in Biology and Medicine, 27,* 361–366.

Lipowski, Z.J. (1984b). What does the word 'psychosomatic' really mean? A historical and semantic inquiry. *Psychosomatic Medicine, 46,* 153–171.

Lipowski, Z.J. (1986). Consultation-liaison psychiatry: The first half century. *General Hospital Psychiatry, 8,* 305–315.

Lipowski, Z.J. (1987). Delirium (acute confusional states). *Journal of the American Medical Association, 258,* 1789–1792.

Lipowski, Z.J. (1988). Somatization: The concept and its clinical application. *American Journal of Psychiatry, 145,* 1358–1368.

Lipowski, Z.J. (1992). Consultation-liaison psychiatry at century's end. *Psychosomatics, 33,* 128–133.

Mendel, W.M., & Solomon, P. (1968). *The Psychiatric Consultation.* New York, NY: Grune & Stratton.

Meyer, W.E., & Mendelson, M. (1961). Psychiatric consultation with patients on medical and surgical wards: Patterns and processes. *Psychiatry, 24,* 197–220.

Olin, H.S., & Hackett, T.P. (1964). The denial of chest pain in thirty-two patients with acute myocardial infarction. *Journal of the American Medical Association, 190,* 977–981.

Pasnau, R.O. (Ed.). (1975). *Consultation-Liaison Psychiatry.* New York, NY: Grune & Stratton.

Schwab, J.J. (1968). *Handbook of Psychiatric Consultation.* New York, NY: Appleton-Century-Crofts.

Shakespeare, W. The Tempest. Act IV, Scene 1.

Snyder, R.W. (2014). *Crossing Broadway: Washington Heights and the Promise of New York City.* Ithaca, NY: Cornell University Press.

Strain, J.J., & Grossman, S. (Eds.). (1975). *Psychological Care of the Medically Ill: A Primer in Liaison Psychiatry.* New York, NY: Appleton-Century-Crofts.

Viederman, M. (1983). A psychodynamic life narrative: A psychotherapeutic intervention useful in crisis situations. *Psychiatry, 46,* 236–246.

Weisman, A.D., & Hackett, T.P. (1958). Psychosis after eye surgery: Establishment of a specific doctor-patient relation and the prevention and treatment of "black patch delirium." *New England Journal of Medicine, 258,* 1284–1289.

Weisman, A.D., & Hackett, T.P. (1961). Predilection to death: Death and dying as a psychiatric problem. *Psychosomatic Medicine, 23,* 232–257.

Appendix Two

PERSONAL REFLECTIONS OF A C-L PSYCHIATRIST

It is a difficult thing to close a train of speech and cut it short once you are under way.
—*Montaigne, 1572 [Frame D., 1942, p. 22]*

As with most scientific writing, my writing in the past has avoided the use of the pronoun "I." It seems awkward to me now, and perhaps too solipsistic, to include myself in this historical account of the subspecialty of consultation-liaison psychiatry. But our work is so rooted in the relations not only of the observed but also of the observer that it seems useful to place myself in its context as a way of highlighting and reacting to the personal idiosyncrasies that influence historical developments. Indeed, history is inevitably intertwined with personalities. Furthermore, as in psychotherapeutic process, attitudes, biases, and experiences of the therapist figure saliently into the dyadic relationship and course of a patient's therapy, referred to as countertransference. So, too, it seems to me, impossible to look at historical events without some modicum of "countertransferential" perception. In many respects, the history of C-L psychiatry is the history of individuals and more. I therefore, apologetically, append these personal reflections in the event my own history is of interest to readers who wish to identify my biases. It may also be of interest (or curiosity) to have an account of one person's career path in consultation–liaison psychiatry.

I beg the indulgence of readers who may be put off by this personal account, but it is my hope that those whose interest spans not just dates and names but also the process by which one chooses a special area of interest and adopts a lifelong commitment to it will find something pertinent to their own objectives here. Hopefully this will not distract from the focus of what has been the foundational trends of the field of C-L psychiatry.

My own career trajectory has spanned almost 60 years, including the period of years described by Lipowski (1986, p. 310) as the "phase of rapid growth" in C-L psychiatry. With a glance in history's rearview mirror, it appears to me that I have always, in some sense, been a C-L psychiatrist, even before I knew what it was or before it was named. I was always interested in how to make people feel better—perhaps even myself. My mother must have tired of hearing me uninvitedly advise her how to take care of the two youngest of us five brothers.

Having little idea of what career pursuits would attract me, I was sampling many paths: writing, music, photography, architecture, reporting. As a physics student, the appeal of nuclear research was strong, but a poor grade in what was probably the only course on nuclear physics in the country at the time prompted my switch to psychology. Why couldn't I get a better grade in nuclear physics?

A part-time job opportunity serving as an interviewer for a community survey with Marie Jahoda and Paul Lazersfeld, both Viennese social psychology émigrés to the United States, seemed like a good way to procrastinate. It introduced me to the essentials of good interviewing, communicating with and listening to the varied complaints and experiences of people in the health care system; in some ways, the angry, reluctant, and sometimes bizarre people I met inoculated me to what might be forthcoming later.

I got through college and the military draft and batted out an application for "office boy" positions with major New York newspapers. There seemed little place else to go but graduate school, continuing with developmental psychology in a teaching track. This held little promise for me as a career track, and, after a master's degree and part of a doctorate, medicine became more to my liking. In preparation, I worked as chief radioisotope technician at Boston University Medical Center (physics again!) for researchers like Arnold "Bud" Relman and Frank Ebaugh, Jr. (son of Frank Ebaugh the psychiatrist) for a year before beginning medical studies at University of Vermont. This was a generally very good experience with not so impressive a rotation in psychiatry, except for the only psychoanalytically trained psychiatrist in town. My earlier interest in psychiatry and psychoanalysis had been nurtured by the books I found on my parents' shelves as well as a course with Edward Bibring during graduate studies before medical school. Milton Greenblatt's course on psychophysiology was an important addition. Later, during residency, Elizabeth Zetzel's psychoanalytic teachings were lucid and relevant to clinical experience.

Following an advanced degree in psychology, medical school and psychiatry seemed a logical choice. Medical school, especially in clinical years, was an adventure and an eye-opener about the health care industry and fundamental doctor-patient relations. Much of what I observed of physicians "at work" in their interactions with patients erased much of my idolatry for physicians. I observed not only what was good about doctors in their interactions with patients but how they "treated" patients (in every sense) and often what I regarded "short of the mark." This was perhaps the beginning of a calling to teach other doctors. The experience culminated in an essay on my observations on such relationships that won me a medical school award.

Following medical school graduation, I chose psychiatry over radiology (another discipline I seriously considered . . . physics again!) because it promised more patient contact and diagnostic challenge. Those who knew me wondered how I could entertain such "disparate" interests; I explained that *both* specialists spent their professional lives trying to make sense of vague shadowy images (this was before MRI) and data.

Once a specialty interest was selected, whether the correct one or not, the medical route was proscribed; few decisions had to be made: Internship, residency, possibly military service, and then who knows what? With psychology, medical school, and psychiatry, perhaps psychoanalysis should follow. I would later appreciate, even before reading Renee Fox's (1957) important paper on training for uncertainty, that uncertainty was an important attribute of C-L work. I had already had a large experience with uncertainty: I was born before my parents had selected a name, and thus I was called Nemo briefly. In the yearbook at graduation from prep school, where captions indicated next steps for graduates, under my picture was the word "uncertain." And the college yearbook misplaced my picture over someone else's name. And for some time after college, I wasn't at all sure what I wanted to do, awaiting call-up by the draft. I was deferred because of my studies in physics, and the war would end before I was needed.

The die was finally cast following medical school! My intent was to explore ways we offered help and support to individuals who suffered all manner of ills, whether of mind or body, and how they could be improved. Internship and residency experiences were selected for their relationship to the larger body of medical science and practice. A "rotating" internship at Albert Einstein Medical Center (Bronx, NY) offered the broadest immersion in a wide variety of experiences including delivering babies, doing surgery, sitting with dying patients in medicine and neurology, and other highly privileged activities. It reinforced my belief that apart from technology, drugs, and other marvels of modern medicine, what we *did* and *said* to patients had a profound effect on the course of illness and disease. And I was dumbstruck at how quickly and eagerly patients were ready to expose not only their bodies but also their minds to complete strangers, so hungry were they for personal understanding.

My first residency years at Einstein were stimulating. The department exuded the excitement of a new program with a number of faculty who had trained in Cincinnati with Maurice Levine, the "grandfather" of psychiatric teaching of physicians: Milton Rosenbaum, Morton Reiser, Wagner Bridger, and others. I was privileged to have as advisors, mentors, teachers, and supervisors a number of those who had an abiding interest in psychosomatic medicine, as well as psychoanalysis; they all emphasized the important responsibility of psychiatrists as teachers. Besides Rosenbaum and Reiser, there were Herbert Weiner, Jose Barchilon, Ed Hornick, and Harris Peck at Einstein as well as Ralph Kahana, Benson Snyder, Grete Bibring,

John Nemiah, Peter Sifneos, Dorothy Huntington, Arthur Valenstein, and Henry Wermer at Beth Israel Hospital, most with interests and experience in psychosomatic medicine and psychoanalytic application to medicine. At Einstein, from time to time, visiting professors included Margaret Mahler, Peter Blos, Sr., Thomas Szasz, and John Rosen, offering a spectrum of psychotherapeutic viewpoints. Our text was Otto Fenichel's (1945) *Psychoanalytic Theory of Neurosis*, a dense but highly informative volume. But we were discouraged from reading, rather to spend most time sitting with patients, with the dictum that "if you can spend one year sitting with a patient, you can learn almost all there is to know about psychiatry" (with extensive supervision, of course!)

A stint at the National Institute of Mental Health's (NIMH) Center for Clinical Neuropharmacological Research, directed by Joel Elkes, later the chair of psychiatry at Johns Hopkins, provided good resources in the science and pharmacology of mental illness. And study of a broad spectrum of patients committed to the large federal mental hospital in Washington (St. Elizabeths [*sic*]) opened vistas into the synergistic, symbiotic, interdependent ways patients and institutions functioned, often to the patient's detriment. Goffman's (1961) study of asylums contained resonating insights as did Caudill's (1958) book on hospitals as small societies. Of my hospital experience, I subsequently published a paper (Lipsitt, 1962)—"Dependency, depression and hospitalization: Toward an understanding of a conspiracy"—on how the hospital and its staff detrimentally establish codependent relationships; published after I left the institution, it did not win me many admirers among hospital staff!

"Finishing" residency training at Beth Israel Hospital in Boston was "frosting on the cake." The experience exposed me to Grete Bibring's tutelage; she was known for her fervent interest in psychotherapy training and application of psychological and psychoanalytic knowledge to the care of "medical/surgical" patients, especially during their hospitalized experience. Publication (1956) of her seminal article in the premier *medical* journal taught both psychiatrists and nonpsychiatrists that psychoanalytic understanding could be practically applied without jargon to typical medical situations. This was my first experience in a defined consultation service (called medical psychology at the time, a holdover from European psychiatry). It was an exhilarating experience, with supervision mainly by psychoanalytically trained physicians like Ralph Kahana, Jack Vorenberg, and John Reichard, committed to working and teaching in the general hospital setting. I was struck by the facility with which Reichard, a psychoanalyst, could translate psychoanalytic and psychological concepts into simple messages for the nonpsychiatrist trainee. "If you see a man (read: doctor) digging a hole with his hands, wouldn't it make sense to offer him a shovel (consultation)?" was a memorable sample.

I vividly recall my first enlightening experience of consulting to nonpsychiatrist physicians and trainees. My supervisor virtually took me by the hand, showing me the value of carefully perusing a patient's chart (especially the copious data that accrued from examination of just the chart's face sheet—I was impressed with how much one could know of a patient with very few bits of information like birth date, marital status, insurance coverage, and other face-page notations), culling important information from the patient's nurse(s), and inviting the assigned house officer to "sit-in" on a brief consultative interview with the patient (a practice seldom observed in more recent times).

Eventually, I assumed the position of director of medical psychology (renamed consultation-liaison service), and my opportunity had come to have some influence over how medicine was practiced, at least in one institution. I had become the hospital's "expert" (meaning referral source) on "problem patients" of all stripes. Instructing house staff and others in the "care of patients" was a small but open window into affecting how doctors behaved with patients, with "medical rounds" shared by myself and the chief of medicine (an invaluable ally) (Lipsitt, 2013).

Proving the adage that necessity is the mother of invention, I had become aware that many patients referred from medical and surgical clinics to our psychoanalytically oriented therapy clinic were often "unsuited for psychotherapy." A brief study demonstrated that patients who did not keep appointments to "Psychiatry Clinic" would come for therapy to a clinic called something other than "psychiatry" or "mental health." And so, the Integration Clinic (IC) was born, to which interesting (if "difficult") patients who had previously refused referral to psychiatry or rejected psychotherapy came without hesitation (Lipsitt, 1964). Many IC patients could be described as alexithymic, a concept originated by Nemiah and Sifneos in the department.

Noting that many of the IC patients had been marginalized as "problem patients" or "crocks" by their physicians, I wrote a paper (Lipsitt, 1970) on the subject that my colleagues liked but felt would be rejected for its (offensive?) use of the word "crock." Because a search for a journal interested predominantly in C-L topics came up short, I had the chutzpah to found one that would dedicate itself to C-L topics. With Dr. Bibring's help, I began putting together an editorial board intended to be broad and inclusive, so that, for example, prominent as an executive editorial committee were professors of the three major specialties at Harvard: Hermann Blumgart from medicine, Oliver Cope from surgery, and Grete Bibring from psychiatry (I was not concerned about "overburdening" with Harvard members!). The advisory board included prominent academics, psychoanalysts, and C-L psychiatrists. Putting together a first issue, including my hand at drawing a logo (in continuous use today), engaging a publisher, and soliciting, sending for peer review, and collating manuscripts for publication was painstaking but exciting work and a way to keep informed at the cutting edge of the field.

Without funding, the search for a publisher was discouraging, with few publishers willing to incur the expense of a new journal in a field where potential subscribers were not easily identified. In the process of my search, I sought the advice of Morton Reiser, who had been my teacher during residency at Einstein

Medical Center (Bronx) and was, at the time, editor of *Psychosomatic Medicine* (PM). He was very interested and supportive and suggested that the journal might be a supplement to PM, with its focus on C-L topics counterbalancing the more experimental subject matter of the journal. He invited me to an editorial board meeting of PM in Philadelphia, to join him in presenting the proposal to the board. I was very anxious at the prospect of presenting to stalwarts and a young resident's idols like Carl Binger, Roy Grinker, Don Oken, and others, even with Reiser's supportive endorsement. As written elsewhere in the book, I experienced unanticipated contumely unlike anything I had experienced before. Most board members were enthusiastic about the idea, and some very wary that addition of *Psychiatry in Medicine* might dilute the core focus of PM, with one eminent emotionally distraught member erupting with "We don't need one more memorial to [name omitted of a prominent board member]," a sentiment that shocked me but also seemed seriously misplaced since I had considered myself founder of the journal. Perhaps if I had been more cognizant of the tumultuous history, rivalries, and organizational disagreements of the society and its journal, I might have been more prepared for the onslaught. The board decided against the idea, and I continued to pursue an interested publisher, finally convincing Greenwood Press to take a chance, in just a few years selling the rights to Baywood Publishing, who continues to produce the journal. When the board felt the journal had grown sufficiently, they recommended transferring to a larger publisher, a proposal declined by Baywood, resulting in my suggestion that we submit a proposal to Elsevier Science Publishing for a journal with larger scope, focusing not only on C-L but on all aspects of psychiatry in its role in the general hospital. Thus was born *General Hospital Psychiatry*, subtitled *Psychiatry, Medicine and Primary Care*, to reflect its focus on clinical application in those three fields, with the interrelatedness of each to the others.

The first journal published the crock paper (after collegial review) in the inaugural issue, sparking considerable attribution among physicians for whom the topic resonated with their personal experience with "difficult patients" but were previously reluctant to acknowledge. One physician wrote to me saying that my paper had relieved him of his guilt about charging a fee to manage these "problem patients."

In 1969, the opportunity presented itself to start a department from scratch and to weave into it an appreciation of psychiatry's relationship to medicine. Recruited by Mount Auburn Hospital with the "offer" to bill privately for all patient contacts, I declined and persuaded them that, with a salary, I would be free to provide greater and more extensive service to the hospital, its staff, and its patients (a guideline for use by others in similar circumstances dealing with administrators!) I had not anticipated the 12-hour days that would follow.

As the only consultant to the medical, surgical, and emergency services, I quickly persuaded the hospital's administration that there was benefit to the hospital's staff, patients, and community to offer "complete, comprehensive" care, and to do so would require at least one other staff psychiatrist. In very few years, what began as a subdivision of the department of medicine became a full-service psychiatry department with all divisions except child and adolescent psychiatry, and a clearly defined C-L service staffed by a full-time director, liaison psychiatric nurse, and social worker, one more teaching service of Harvard Medical School. A dedication to "team" effort in C-L was promptly apparent, although one hoary internist on the staff brought me before the board for "allowing a nurse" to consult on a patient, recommending that I be fired! I wasn't, and nurses continued to be part of the C-L team.

At the time, a number of "beginners" were establishing psychiatric departments in community hospitals in the greater Boston area. Regular meetings of John Reichard, Jerry Wacks, John Merrifield, Arthur Berg, and myself offered mutual support and suggestions over the challenges and uncertainties of negotiating with reluctant administrators. Special focus on C-L developments was assisted by Fred Guggenheim, at the time director of the private consulting service at Massachusetts General Hospital. Fred's enthusiasm knew no bounds as we discussed the timeliness for inaugurating a national C-L organization, a gesture not met entirely with unbridled enthusiasm among colleagues. The rest, as noted in this text, is "history."

Membership of the C-L psychiatrist in relevant organizations is important for personal and professional growth. Participation in organizations like the American Psychosomatic Society (APS), which I was encouraged to join by John Nemiah; the Academy of Psychosomatic Medicine; the American Psychiatric Association, through its sometimes fruitless committee work; the local district branch, of which I was a future president; and the Association for Academic Psychiatry, supportive of C-L psychiatry, were all invaluable learning experiences for a C-L psychiatrist. Annual meetings of APS were richly informative, with individuals presenting their ideas to a cadre of expert evaluators like George Engel, Arthur Schmale, William Greene, John Mason, Richard Rahe, and other researchers in the field. Much dealt with experimental methodology and was usually over my head, but it fostered an appreciation of clinical discipline and astute observation. Colleagues of my own generation were available to "jaw" with and to compare experiences. And membership (eventual presidency) in an international group, the International College of Psychosomatic Medicine, kept me connected with what was taking place in C-L psychiatry in other parts of the world. Editing two journals was a labor of love and a special way to keep informed about and in touch with most of those who were productively active in the field, whether writers, reviewers, board members, or readers. I would recommend to aspiring C-L psychiatrists that they consider the importance of writing in their profession since it enhances observational power, clinical curiosity, and pleasure to their profession. Honing interviewing skills and teaching should also become comfortable aspects of their work. The C-L psychiatrist can enjoin Montaigne's confession that "there is a certain satisfaction which tickles me when I do a just action and make others content" (Frame, D., 1942, p. 43).

Finally retiring from the chairmanship of the department I founded, I count myself an inveterate C-L psychiatrist. What began in uncertainty concludes with that much certainty! I would urge any young psychiatrist to pursue a similar path for its great rewards. We may even possibly influence some nonpsychiatrist physicians to adopt a different view of psychiatry and ways of caring for patients!

References

Bibring, G.L (1956). Psychiatry and medical practice in a general hospital. *New England Journal of Medicine, 254,* 366–372.

Caudill, W. (1958). *The Psychiatric Hospital as a Small Society.* Oxford, UK: Harvard University Press.

Fenichel, O. (1945). *The Psychoanalytic Theory of Neurosis.* New York, NY: W.W. Norton & Co.

Fox, R.C. (1957). Training for uncertainty. In R.K Merton, G. Reader, & P.L. Kendall (Eds.). *The Student-Physician: Introductory Studies in the Sociology of Medical Education.* (pp. 207–241). Cambridge, MA: Harvard University Press.

Frame, D.M. (1942). *The Complete Works of Montaigne: Essays, Travel, Journal, Letters.* (Translated by D.M. Frame from original, 1572). Stanford, CA: Stanford University Press.

Goffman, E. (1961). *Asylums: Essays on the Social Situation of Mental Patients and Other Inmates.* New York, NY: Penguin Random House.

Lipowski, Z.J. (1986). Consultation-liaison psychiatry: The first half century. *General Hospital Psychiatry, 8,* 305–315.

Lipsitt, D.R. (1962). Dependency, depression, and hospitalization: Toward an understanding of a "conspiracy." *Psychiatric Quarterly, 36,* 537–554.

Lipsitt, D.R. (1964). Integration clinic: An approach to the teaching and practice of medical psychology in an outpatient setting. In N.E. Zinberg (Ed.). *Psychiatry and Medical Practice in a General Hospital.* (pp. 231–249). New York, NY: International Universities Press.

Lipsitt, D.R. (1970). Medical and psychological characteristics of "crocks." *International Journal of Psychiatry in Medicine, 1,* 15–25.

Lipsitt, D.R. (2013). Partners at the interface. *American Journal of Psychiatry, 170,* 1401–1402.

INDEX